Clinical Applications of Linguistics to Speech–Language Pathology

Clinical Applications of Linguistics to Speech-Language Pathology is a practical guide that provides linguistically grounded approaches to clinical practice. It introduces key linguistic disciplines and discusses how they form a basis for assessment and treatment of individuals with communication differences or disorders.

Written by experts in linguistics and communication disorders, each chapter provides clinicians with a foundational understanding of linguistics as it applies to spoken and signed languages and underscores the importance of integrating linguistic theories into clinical decision-making. The book is divided into two parts that focus on the applications of linguistics to speech and language differences and disorders in both children and adults. The chapters cover the full range of linguistic domains, including phonetics, phonology, morphology, syntax, semantics, pragmatics, and sociolinguistics. Applications to a wide range of populations, including childhood apraxia of speech, aphasia, dysarthria, traumatic brain injury, and accent modification clients, are also discussed. Many chapters include assessment and treatment resources that can be used by practicing clinicians.

This highly accessible and comprehensive book is an indispensable resource for practicing speech-language pathologists and other members of the profession, including instructors with minimal exposure to linguistics. It will also be beneficial for students of Linguistics, Speech and Hearing Sciences, and Audiology and Speech Language Pathology who are seeking practical knowledge of the fields.

Naomi Gurevich, PhD, CCC–SLP, is Assistant Professor in the Department of Communication Sciences and Disorders at Purdue University Fort Wayne, USA. Her research interests combine her background in phonology with acquired language disorders. She has previously authored two books in these areas.

Christopher M. Grindrod, PhD, is Assistant Professor in the Department of Communication Sciences and Disorders at Purdue University Fort Wayne, USA. His research focuses on investigating language impairments in aphasia, and cognitive-communication disorders associated with right hemisphere brain injury. He has published extensively in these areas for over 20 years.

Clinical Applications of Linguistics to Speech-Language Pathology

A Guide for Clinicians

**Edited by Naomi Gurevich
and Christopher M. Grindrod**

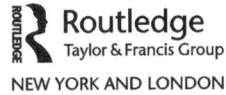

Routledge
Taylor & Francis Group

NEW YORK AND LONDON

Cover image: © Hava Gurevich Art

First published 2023
by Routledge
605 Third Avenue, New York, NY 10158

and by Routledge
4 Park Square, Milton Park, Abingdon, Oxon, OX14 4RN

Routledge is an imprint of the Taylor & Francis Group, an informa business

Library of Congress Cataloging-in-Publication Data
Names: Gurevich, Naomi, 1966– editor. | Grindrod, Christopher M., editor.
Title: Clinical applications of linguistics to speech-language pathology : a guide for clinicians / edited by Naomi Gurevich & Christopher M. Grindrod.
Description: New York, NY : Routledge, 2022. | Includes bibliographical references and index.
Identifiers: LCCN 2022021187 (print) | LCCN 2022021188 (ebook) | ISBN 9780367492489 (paperback) | ISBN 9780367492915 (hardback) | ISBN 9781003045519 (ebook)
Subjects: MESH: Language Disorders—therapy | Linguistics—methods | Speech Therapy | Language Therapy | Speech-Language Pathology—methods
Classification: LCC RC428 (print) | LCC RC428 (ebook) | NLM WL 340.2 | DDC 616.85/5—dc23/eng/20220902
LC record available at https://lccn.loc.gov/2022021187
LC ebook record available at https://lccn.loc.gov/2022021188

ISBN: 978-0-367-49291-5 (hbk)
ISBN: 978-0-367-49248-9 (pbk)
ISBN: 978-1-003-04551-9 (ebk)

DOI: 10.4324/9781003045519

Typeset in Bembo
by Apex CoVantage, LLC

Contents

Contributors

Claudia I. Abbiati is completing her PhD in the Interprofessional Health Sciences program at the University of Vermont, USA. Her research focuses on speech sound development, differences, and disorders in neurodiverse populations, including childhood apraxia of speech.

Roelien Bastiaanse is Professor Emeritus of Neurolinguistics at the Center for Language and Cognition at the University of Groningen, the Netherlands. Her research focuses on cross-linguistic aspects of agrammatic aphasia with an emphasis on verb production. She has developed many influential assessment and treatment programs for aphasia in various languages.

Jessica R. Berry is Assistant Professor in the Department of Speech Pathology and Audiology at South Carolina State University, USA. Her research focuses on child language with an emphasis on the grammar of children with Gullah Geechee heritage.

Stacy K. Betz is Associate Professor in the Department of Communication Sciences and Disorders at Purdue University Fort Wayne, USA. Her research focuses on identifying the most accurate measures for diagnosing language impairments in preschool and elementary school age children.

Talia Bugel is Professor of Spanish in the Department of International Language and Culture Studies at Purdue University Fort Wayne, USA. She specializes in sociolinguistics and second language acquisition. She is a professional translator and interpreter, working with English, French, Portuguese, and Spanish.

Michael S. Cannizzaro is Associate Professor in the Department of Communication Sciences and Disorders at the University of Vermont, USA. He investigates brain and behavior relationships in typical and brain-injured populations. His research on discourse processing incorporates behavioral, linguistic, computational, and neuroimaging methodologies.

Carl Coelho is Professor Emeritus in the Department of Speech, Language and Hearing Sciences at the University of Connecticut, USA. He is widely known for his research on discourse and communication disorders in adults with traumatic brain injury.

Jennifer Cole is Professor in the Department of Linguistics at Northwestern University, USA. Her research uses experimental and computational methods to study the sound structure of language. She was the founding General Editor of Laboratory Phonology and a founding member of the Association for Laboratory Phonology.

Kyomi D. Gregory-Martin is Associate Professor in the Department of Communication Sciences and Disorders at Pace University, USA. She specializes in child language development with an emphasis on culturally and linguistically diverse populations.

Christopher M. Grindrod is Assistant Professor in the Department of Communication Sciences and Disorders at Purdue University Fort Wayne, USA. His research focuses on investigating language impairments in aphasia, and cognitive-communication disorders associated with right hemisphere brain injury.

Naomi Gurevich is Assistant Professor in the Department of Communication Sciences and Disorders at Purdue University Fort Wayne, USA. Her research interests combine her background in phonology with acquired language disorders.

Allison Hilger is Assistant Professor in the Department of Speech, Language, and Hearing Sciences at the University of Colorado Boulder, USA. Her research investigates impaired speech production in motor speech disorders. More specifically, she looks at how prosody is affected in neurological disease or impairment.

Lauren E. Kelley is a school-based Speech-Language Pathologist in Houston, TX, USA. Her current clinical and research interests include language deprivation, pediatric language disorders, sign language disorders, and aural re/habilitation.

Heejin Kim is Research Assistant Professor in the Department of Linguistics at the University of Illinois at Urbana-Champaign, USA. She investigates the acoustic and perceptual correlates of segmental and prosodic categories in motor speech disorders and explores an optimal training protocol for perceptual learning of dysarthric speech.

James McCann is Assistant Professor in the Department of Hearing, Speech, and Language Sciences at Gallaudet University, USA. His research interests include identifying language disorders in deaf children acquiring visual language and identifying evidence-based practice for language instruction and intervention with deaf children.

Janna B. Oetting is Professor in the Department of Communication Sciences and Disorders at Louisiana State University, USA. Her research focuses on language development and disorders across dialects of English to reduce disparities in health and education among children. She is a Fellow of the American Speech-Language-Hearing Association.

Shivani Patel is Speech-Language Pathologist at Lucile Packard Children's Hospital, Stanford Children's Health in Palo Alto, CA, USA. Her areas of clinical expertise include autism spectrum disorder and related developmental disorders, childhood apraxia of speech, and early intervention.

David Quinto-Pozos is Associate Professor in the Department of Linguistics at the University of Texas at Austin, USA. His research includes signed language acquisition, developmental signed language disorders, constructed action, signed language contact and language change, and signed-spoken language interpretation.

Shaun R. Stephens is Speech-Language Pathologist at the Stern Center for Language and Learning in Williston, Vermont, USA. He specializes in treating social cognition and discourse-level language impairments, and in using hands-on and experiential learning among children and adults.

Jill Thorson is Assistant Professor in the Department of Communication Sciences and Disorders at the University of New Hampshire, USA. Her research focuses on the perception and production of prosody at different stages in development, and how these early language processes impact successful communication.

Shelley L. Velleman is Professor in the Department of Communication Sciences and Disorders at the University of Vermont, USA. Her research focuses on speech sound development in typically developing children and in children with motor speech disorders, including childhood apraxia of speech.

Preface

Speech-language pathologists assess and treat clients with language disorders, often without any formal education in linguistics. In the United States, training for clinical certification and licensure requires coursework in speech and hearing sciences, but surprisingly not in language science or linguistics. Clinicians are expected to follow principles of evidence-based practice, but when the support for intervention is based in linguistic theories, they are rarely in a position to fully understand the evidence on which they are basing their clinical decisions. Our goal for this book is to facilitate the clinical implementation of linguistic theory by making it accessible. This book is meant to serve the needs of clinicians by introducing key linguistic disciplines and how these areas form a basis for assessment and intervention. To ensure that the book is maximally useful to clinicians, linguistic concepts are discussed in clear, accessible language, all terminology is well defined, and content is directly tied to its clinical application. Our hope is that this book provides foundational linguistics knowledge to clinicians and empowers them to better integrate it into their clinical decision-making. We also hope that this book will highlight the importance of including linguistics in the curriculum of undergraduate and graduate programs in communication disorders.

The book focuses on child and adult populations, with chapters on foundational linguistic domains relevant to communication disorders and differences. Each chapter starts with a short statement to the clinician to clarify how the information can be applied in clinical practice. Some chapters also include ready-to-use clinical-linguistic resources. Part One focuses on applications of linguistics to child speech and language differences and disorders. In Chapter 1, Shelley L. Velleman and Claudia I. Abbiati review structural aspects (phonotactics) of syllables and words, along with the primary aspects of prosody that interact with phonotactics. They then examine how this knowledge can be applied to the assessment and treatment of childhood apraxia of speech and autism spectrum disorders. In Chapter 2, Stacy K. Betz provides an overview of the interaction between morphology and syntax with a specific emphasis on tense, agreement, and finiteness marking. She then discusses strategies to assess and treat morphosyntax in children with Developmental Language Disorders.

In Chapter 3, Jill Thorson focuses on prosody or the melodic and rhythmic variation of speech. After reviewing prosodic development in typically developing children, she then considers how prosody can be assessed and treated in autism spectrum disorders and childhood apraxia of speech. In Chapter 4, Janna B. Oetting, Jessica R. Berry, and Kyomi D. Gregory-Martin focus on finiteness marking in dialectal variations of English, specifically African American English. They provide key insights into impairments in Developmental Language Disorders in African American English and then discuss how this information can inform best practices in clinical intervention. Finally, in Chapter 5, James McCann, Lauren E. Kelley, and David Quinto-Pozos provide an overview of structural aspects of sign language, including phonology, nonmanual markers, verb inflection, classifiers, and referential shift, while also considering typical development in these areas. They then discuss guidelines to inform selection of treatment targets for intervention in Developmental Signed Language Disorders.

Part Two focuses on applications of linguistics to adult speech and language differences and disorders. In Chapter 6, Naomi Gurevich and Heejin Kim introduce a conceptual hierarchy of functional importance to intelligibility based on four phonological properties of sounds (i.e., contrast, context, frequency, and functional load). They then explain the use of this framework in clinical practice to both diagnose and treat intelligibility disorders in dysarthria. In Chapter 7, Roelien Bastiaanse reviews key aspects of verb argument structure to highlight its pivotal role in sentence production. She then discusses the implications for assessment and treatment of verb and sentence production in aphasia. In Chapter 8, Christopher M. Grindrod provides an overview of lexical semantics with a focus on semantic ambiguity, and how word meaning varies depending on the surrounding linguistic context. He then discusses how context can be incorporated into various treatments to target difficulties in understanding ambiguity associated with aphasia and right brain injury. In Chapter 9, Shaun R. Stephens, Carl Coelho, and Michael S. Cannizzaro introduce techniques to elicit discourse as well as approaches to discourse analysis. They then provide suggestions for the assessment and treatment of discourse impairments following traumatic brain injury. In Chapter 10, Jennifer S. Cole, Allison Hilger, and Shivani Patel review the function of prosody in marking juncture between words and phrases, and in conveying pragmatic meaning related to reference and speech acts. They also propose strategies for the assessment and treatment of prosody in dysarthria, apraxia of speech, right hemisphere disorder, and autism spectrum disorders in adults. Finally, in Chapter 11, Naomi Gurevich and Talia Bugel outline the phonetic and phonological bases of accentedness, as well as the sociolinguistic factors that contribute to its impact on speakers. They then address implications for clinical practice and provide suggestions for a culturally aware paradigm for the assessment and treatment of accent modification clients.

We are extremely grateful that such an outstanding group of colleagues accepted the challenge we posed to write about these linguistically and clinically important topics. Each author possesses considerable theoretical and clinical expertise in their respective fields. Their competence and hard work shines through the pages. We are deeply indebted to all of them for the time and expertise they each committed to the book. We sincerely hope that clinicians will benefit from this collective effort.

Naomi and Chris

Part I

Applications to child speech and language differences and disorders

1 Phonetics and Phonology

Beyond the phoneme

Shelley L. Velleman and Claudia I. Abbiati

Abstract

Phonetics courses and the tests that are most commonly administered to children with speech sound disorders focus heavily on segments. Little attention is paid to the structures that these consonants and vowels combine to create—syllables, words, and beyond. Prosody, the pitch, loudness, and duration patterns of speech, is similarly given little emphasis in both domains. Yet, these two aspects of phonology integrate to provide the foundation for spoken language. Children with speech sound disorders, such as Childhood Apraxia of Speech (CAS), may have particular difficulty with complex speech structures despite being able to produce the individual sounds. Similarly, certain aspects of prosody may be especially challenging for children on the autism spectrum, while other aspects may be most difficult for those with CAS. In this chapter, we review key aspects of phonotactics as well as the components of prosody that interact the most with phonotactics. Then we describe phonotactic and prosodic development and disorders with suggestions for assessment and intervention.

Statement to the reader

As a clinician, you know the ages at which English consonants are acquired. You are probably aware that some consonants are mastered first in certain word positions. However, consonants in isolation are meaningless. You are probably less familiar with the scaffolds into which consonants and vowels are slotted to create syllables, words, and phrases. Without these structural aspects (phonotactics) of syllables and words, along with the primary aspects of prosody that interact with phonotactics, oral language is unintelligible. Certain child populations are especially likely to have phonotactic and/or prosodic deficits. We present the key concepts and what is known about typical and atypical

DOI: 10.4324/9781003045519-2

development of phonotactics and prosody. We end the chapter with clinical implications by reviewing assessment and intervention approaches.

Introduction

Just as the components of an engine must be put together in a certain way for that engine to function, the consonants and vowels of each language must be assembled according to conventions specific to that language. Each language has two types of frameworks within which consonants and vowels are assembled into syllables, words, phrases, and beyond: phonotactics and prosody. Many speech tests, guidelines, and textbooks focus primarily on delays and disorders in the development of consonants and sometimes vowels. Syllable and word shapes (phonotactics) and the melody, loudness, and rhythm of language (prosody) are often neglected. Yet, these two aspects of speech production, and the interactions between them, are critical for successful oral communication. Segments (consonants and vowels) cannot truly be mastered unless they are practiced in a variety of phonotactic and prosodic contexts.

There are several reasons for focusing on phonotactics in our clinical assessments and interventions. First of all, many speech sound error patterns actually affect the structure of the syllable or word rather than the consonants or vowels per se. These include final consonant deletion (e.g., [kæ] for *cat*), cluster reduction (e.g., [mæk] for *mask*), reduplication (e.g., [wawa] for *water*), metathesis (e.g., [gʌb] for *bug*), and the like. Others only operate at the syllable or word level. For example, consonant harmony (e.g., [gɔgi] for *doggie*) cannot be detected if we only look at one consonant at a time; we must refer to the whole syllable or word to determine whether error patterns such as these are occurring. We also know that the development of many consonant and vowel segments varies depending on their placement within the word. In English, for instance, most consonants develop first in the initial position, although some (velars and fricatives) may appear first in the final position (Dinnsen, 1996; Farwell, 1977; Ingram, 1974). Research has shown that segmental complexity interacts with structural complexity; late-mastered speech sounds may be more difficult to produce in complex syllable or word shapes. Furthermore, in childhood apraxia of speech (CAS), the phonotactic complexity of the target word, the phonotactic frequency of the target syllables (i.e., how often each syllable occurs in the language), and the child's phonotactic accuracy determine a child's phonetic accuracy (Jacks et al., 2006). Finally, morphology interacts significantly with phonotactics in English. Most plural (*bricks*), possessive (*Kim's*), third person singular (*jumps*), and past tense (*walked*) forms in English include final consonant clusters. In short, syllable and word structures provide key frameworks for the consonants and vowels in our languages and therefore must be considered whenever we are planning speech sound intervention. We explore these structural aspects of phonology and delve into these phonetic–phonotactic interactions in much more depth in this chapter.

Prosody, the pitch, loudness, and duration patterns of speech, provides another key framework for consonants, vowels, syllables, words, and well beyond. Prosody is the rhythmic pattern of words, phrases, and beyond. In English, intonation plays an important role in helping a listener to determine whether an utterance is a yes/no question, a wh-question, or a statement. It also facilitates parsing the grammar of a sentence. In other languages, tone changes the meanings of words. In yet another set of languages, duration determines lexical meanings. One of the most complex aspects of prosody in English is stress, which serves multiple functions, including content, form, and use. It differentiates noun phrases versus compound words (content) and parts of speech (form), as well as adding emotional meaning to sentences (use). Without prosody, words and sentences would be lacking several cues that are vitally important for the listener who is trying to process the utterance.

In this chapter, we focus on phonotactics, prosody, and how prosody and phonotactics interact, both in typical speech production and in children with various types of speech sound disorders. We describe methods for assessing these key areas of phonological development and strategies for intervening when deficits are detected.

Phonotactics

Introduction

Consonants and vowels are the building blocks for words. However, they cannot be, and are not, combined any which way. There are both universal and language-specific restrictions on the types of syllable and word shapes that are formed. In addition, there are both universal and language-specific tendencies with respect to the order in which these formations are mastered in young children. Furthermore, there are specific patterns of difficulty that are often exhibited by children with speech sound delays and disorders.

In this section, we first consider the components used to build syllable and word shapes and the structures that result. Then we review the typical course of phonotactic development, with a focus primarily on English but with examples from other languages for contrast. Finally, we review the error patterns associated with specific speech sound disorders.

Key concepts

Each syllable comprises two key components: the onset and the rhyme (sometimes spelled "rime"). The onset is the consonant or consonants at the beginning of the syllable. In the languages of the world, there is no known language that does not allow syllables or words to begin with a consonant onset. In fact, consonant + vowel ("CV") is the only syllable type that occurs in every single known language in the world. For that reason, CV is often referred to as a "canonical" or universal syllable type.

Some languages do not allow complex onsets—that is, onset consonant clusters—at all. In English, up to three consonants may be included within one onset, as in the word *splash*. If there are three, the first one will always be [s], the second will be a stop ([p], [t], or [k]), and the third will be a liquid ([l] or [ɹ]) or a glide [w] or [j]). This pattern doesn't completely follow the universal "sonority hierarchy" in which the most closed elements (stops) fall at the periphery of the syllable, while the most open ones (vowels) are in the heart of the syllable (Goldsmith, 1990). Fricatives and stops are obstruents—they stop or squeeze the air flow—so they occur at syllable edges, while liquids and glides are approximants—they shape the air flow—so they occur closer to the middle of the syllable. However, English violates this universal tendency in the sense that [s] can occur either at the beginning of a word, even <u>before</u> more-closed stops, or at the very end of a word, even <u>after</u> more-closed stops. In some languages clusters such as sp-, st-, sk- and -ps, -ts, -ks are not possible as they are in English. Some languages, such as Russian, have even more complex clusters than English (e.g., Russian *fspl-* as in *fsplesk* meaning *splash*, and *vzgl-* as in *vzglat* meaning *glance*; Trapman & Kager, 2009).

The remainder of the syllable is the rhyme, composed of a nucleus and a coda.

The heart of every syllable is its nucleus. English nuclei are most often vowels, although some consonants can also play this role. For example, in the word "little" the nucleus of the second syllable is a syllabic [l]: [lɪɾl]. In some languages, such as English, the nucleus can be complex (that is, a diphthong, such as [ɔɪ] in *oil*, or even a triphthong, like [aɪɚ] in *fire*). Syllables with tense vowels, like [i] in *beet*, [u] in *boot*, and [o] in *boat*, or complex nuclei (diphthongs or triphthongs) are "heavy." In contrast, syllables with a single lax vowel, such as [ɪ] in *little*, are "light." The nucleus, as the most resonant part of the syllable, bears most of the acoustic prosodic features of the syllable: pitch, duration, and loudness.

The final edge of a syllable, if there is one, comprises the coda consonant(s). Some languages, such as Hawaiian, do not allow final consonants. Others allow only very limited codas; in Japanese, for example, only nasals are permitted in coda position. In English, having a coda is another way for a syllable to be heavy. English is generous with respect to codas: up to 4 consonants can occur in a single coda, as in the word *strengths* ([stɹɛŋkθs]—in some English dialects). Once again, the sonority hierarchy typically determines coda clusters, but English violates this guideline in one respect, by allowing [s] to occur after stops, such that clusters such as -ps, -ts, and -ks occur.

The resultant English syllable shape is as shown in Figure 1.1. Note that items in parentheses are optional.

For syllables in English (and many other languages), the nucleus and coda are grouped together in the rhyme, while the onset stands alone. This reflects several facts about the psychological reality of syllable shapes. First, in poetry in English (and many other languages), we match the rhymes of syllables— nucleus and coda together ("The **rose** tickled my n**ose**"). In alliteration (e.g., "six slimy snakes slithered slowly"), on the other hand, the onsets alone match. Similarly, in the majority of slips of the tongue, onsets are repeated or switched with each other (e.g., "a leading list" for "a reading list" or "heft lemisphere"

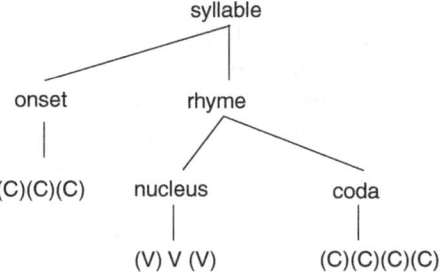

Figure 1.1 English syllable shape.

for "left hemisphere"; Fromkin, 1973, p. 114). Codas rarely switch or persever-ate with each other and never switch with onsets.

At the word level, a new possibility arises of intersyllabic consonant sequences. Consonants that could not occur together in a certain order in a cluster can do so when they are in adjoining syllables. For example, [k] and [n] cannot combine in that order as either an onset cluster (kn-) or a coda cluster (-kn). However, they are fine in adjacent syllables (e.g., *picnic* [pɪknɪk]).

Languages also differ with respect to word lengths. Although no language has an upper limit on the number of syllables that can occur per word, the mono-syllabic word shapes that are extremely common in English (e.g., CV, CVC) are quite rare in some other languages, such as the Indian language Kannada, in which the vast majority of words are at least disyllabic (Rupela & Manjula, 2006). Some languages with few possible syllable shapes, such as Hawaiian, which allows no clusters and no codas and as a result has only 162 possible syl-lables, have many very long multisyllabic words (Crystal, 1987).

Within syllables and words, and even across words, the components of one syllable or word can influence the components of another. When articulatory postures or movements overlap or "coarticulate," the segments become more alike; they "assimilate." This coarticulation may be "anticipatory": getting ready for a sound that's coming up. In English, for example, vowels are nasalized before a nasal consonant, as in the word *candy* [ˈkæ̃ndi]. This occurs because the velum must be lowered in order to allow air to flow through the nasal cav-ity. The speaker begins lowering it during the vowel, because the velum moves relatively slowly. In other cases, coarticulation is perseverative: hanging onto the characteristics of one sound into the next sound. For instance, this affects the pronunciation of the plural "s" (and also third person singular "s," possessive "s," and past tense "d"); it is voiced when the final consonant in the word is voiced (e.g., *dogs* [dɔgz], *pulled* [pʊld]), but voiceless when the final consonant is voiceless (e.g., *cats* [kæts], *kissed* [kɪst]). This occurs because it's easier to keep the vocal folds vibrating if they already are doing so, and easier not to have to restart the vibrations if they have ceased.

Within syllables and words, coarticulation usually doesn't alter the structure of the syllable or word. However, coarticulation also happens between words, such as when /d/ is pronounced as [dʒ] right before a /j/ (e.g., *Did you?* pronounced as [dɪdʒu]). In this case, two phones ([d] + [j]) have been merged into one ([dʒ]). Deletion of consonants also occurs when the coda of one word is the same as the onset of the next word: /bæd dɔg/ *bad dog* becomes [bæd:ɔg] because there's no sense in saying [d] twice in a row. Onset /h/s also tend to be omitted when they are preceded by a coda consonant. Thus, *give him* might be pronounced [gɪvɪm] and *It's his* as [ɪtsɪz]. Use of a coda to serve as the onset of the next word is called "ligature."

Coarticulation allows us to speak more quickly and fluidly. Although it often makes comprehension more challenging for second language learners, it actually improves comprehension in native speakers of a language.

Typical phonotactic development

By definition, all infants produce CV syllables from the onset of canonical babbling, between 8 and 12 months. English-learning infants produce at least some codas by 2 years. They also produce two-syllable as well as monosyllabic words at that age (Stoel-Gammon, 1987). Three-syllable words should occur by age 4 at the latest (Shriberg, 1993). Some children expand first from one-syllable open syllables (CV) to two-syllable open syllables (CVCV), while others produce closed monosyllabic words (CVC) before bisyllabic words with open syllables (Demuth & Fee, 1995).

There are various ways in which phonotactics may interact with phonetics. At a basic level, harmony, which is the use of the same consonant, as in *baby* [beɪbi] or *mom* [mɑm], or the same vowel, as in *bow-wow* [baʊwaʊ], can facilitate the child's productions. This is the same principle that differentiates reduplicated babble ([babɑbɑ], [dididi], [gugugu], etc.) from variegated babble ([bɑdigu]). In either stage—babble or early words—a child may be beyond harmony yet still have restrictive patterns. For example, Christopher (Priestly, 1977) used [j] as his default medial consonant (e.g., [dɑjɑk] for *dragon*). Shelli (Berman, 1977), on the other hand, always moved the velar to the initial position (e.g., [kibi] for *piggie*, [god] for *dog*). This is called "metathesis," and it refers to sounds trading places. Errors of this type are very difficult to identify unless we look at the word as a whole. Otherwise, we would say that Shelli produced [k] for /p/, [b] for /g/, [g] for /d/, and [d] for /g/—a very confusing pattern of errors! Migration is a similar type of movement in which only one consonant moves. For instance, a child might say [noʊs] for *snow* because she cannot produce sn-clusters but she can produce [s] in coda position. Again, if we don't consider the whole word, we have a very strange error of cluster reduction ([sn] → [n]) plus adding an [s] where it doesn't belong.

Phonotactics interacts with phonetics as well in the sense that young children learning English appear to be aware of syllable weights (Redford & Oh, 2016) and that light syllables are disfavored. They are more likely to produce the coda of a word that contains a lax vowel (e.g., *sit* [sɪt]) than the coda of a word that contains a tense vowel or a diphthong (e.g., *seat* [sit]), since adding the coda after the lax vowel makes it a preferred, heavy syllable. The word with the tense vowel is already a heavy syllable, so it doesn't need the coda (Demuth et al., 2006; Kehoe & Stoel-Gammon, 2001).

Clusters emerge by 2 years in many although not all English-learning children (Stoel-Gammon, 1987). The clusters that occur first, in English, tend to be of two types. In initial position, the first clusters are usually those that have the most constriction contrast, following the sonority hierarchy: stop + glide (especially tw-; Smit et al., 1990) or perhaps stop + [l] (McLeod et al., 2001). In final position, the first ones tend to be "homorganic" nasal + stop clusters: those in which the nasal and the stop have the same place of articulation (e.g., -mp, -nd, -ŋk; Kirk & Demuth, 2003; McLeod et al., 2001) so that the tongue position does not change from one consonant to the next. Contrary to popular belief, these final clusters often precede the initial ones in children learning English or several other languages (Lleo & Prinz, 1996; McLeod et al., 2001). One might expect that English clusters that violate the sonority hierarchy (e.g., [s] + stop initial clusters) would be acquired later. On the contrary, on average, they are mastered at about the same time as other fricative clusters (Smit et al., 1990). However, some children may acquire them later and others may acquire them sooner. In all of these ways, phonotactics (clusters and word positions) interacts with phonetics (the development of specific consonants).

It is important to note that both the phonetics and the phonotactics of individual languages and even dialects will impact acquisition order. For example, Pearson et al. (2009) showed that while children learning African American English (AAE) as a first dialect master certain consonants that are less frequent in their dialect (such as /ð/) later than children learning General American English (GAE), they master other phonemes (such as /s/, /z/, and /ɹ/) and clusters (those with /ɹ/) that are present in both dialects earlier. These differences likely represent learning trade-offs between phonotactic difficulty (fewer codas and coda clusters in AAE) and phonetic difficulty (more challenging phonemes such as /s/, /ɹ/). This finding was verified in children with speech sound disorders as well, although it was less clear cut in that population (Velleman & Pearson, 2010).

With respect to the development of coarticulation, most studies have focused on subtle acoustic influences of one sound on another (e.g., a vowel in one syllable influencing the formants of a vowel in another syllable) rather than on types of coarticulation that have phonotactic impacts. However, some data are available about how early interword phonotactic impacts may begin. Stemberger (1988) reported on his daughter Gwendolyn, who used the coda of one word as the onset of the next, if the next word was vowel-initial (as adult English speakers do) at 29–32 months. For instance, she pronounced *get up and go* as *geh tu pan go* as [da tʌ piːn doʊ] (with velar fronting affecting the [g] in *get* and *go*). From 30 to 33 months, she also, like adult English speakers, deleted [h] in onset position if there was a coda in the preceding word, using that coda as the now-missing initial consonant. For example, for *not out here* she said *na tow tere* [na ta ti:] (with diphthong reduction and omission of the rhotic). These ligature patterns became less evident by 36 months, possibly because her speech became smoother and more adult-like.

Atypical phonotactic development

The most well-studied childhood speech disorder associated with phonotactic deficits is CAS, a motor speech disorder thought to result from deficits in motor programming and/or motor planning. Phonotactic challenges may be apparent even in the prelinguistic babbling period, when infants later diagnosed with CAS are later to produce, and also produce fewer, canonical (CV syllable) babbles (Overby et al., 2020). When they begin to produce words, children with CAS may produce simpler syllable or word shapes (Velleman, 1994). Consonant omissions are even more common in young children with CAS than other youngsters (Lewis et al., 2004; Shriberg et al., 1997). Jacks et al. (2006) carried out a longitudinal study of three children with CAS between 4½ and 7½ years of age. Although the participants deleted final consonants more often than consonants in other positions, all three demonstrated some initial consonant deletion over the entire time span, which is extremely rare in children who are typically developing (TD). Their consonant clusters were accurate a maximum of 48% of the time, well below expected levels. Although the children typically produced the correct number of syllables in monosyllabic and disyllabic words, syllables were sometimes deleted from longer words. In addition, the syllable shapes of even simple monosyllabic words (CV, V, VC, CVC) were incorrect 25% of the time, of disyllabic words about 50% of the time, and of longer words and more complex monosyllables (those with consonant clusters) a little less than two-thirds of the time. Word length predicted consonant accuracy within the word, an example of phonotactics affecting phonetics.

With respect to word-level error patterns, children with CAS may demonstrate more frequent reduplication and harmony than children with other speech sound disorders (Velleman, 2003). Case studies have included children with CAS who demonstrate "distribution restrictions." These include a 4-year-old child who could combine [b] with [ɑ] but not with [i], and [d] with [i] but not [ɑ], so that she pronounced *baby* either as [bɑbɑ] or as [didi] (Velleman, 1994). In another case, a 6-year-old always produced the velar last in a word, so that *cat* was [tæk] and *carrot* was [tɛwɪk] (Velleman, 2016). Several other authors have noted difficulties with consonant sequencing in children with CAS, including metathesis (e.g., Lewis et al., 2004).

Even older children with CAS (aged 7–14 years) may still demonstrate phonotactic error patterns, such as cluster reduction (Shriberg et al., 1997) and weak syllable deletion (Velleman & Shriberg, 1999). Increased difficulty with longer multisyllabic words is a frequently cited symptom at all ages (Jacks et al., 2006), including migration of sounds from their target placement to other positions, such as *Sleeping Beauty* pronounced as [sipɪŋ bluwi]. Thus, phonotactic deficits are an important symptom of CAS over time.

There are some studies of coarticulation in children with CAS. They suggest that the coarticulation of such children is less mature than that of children without speech sound disorders (Maas & Mailend, 2017; Nijland et al., 2002, 2003; Wells, 1994). However, these studies focus primarily on the acoustic impacts of one segment on another, across syllables. The phonotactic impacts of coarticulation—such as ligature—in this population are largely unknown.

Children on the autism spectrum (OAS) are also at risk for phonotactic delays and disorders. According to Schoen et al. (2011), at 18–36 months children who are OAS produced fewer speech-like vocalizations than age- or language-matched children, even though they were over a year older than the language-matched children, on average. They also produced fewer consonant clusters and less complex syllable structures overall than age-matched children. The clusters that they did produce were more likely to be ones that do not occur in their own language (also reported by Nordgren, 2015). In other studies, as well, deficits have been identified in syllable production (Wetherby et al., 1989). Perception of coarticulation has been studied by several authors, but little is known about the production of coarticulation, especially inter-word coarticulation, in people who are OAS.

Prosody

Introduction

Prosody is a multidimensional linguistic phenomenon that is present across all languages. Speakers use prosody to convey and encode linguistic information, including the function (pragmatic), form (grammar and phonology), and content (semantics) of language. As with phonotactics, there are universal and language-specific restrictions and tendencies on how prosody is used based upon a word's syllable structure and lexical class, as well as a speaker's phonological knowledge and the patterns of the language(s) one speaks, including one's accent. There are also specific patterns of difficulty that children who are developing typically exhibit, as well as those with speech sound delays or disorders.

In this section, we review the intersection of stress with lexical class and syllable structure. Then we review the typical course of prosodic development, with a focus primarily on English lexical stress but with examples from other languages for contrast. Finally, we review the prosodic challenges associated with specific speech sound disorders.

Key concepts

English has often been characterized as a stress-timed language (Abercrombie, 1967; Pike, 1945), which means that the timing of an utterance is determined based upon the patterning of stress, specifically the durations of stressed versus unstressed syllables. In English, stress is the property of syllables. Stressed syllables are higher in pitch, longer in duration, and louder relative to unstressed syllables. Whether in words or nonwords, English speakers' use of stress is largely influenced by three factors: lexical class, syllable structure, and the speakers' familiarity with stress patterns in other words (Guion et al., 2003).

Stress and lexical class

Stress patterning often reflects the grammatical functions of words, especially disyllabic words. Consider that the word "present" can be used as a noun, an adjective, or a verb. We place stress on the first syllable to indicate a noun or an adjective (*pre-zuhnt* [ˈpɹɛzənt]) and the second syllable to indicate a verb (*pree-zent* [pɹiˈzɛnt]). Lexical class and stress placement change when a morpheme is added to a word (e.g., the verb *legal* [ˈligəɫ] becomes the noun *legality* [ləˈgælɪɾi]). As demonstrated through these examples, individual words tend to alternate between stressed (strong) and unstressed (weak) syllables in English. Furthermore, most English words do not have two stressed syllables next to each other, with the exception of compound words (e.g., *greenhouse* [ˈgɹinˌhaʊs]). The word *happiness* is more typical: the first syllable is stressed and the last two syllables are unstressed (*happiness* [ˈhæpinɛs]), creating a strong-weak-weak stress pattern. This is different from the word *apology* [əˈpɑlədʒi] whose stress pattern is weak-strong-weak-weak and *premature* [pɹiməˈtʃɝ] whose stress pattern is weak-weak-strong. Although words often have two weak syllables in a row, it's unusual to have more than two weak ones together, as is seen in the word *indefatigable* [ɪndəˈfærɪgəbəɫ].

Words can be described as having either a trochaic stress pattern (strong syllable first, as in *happiness*) or an iambic pattern (weak syllable first, as in *apology* and *premature*; Bhatara et al., 2018). The majority of English nouns have a trochaic stress pattern compared to verbs (Kelly & Bock, 1988); trochaic words are also more common overall. In fact, the trochaic stress pattern is present 3.4 times more often in disyllabic words than the iambic stress pattern in English (Clopper, 2002). Reasons for why this might occur will be reviewed in the section about prosody development.

Stress and syllable structure

The structures of syllables, as reviewed previously, differ from each other by consonant and vowel composition and organization, as well as by syllable weight. Some syllables are "light" and others are "heavy." As noted earlier, in English, syllables are heavy if they contain a tense vowel (e.g., [i] in *bee*), a diphthong (e.g., [aɪ] in *bye*), and/or a coda (e.g., [t] in *bit*). Other syllables are light. Some light syllables, including those ending in lax vowels such as [ɪ], [ɛ], and [ʊ], are not allowed in word-final position; words like [pɪ] or [tʊ] are not possible in English. Heavy syllables are far more likely to be stressed than light syllables (Guion et al., 2003; Redford & Oh, 2016).

The type of vowel within a syllable plays an important role with respect to syllable weight and, thus, stress placement. The second syllable of a disyllabic word will be stressed if it contains a tense vowel or diphthong or at least a two-element consonant cluster (Chomsky & Halle, 1968; Hayes, 1982). The first syllable would contain either an unstressed full or reduced vowel (e.g., *elect* [ə'lɛkt]). Likewise, the first syllable will receive stress if it contains a long vowel, such as a diphthong (e.g., *chowder* ['tʃaʊɾɚ]). The relationship between stress placement and vowel type can be observed between the schwa [ə] and wedge [ʌ]. Each corresponds to the same audible sound and distinctive vowel features, except the schwa occurs in unstressed syllables and the wedge occurs in stressed syllables (e.g., *abut* [ə'bʌt]). Furthermore, when a morpheme is added to a word, stress placement and the vowel within the stressed syllable change. Consider again the *legal* ['ligəɫ] to *legality* [lə'gælɪɾi] example. When the stress placement changes to the second syllable, the vowels in the first and second syllables change. Even if the vowel phoneme itself doesn't change, it can go through vowel reduction. Consider *electric* [i'lɛ:ktɹɪk] and *electricity* [ilɛk'tɹɪsəti]. Due to moving the stress to the third syllable, the length of the [ɛ] in the second syllable of *electricity* is reduced compared to when it is stressed and, thus, lengthened in *electric*.

Typical development of phonotactic–prosodic interface

Between 7 and 10 months of age, infants whose native language is stress-timed attend more to words that have trochaic stress patterns (Houston et al., 2000; Jusczyk et al., 1999). English-speaking infants display a preference for trochaic words compared to iambic words (Jusczyk et al., 1993; Mehler et al., 1988), and they produce them even in their non–linguistic vocalizations (Davis et al., 2000; Vihman et al., 2006). At 10 months of age, English-speaking infants begin to perceptually segment words with iambic stress patterns as well (Jusczyk et al., 1999). As early as 2 years of age, English-learning children use duration to differentiate stressed and unstressed syllables, allowing them to use lexical stress patterns (Kehoe et al., 1995; Pollock et al., 1993). By 3 years of age, children's productions of trochaic stress patterns become adult-like, with the acquisition of iambic patterns developing more slowly (up to 7 years of age; Ballard et al., 2012). This challenge is thought to be related to weak syllable deletion (Gerken, 1994, 1996; Kehoe & Stoel-Gammon, 1997). Children as young as 2 years are more likely to omit a weak syllable that occurs before a stressed syllable (e.g., *banana* /bə'nænə/ said as *nana* ['nænə]) than one that occurs afterward (e.g., *banana* /bə'nænə/ said as *banah* [bə'næ]). This probably reflects the preference for trochaic stress patterns. It also relates to prosodic foot structure, which is described in detail in Chapter 3.

Similarly, in languages with geminates ("double" consonants) in medial position, such as Finnish and Japanese, or with word-final stress such as French, children are more likely to omit initial consonants, presumably because the child's attention is drawn away from initial position to medial or final positions by the prosody of the language (Velleman & Vihman, 2002; Vihman & Croft, 2007; Vihman & Velleman, 2000). In contrast, stress in English is far more likely to be on the initial syllable and word-initial consonant deletion is far less common.

As with phonotactics and phonetics, individuals with particular English accents or dialects may produce stress patterns differently. Speakers of AAE mark lexical stress on some words differently than speakers of GAE, a phenomenon known as forestressing (Thomas, 2015). For example, in GAE stress falls on the second syllable in the words "guitar" [gə'tɑɚ], "police" [pə'lis], and "July" [dʒə'laɪ], whereas in AAE stress is on the first syllable (i.e., ['gi.tɑɚ], ['poʊlis], and ['dʒulaɪ]). This same phenomenon also occurs in some regional dialects in the southern United States. According to Thomas (2015), more research is needed on AAE prosody (e.g., fundamental frequency, speech rate) in order to understand the impacts of social, generational, and regional influences. Speech-language pathologists (SLPs) must engage in activities related to cultural and linguistic competency and respect the unique identities and experiences of each client. Refer to Chapter 4 for more information on AAE. More details about prosodic development are provided in Chapter 3.

Atypical phonotactic-prosodic development and use

Individuals with neurodevelopmental conditions may present with dysprosody or prosodic impairment. Dysprosody is a phonetic impairment due to a physiological inability to use pitch, duration, and loudness. In contrast, a prosodic impairment is when pitch, duration, and/or loudness are misused linguistically or paralinguistically despite the speaker's physiological ability to produce these features (Velleman, 2016). Individuals with Williams syndrome (WS) (Mervis & Velleman, 2011) or Down syndrome (Kumin, 2001) present with muscle tone anomalies. Differences in muscle tone mean that the tension of one's muscles is too much (high muscle tone) or not enough (low muscle tone) when speaking. This can impact the use of prosody.

Toddlers with WS aged 9–39 months produced fewer syllables per utterance on average relative to age expectations during 30-minute play sessions (Velleman et al., 2006). English-speaking toddlers with WS between 15 and 48 months of age can perceptually segment words with a trochaic stress pattern from a speech stream, but not words with an iambic stress pattern (Nazzi et al., 2003). With respect to older children, English-speaking adolescents with WS exhibited significantly more stress errors (i.e., reduced, excessive, equal, and/or misplaced stress) than age- and sex-matched typically-developing (TD) adolescents (Hargrove et al., 2013). Spanish-speaking adolescents and young adults with WS perform more poorly on tests of expressive and receptive syntactic chunking and expressive contrastive stress compared to age-matched, typically developing peers, even while controlling for IQ (Martínez-Castilla et al., 2011).

In individuals with Down syndrome (DS), perceptual phonological issues have been associated with prosodic abnormalities, specifically challenges identifying syllable, word, and phrase-level boundaries and other prosody comprehension skills (Bray et al., 1995; Heselwood et al., 1995). With respect to production, individuals with DS have difficulties producing the grammatical functions of prosody, including lexical stress (Pettinato & Verhoeven, 2008), contrastive stress (Stojanovik, 2011), and question intonation (Zampini et al., 2016). Thus, it is currently thought that people with DS have limitations on prosodic features with respect to perception, imitation, and spontaneous production (Kent & Vorperian, 2013).

While individuals who are OAS may also present with muscle tone anomalies, research often characterizes their prosody as being related to prosodic impairment. Before 6 months of age, infants later diagnosed as being OAS produce significantly fewer complex pitch contours and significantly more simple pitch contours relative to infants developing typically (Brisson et al., 2014). Children who are OAS misplace stress when producing utterances (Peppé et al., 2007), including atypical lexical stress patterns and weak syllable deletion in addition to sound substitutions in multisyllabic words (Arciuli & Bailey, 2019; McAlpine et al., 2014). For instance, they have been shown to produce stressed syllables with increased duration compared to TD speakers during a sentence completion task (Grossman et al., 2010); this results in longer word durations. Similarly, Paul et al. (2005) found that children who are OAS exhibit difficulties on prosody tasks involving stress, including the grammatical, lexical, and pragmatic functions of stress.

One of the key characteristics of CAS is difficulty with lexical stress. In particular, children with CAS tend to overstress the syllables that should be unstressed in words such that it sounds like every syllable is stressed ("excess equal stress"), although there actually are acoustic differences between their productions of stressed and unstressed syllables (Munson et al., 2003). For obvious reasons, this deficit is exacerbated in longer words, especially those with less typical stress patterns (e.g., iambic stress). They also tend to delete unstressed syllables from multisyllabic words at later ages than TD children or children with other SSDs do (Velleman & Shriberg, 1999). More information about prosodic difficulties in children with CAS is provided in Chapter 3.

Summary

As we have seen, phonotactics and prosody work together to provide a scaffold onto which consonants and vowels can be placed to create syllables, words, phrases, and beyond. Both can influence the child's use of certain error patterns, such as final consonant deletion, cluster reduction, and weak syllable deletion. The aspects of these two linguistic components that we have emphasized here can be summarized with respect to how they interact with syllable shapes, word shapes, and longer structures (phrases, sentences) as shown in Table 1.1. Later, we organize the clinical implications of these two aspects of the phonology of English in this same way, with respect to assessment and intervention.

Table 1.1 English phonotactics-prosody summary.

	Phonotactics	Prosody	Comments

Syllable shape	Structure of syllable:
	• onset
	  ○ singleton (1 C)
	  ○ cluster (2-3 Cs)
	• rhyme
	  ○ nucleus
	  ○ coda
	
	• Error patterns:
	  ○ final consonant deletion
	  ○ cluster reduction
	  ○ initial consonant deletion (atypical)
		Stress placement impacted by syllable weight:
		• light syllable
		  ○ rhyme = lax vowel
		  ○ likely unstressed
		• heavy syllable
		  ○ tense vowel and/or diphthong and/or coda
		  ○ likely stressed
		
		Error patterns:
		• vowel reduction
		• excess equal stress (atypical)
			• CV—universal syllable shape
			• Many different stress patterns in other languages (including no stress)

Word shape	• 1+ syllables (no limit)
	• intersyllabic consonant sequences
	
	Error patterns:
	• weak syllable deletion
	• harmony
	• metathesis, migration
	• medial consonant deletion (atypical)
		• stress-timed
		• often alternating stress
		• trochaic (strong first)
		• iambic (weak first)
		• stress may shift when suffix morphemes added
		
		Error patterns:
		• weak syllable deletion
		• stress shifts (atypical)
		• monostress (atypical)
			• Monosyllabic words common in English; rare in some other languages
			• Trochaic most common in English words:
			  ○ trochaic learned first
			  ○ iambic developing up to age 7

Beyond		• compound words versus adjectival phrases • emphatic (sentence-level) stress	• Between-word coarticulation, including deletion and ligature, in English and other languages

Phonotactics and prosody: clinical implications

Because there is considerable overlap in assessment approaches for identifying phonotactic and prosodic error patterns, and some overlap in intervention strategies, both will be reviewed together in this final section. For children who are young or whose speech sound disorders are more severe, we focus on assessing and treating the production of very simple syllable and word shapes, including the inclusion of onsets, complex nuclei (diphthongs), and codas and the production of two-syllable words with trochaic and (later) iambic stress patterns. These provide a variety of environments that may prove more or less challenging for consonant production. For children who are older or whose speech sound disorders are less severe, multisyllabic words allow us to assess and treat longer, more complex structures with a variety of stress patterns.

Furthermore, both simple and complex words can be combined into phrases and sentences, with various different types of stress. For true communicative success, phonetic learning (of consonants, primarily) must be embedded within this wide variety of phonotactic and prosodic contexts.

Assessment

Assessment of simple syllables and words can be achieved through a speech sample (e.g., a parent–child play session) or administration of a single-word articulation test (such as the Goldman-Fristoe Test of Articulation—3rd Edition [Goldman & Fristoe, 2015] and many other, similar tests). However, neither a speech sample nor an articulation test is controlled for syllable and word shapes. Therefore, using that approach would require taking the child's productions and analyzing them afterward with respect to the syllable and word shapes targeted and produced, remembering to watch for immature error types such as harmony, metathesis, and migration (see Velleman, 2016).

Luckily, there are some tests that control for syllable and word shapes. The Dynamic Evaluation of Motor Speech Skill (DEMSS; Strand & McCauley, 2019) is organized based upon word shape and stress pattern with several words per shape. Word shapes range from ten CV words (e.g., *me, hi, bye*) through VC, CVCV, and CVC, to six three-syllable words with different stress patterns (e.g., ba**na**na, **pee**kaboo, lemo**nade**). The words are controlled for whether or not they include reduplication or harmony. The Toddler Polysyllable Test (T-POT; Baker, 2018) allows for the assessment of complex word shapes, specifically tri- and quadrisyllabic words. Similar to the DEMSS, the stress patterning of these complex word shapes varies. However, it includes some longer words than the DEMSS. For children who are suspected of having distribution restrictions (such as harmony), the criterion-referenced Test of Syllable Sequencing Skills that is packaged with the intervention material Moving across Syllables (Kirkpatrick et al., 1990) may be helpful. Finally, the Profiling Elements of Prosody in Speech-Communication test (PEPS-C; Peppé, 2015) is a measure used to examine prosodic forms and functions in older children. It allows clinicians to examine clients' lexical stress patterns and also phrase-level stress, prosodic boundaries, and contrastive stress.

Unfortunately, none of these tests are organized in such a way as to assess a variety of clusters in all positions (see Chapter 6). Single-word articulation tests often include just a small number of clusters, especially in initial position. Therefore, an informal assessment of words with specific cluster types that seem relevant for the client at a particular time may be needed (see Velleman, 2016, for analysis forms).

Intervention

It's tempting when working with children with severe speech sound disorders to model words and phrases unnaturally slowly, without the appropriate prosody or allophones (e.g., pronouncing *pretty* as [ˈpʰɹɪtʰi], with an aspirated [t], instead of [ˈpʰɹɪɾi], with a flap/tap). Many SLPs also view prosody as "the frosting on the cake" (i.e., as a less key aspect of speech that can be added later, once the child is producing all segments accurately). However, a primary goal of therapy is to teach the client to speak in a way that will sound natural. It's very difficult to add naturalness, especially natural prosody, later. Furthermore, because prosody impacts many other aspects of communication, including pragmatics as well as morphology and syntax, it is critical for intelligibility and for social interactions. Therefore, prosody intervention should begin immediately, at the same time as treatment for segmental and phonotactic aspects of speech. Phonotactic and phonotactic-prosodic interventions should be individualized given the client's speech profile (consonant/vowel segments, syllable/word shapes, and prosodic repertoire). This includes collaborating with families to ensure accentual and dialectal features of the client's speech profile are recognized, respected, and appropriately integrated into intervention plans.

For young children or those with more severe speech sound disorders, early goals are likely to focus on simple syllable and word shapes with appropriate prosodic contours, including production of two-syllable words as well as monosyllables. For those who have difficulty combining segments at all, there are many very simple vowel-heavy emotion words that provide communicative power and practice with salient prosodic patterns despite low articulatory complexity. These include monosyllables like *ow, ooh, whee,* and *whoa* as well as disyllabic words such as *uh-oh, uh-uh,* and *uh-huh.* As soon as possible, more constricted consonants (stops, nasals) should be targeted in simple monosyllables (i.e., CV, VC, CVC) and disyllables (i.e., VCV, CVCV). For disyllables, it's often effective to start with words that are reduplicated (e.g., *mama, boo-boo*) or have consonant harmony (e.g., *daddy, baby*) or vowel harmony (e.g., *bow-wow, boo-hoo*). For addressing codas, it's important to remember that consonant harmony (as in *mom* and *dad*) and/or lax vowels (as in *bit* and *cut* but not *beat* and *coot*) may be helpful. For those who can speak in phrases, adjacency can also facilitate coda production (e.g., *goo**d d**og* to teach final [d]). It's also helpful to consider that velars and fricatives may be easier to achieve in final position than other consonant classes or than in initial position (Velleman, 2016). Visual representations and even movement activities (e.g., acting out the coda as the caboose on a train) may also convey the concept of closing the syllable with a consonant (Bernhardt, 2015).

Once the child is producing two-syllable words or two-word phrases, therapy should include a focus on appropriate stress patterns and smooth, fluent production. Strategies that are helpful here include a great deal of repetition to facilitate fluency and embedding practice within meaningful activities that elicit emphasis, questions as well as statements, and emotional intonation. Visual representations of stress patterns (e.g., a large block for a stressed syllable and a smaller block for an unstressed syllable) may be useful.

For older children or those with less severe speech sound disorders, more sophisticated word shapes and prosodic patterns are the targets. This includes clusters and multisyllabic words; the latter require attention to lexical stress as well as phonotactic accuracy. Although children with CAS may not follow typical developmental patterns, it's important to keep those in mind, including the fact that whether or not clusters are homorganic (as are *st-* and *-mp*) and whether or not they follow the sonority hierarchy (as stop + liquid clusters do, but [s] + stop clusters don't) may matter to some children. For children who have distribution restrictions, an approach such as Moving Across Syllables (Kirkpatrick et al., 1990), which is organized by place of articulation, may be useful.

When teaching multisyllabic words, many of us instinctively break them down and practice them from front to back (in-stinc-tive-ly). However, because of the prosody and the morphology of English, it's actually more appropriate to use "backward build-ups" (Velleman, 2003). When we produce words syllable by syllable from beginning to end, our pitch goes down and we use phrase-final lengthening at the end of each syllable. But these features are not appropriate when the word is produced as a whole; they would make the word sound segmented (choppy). Backward build-ups are a bit challenging to learn, but they are very effective at facilitating natural-sounding, appropriately stressed multisyllabic words. The steps are the following:

1. Write the word, phrase, sentence, syllable by syllable or word by word, with the stressed syllables in caps to help you (and the child if they are literate). Start each syllable with a consonant, if possible (e.g., *BU-tton*, not *BUTT-on*).
   HI po **PO** ta mus
2. Have the child practice the last syllable several times until it's smooth. If the child can read, you might want to cover up the other syllables.
3. Have the child practice the last two syllables several times until they're smooth. Remember to say these syllables the way that they will sound when you pronounce the whole word. In this example, that would be *duh-MUSS* [də‿mʌs] (with a little more stress on *muss*), not *TAYmuss* ['tʰeɪ̃məs]. The letter *t* is pronounced as [d] because, within the context of the whole word, it is flapped/tapped.
4. Have the child practice the last three syllables several times until they're smooth. Remember to say these syllables the way that they will sound when you pronounce the whole word (['**pʰɑ:**rəməs]).
5. Have the child practice the last four syllables several times until they're smooth. Remember to say these syllables the way that they will sound when you pronounce the whole word ([pə'**pʰɑ:**rəməs]).
6. Have the child practice the whole word several times until it's smooth. Remember to say it naturally, with the correct stress and allophones ([ˌhɪpə'**pʰɑ:**rəməs]).

If at any time the child begins to have trouble, go back to the previous step and practice several more times at that level before moving forward again. As in Dynamic Temporal and Tactile Cueing (DTTC) therapy (Strand, 2020), it may be helpful to practice the sequence simultaneously before using a model–imitation strategy. This same approach can be used at the phrase or sentence level.

A useful strategy for practicing sentential (emphatic stress), also first proposed by Velleman (2003), can go hand in hand with practicing wh-questions for children who have language difficulties as well. In this case, the child will produce the same response to each question, but vary the stress depending on the question that was asked. For example, the sentence might be: *The white mouse ate the cheese in the kitchen yesterday.* Different wh-questions should elicit different emphatic stress patterns:

Q: Who ate the cheese in the kitchen yesterday?
A: The **white** **mouse** ate the cheese in the kitchen yesterday.

Q: What did the white mouse eat in the kitchen yesterday?
A: The white mouse ate **the** **cheese** in the kitchen yesterday.

Q: Where did the white mouse eat the cheese yesterday?
A: The white mouse ate the cheese **in the kitchen** yesterday.

Q: When did the white mouse eat the cheese in the kitchen?
The white mouse ate the cheese in the kitchen **yesterday**.

Q: Which mouse ate the cheese in the kitchen?
A: The **white** mouse ate the cheese in the kitchen yesterday.

A similar strategy involves providing contradictory answers. For example, the adult says, *Mary took a **train** to Boston* and the child replies, *No, Mary took a **plane** to Boston* and so on (Fish, 2015). Of course, the length and complexity of the sentences and the words therein should be tailored to the child's pronunciation ability.

For resilient school-aged children who have difficulty producing multisyllabic words with the correct stress, rhythm, segments, and number of syllables, Rapid Syllable Transition Training (ReST; McCabe et al., 2017) can be very helpful. In this approach, nonsense words are selected to have a certain length (number of syllables) and certain target phonemes that are somewhat of a challenge to the child's abilities at that time. Each word is modeled by the SLP. The child repeats, then judges their own productions with respect to "smoothness" (no inappropriate pauses or groping), beats (all syllables present and correctly stressed), and sounds (sounds produced accurately). Schedules of training and feedback follow a particular protocol; details, self-training materials, and therapy materials are available at https://rest.sydney.edu.au/. Additional information about ReST is provided in Chapter 3.

Conclusion

Phonotactics and prosody provide the foundation for the sequences of consonants and vowels that form words, phrases, and sentences. Prosody additionally provides grammatical cues and insight into the speaker's emotional meaning. Furthermore, certain word and syllable shapes and prosodic patterns impact a speaker's ability to accurately produce the phones. Children with CAS and those with neurodevelopmental conditions, including autism, are at special risk of difficulties in these areas. Therefore, these aspects of phonology are at least as important to assess and treat as the segments themselves. They should and can be targeted from the earliest stages of intervention. Furthermore, segmental practice should always be embedded within a variety of phonotactic and prosodic contexts.

References

Abercrombie, D. (1967). *Elements of general phonetics*. Edinburgh University Press.

Arciuli, J., & Bailey, B. (2019). An acoustic study of lexical stress contrastivity in children with and without autism spectrum disorders. *Journal of Child Language, 46*(1), 142–152.

Baker, E. (2018). *Toddler polysyllable test for GAE (T-POT for GAE)*. www.e.baker2@westernsydney.edu.au

Ballard, K. J., Djaja, D., Arciuli, J., James, D. G., & van Doorn, J. (2012). Developmental trajectory for production of prosody: Lexical stress contrastivity in children ages 3 to 7 years and in adults. *Journal of Speech, Language, and Hearing Research, 55*, 1822–1835.

Berman, R. A. (1977). Natural phonological processes at the one-word stage. *Lingua, 43*, 1–21.

Bernhardt, B. M. (2015, September 22). Phonology and fun-ology website: Free assessment tools, tutorials, and activities. *Communique*. https://blog.sac-oac.ca/phonology-and-fun-ology-website-free-assessment-tools-tutorials-and-activities/

Bhatara, A., Boll-Avetisyan, N., Höhle, B., & Thierry, N. (2018). Early sensitivity and acquisition of prosodic patterns at the lexical level. In P. Prieto & N. Esteve-Gibert (Eds.), *The development of prosody in first language acquisition* (pp. 37–57). John Benjamins Publishing Company.

Bray, M., Heselwood, B., & Crookston, I. (1995). Down's syndrome: Linguistic analysis of a complex language difficulty. In M. Perkins & S. Howard (Eds.), *Case studies in clinical linguistics* (pp. 123–145). Whurr.

Brisson, J., Martel, K., Serres, J., Sirois, S., & Adrien, J. L. (2014). Acoustic analysis of oral productions of infants later diagnosed with autism and their mother. *Infant Mental Health Journal, 35*, 285–295.

Chomsky, N., & Halle, M. (1968). *The sound pattern of English*. Harper & Row.

Clopper, C. G. (2002). Frequency of stress patterns in English: A computational analysis. *Indiana University Linguistics Club Working Papers, 2*, 1–9.

Crystal, D. (1987). *The Cambridge encyclopedia of language*. Cambridge University Press.

Davis, B. L., MacNeilage, P. F., Matyear, C. L., & Powell, J. K. (2000). Prosodic correlates of stress in babbling: An acoustical study. *Child Development, 71*, 1258–1270.

Demuth, K., Culbertson, J., & Alter, J. (2006). Word-minimality, epenthesis, and coda licensing in the early acquisition of English. *Language and Speech, 49*(2), 137–174.

Demuth, K., & Fee, E. J. (1995). *Minimal words in early phonological development* [Unpublished manuscript]. Brown University and Dalhousie University.

Dinnsen, D. A. (1996). Context effects in the acquisition of fricatives. In B. Bernhardt, J. Gilbert, & D. Ingram (Eds.), *Proceedings of the UBC international conference on phonological acquisition* (pp. 136–148). Cascadilla Press.

Farwell, C. B. (1977). Some strategies in the early production of fricatives. *Papers and Reports in Child Language Development, 12*, 97–104.

Fish, M. (2015). *Here's how to treat childhood apraxia of speech* (2nd ed.). Plural Publishing.

Fromkin, V. (1973). Slips of the tongue. *Scientific American, 229*(6), 110–117.

Gerken, L. A. (1994). The metrical template account of children's weak syllable omissions from multisyllabic words. *Journal of Child Language, 12*, 565–584.

Gerken, L. A. (1996). Phonological and distributional information in syntax acquisition. In J. L. Morgan & K. Demuth (Eds.), *Signal to syntax: Bootstrapping from speech to grammar in early acquisition* (pp. 411–425). Lawrence Erlbaum Associates.

Goldman, R., & Fristoe, M. (2015). *Goldman-Fristoe test of articulation-3 (GFTA-3)*. Pearson Assessments.

Goldsmith, J. A. (1990). *Autosegmental and metrical phonology*. Blackwell.

Grossman, R., Bemis, R., Skwerer, D., & Tager-Flusberg, H. (2010). Lexical and affective prosody in children with high-functioning autism. *Journal of Speech, Language, and Hearing Research, 53*(3), 778–793.

Guion, S. G., Clark, J. J., Harada, T., & Wayland, R. P. (2003). Factors affecting stress placement for English nonwords include syllabic structure, lexical class, and stress patterns of phonologically similar words. *Language and Speech, 46*, 403–427.

Hargrove, P. M., Pittelko, S., Fillingane, E., Rustman, E., & Lund, B. (2013). Perceptual speech and paralinguistic skills of adolescents with Williams syndrome. *Communications Disorders Quarterly, 34*(3), 152–161.

Hayes, B. (1982). Extrametricality and English stress. *Linguistic Inquiry, 13*, 227–276.

Heselwood, B. C., Bray, M., & Crookston, I. (1995). Juncture, rhythm and planning in the speech of an adult with Down's syndrome. *Clinical Linguistics & Phonetics, 9*(2), 121–137.

Houston, D. M., Jusczyk, P. W., Kuijpers, C., Coolen, R., & Cutler, A. (2000). Cross-language word segmentation by 9-month-olds. *Psychonomic Bulletin & Review, 7*(3), 504–509.

Ingram, D. (1974). Fronting in child phonology. *Journal of Child Language, 1*, 233–241.

Jacks, A., Marquardt, T. P., & Davis, B. L. (2006). Consonant and syllable structure patterns in childhood apraxia of speech: Developmental change in three children. *Journal of Communication Disorders, 39*, 424–441.

Jusczyk, P. W., Cutler, A., & Redanz, N. J. (1993). Infants' preference for the predominant stress patterns of English words. *Child Development, 64*, 675–687.

Jusczyk, P. W., Houston, D. M., & Newsome, M. (1999). The beginnings of word segmentation in English-learning infants. *Cognitive Psychology, 39*(3–4), 159–207.

Kehoe, M., & Stoel-Gammon, C. (1997). Truncation patterns in English-speaking children's word productions. *Journal of Speech Language and Hearing Research, 40*(3), 526–541.

Kehoe, M. M., & Stoel-Gammon, C. (2001). Development of syllable structure in English-speaking children with particular reference to rhymes. *Journal of Child Language, 28*(2), 393–432.

Kehoe, M., Stoel-Gammon, C., & Buder, E. H. (1995). Acoustic correlates of stress in young children's speech. *Journal of Speech, Language, and Hearing Research, 38*, 338–350.

Kelly, M. H., & Bock, J. K. (1988). Stress in time. *Journal of Experimental Psychology: Human Perception and Performance, 14*, 389–403.

Kent, R. D., & Vorperian, H. K. (2013). Speech impairment in Down syndrome: A review. *Journal of Speech, Language, and Hearing Research, 56*, 178–210.

Kirk, C., & Demuth, K. (2003). Onset/coda asymmetries in the acquisition of clusters. In B. Beachley, A. Brown, & F. Conlin (Eds.), *Proceedings of the 27th Boston University conference on language development* (pp. 437–448). Cascadilla Press.

Kirkpatrick, J., Stohr, P., & Kimbrough, D. (1990). *Moving across syllables*. Communication Skill Builders.

Kumin, L. (2001). Speech intelligibility in individuals with Down syndrome: A framework for targeting specific factors for assessment and treatment. *Down Syndrome Quarterly, 6*, 1–8.

Lewis, B. A., Freebairn, L. A., Hansen, A. J., Iyengar, S. K., & Taylor, H. G. (2004). School-age follow-up of children with childhood apraxia of speech. *Language, Speech, and Hearing Services in the Schools, 35*(2), 122–140.

Lleo, C., & Prinz, M. (1996). Consonant clusters in child phonology and the directionality of syllable structure assignment. *Journal of Child Language, 23*, 31–56.

Maas, E., & Mailend, M. L. (2017). Fricative contrast and coarticulation in children with and without speech sound disorders. *American Journal of Speech Language Pathology, 26*, 649–663.

Martínez-Castilla, P., Sotillo, M., & Campos, R. (2011). Prosodic abilities of Spanish-speaking adolescents and adults with Williams syndrome. *Language and Cognitive Processes, 26*, 1055–1082.

McAlpine, A., Plexico, L. W., Plumb, A. M., & Cleary, J. (2014). Prosody in young verbal children with autism spectrum disorder. *Contemporary Issues in Communication Science and Disorders, 41*, 120–132.

McCabe, P., Murray, E., Thomas, D. C., & Evans, P. (2017). Clinical manual for Rapid Syllable Transition Treatment. http://sydney.edu.au/health-sciences/rest-media/rest-clinician-manual.pdf

McLeod, S., van Doorn, J., & Reed, V. A. (2001). Normal acquisition of consonant clusters. *American Journal of Speech-Language Pathology, 10*, 99–110.

Mehler, J., Jusczyk, P., Lambertz, G., Halsted, N., Bertoncini, J., & Amiel-Tison, C. (1988). A precursor of language acquisition in young infants. *Cognition, 29*, 143–178.

Mervis, C. B., & Velleman, S. L. (2011). Children with Williams syndrome: Language, cognitive, and behavioral characteristics and their implications for intervention. *Perspectives on Language Learning and Education, 18*(3), 98–107.

Munson, B., Bjorum, E. M., & Windsor, J. (2003). Acoustic and perceptual correlates of stress in nonwords produced by children with suspected developmental apraxia of speech and children with phonological disorder. *Journal of Speech Language and Hearing Research, 46*(1), 189–202.

Nazzi, T., Paterson, S., & Karmiloff-Smith, S. (2003). Early word segmentation by infants and toddlers with Williams syndrome. *Infancy, 4*(2), 251–271.

Nijland, L., Maassen, B., Van Der Meulen, S., Gabreels, F., Kraaimaat, F. W., & Schreuder, R. (2002). Coarticulation patterns in children with developmental apraxia of speech. *Clinical Linguistics and Phonetics, 16*(6), 461–483.

Nijland, L., Maassen, B., Van Der Meulen, S., Gabreels, F., Kraaimaat, F. W., & Schreuder, R. (2003). Planning of syllables in children with developmental apraxia of speech. *Clinical Linguistics & Phonetics, 17*(1), 1–24.

Nordgren, P. M. (2015). Phonological development in a child with autism spectrum disorder: Case study of an intervention. *Journal of Interactional Research in Communication Disorders, 6*(1), 25–51.

Overby, M., Belardi, K., & Schreiber, J. (2020). A retrospective video analysis of canonical babbling and volubility in infants later diagnosed with childhood apraxia of speech. *Clinical Linguistics & Phonetics, 34*(7), 634–651.

Paul, R., Augustyn, A., Kin, A., & Volkmar, F. (2005). Perception and production of prosody by speakers with autism spectrum disorders. *Journal of Autism and Developmental Disorders, 35*(2), 205–220.

Pearson, B. Z., Velleman, S. L., Bryant, T. J., & Charko, T. (2009). Phonological milestones for African American English-speaking children learning Mainstream American English as a second dialect. *Language, Speech, and Hearing Services in the Schools, 40*, 229–244.

Peppé, S. (2015). Profiling Elements of Prosody in Speech Communication (PEPS-C). http://www.peps-c.com/peps-c-2015.html

Peppé, S., McCann, J., Gibbon, F., O'Hare, A., & Rutherford, M. (2007). Receptive and expressive prosodic ability in children with high-functioning autism. *Journal of Speech Language and Hearing Research, 50*, 1015–1028.

Pettinato, M., & Verhoeven, J. (2008). Production and perception of word stress in children and adolescents with Down syndrome. *Down Syndrome Research and Practice*. Advance online publication. https://assets.cdn.down-syndrome.org/pubs/a/reports-2036.pdf

Pike, K. (1945). *The intonation of American English*. University of Michigan Press.

Pollock, K., Brammer, D., & Hageman, C. (1993). An acoustic analysis of young children's productions of word stress. *Journal of Phonetics, 21*, 183–203.

Priestly, T. M. S. (1977). One idiosyncratic strategy in the acquisition of phonology. *Journal of Child Language, 4*, 45–65.

Redford, M. A., & Oh, G. E. (2016). Children's abstraction and generalization of English lexical stress patterns. *Journal of Child Language, 43*(2), 338–365.

Rupela, V., & Manjula, R. (2006). Phonotactic development in Kannada: Some aspects and future directions. *Language Forum: A Journal of Language and Literature, 32*(1–2), 83–93.

Schoen, E., Paul, R., & Chawarska, K. (2011). Phonology and vocal behavior in toddlers with autism spectrum disorders. *Autism Research, 4*, 1–12.

Shriberg, L. D. (1993). Four new speech and voice-prosody measures for genetics research and other studies in developmental phonological disorders. *Journal of Speech Language and Hearing Research, 36*, 105–140.

Shriberg, L. D., Aram, D. M., & Kwiatkowski, J. (1997). Developmental apraxia of speech: II. Toward a diagnostic marker. *Journal of Speech Language & Hearing Research, 40*(2), 286–312.

Smit, A. B., Hand, L., Freilinger, J. J., Bernthal, J. E., & Bird, A. (1990). The Iowa articulation norms project and its Nebraska replication. *Journal of Speech and Hearing Disorders, 55*(4), 779–798.

Stemberger, J. P. (1988). Between-word processes in child phonology. *Journal of Child Language, 15*, 39–61.

Stoel-Gammon, C. (1987). Phonological skills of 2-year-olds. *Language Speech and Hearing Services in the Schools, 18*, 323–329.

Stojanovik, V. (2011). Prosodic deficits in children with Down syndrome. *Journal of Neurolinguistics, 24*(2), 145–155.

Strand, E. A. (2020). Dynamic temporal and tactile cueing: A treatment strategy for childhood apraxia of speech. *American Journal of Speech-Language Pathology, 29*, 30–48.

Strand, E. A., & McCauley, R. J. (2019). *The dynamic evaluation of motor speech skill (DEMSS)*. Brookes.

Thomas, E. R. (2015). Prosodic features of African American English. In A. Lanehart (Ed.), *The Oxford handbook of African American language* (pp. 420–435). Oxford University Press.

Trapman, M., & Kager, R. (2009). The acquisition of subset and superset phonotactic knowledge in a second language. *Language Acquisition, 16*(3), 178–221. https://www.jstor.org/stable/40645783?seq=1#metadata_info_tab_contents

Velleman, S. L. (1994). The interaction of phonetics and phonology in developmental verbal dyspraxia: Two case studies. *Clinics in Communication Disorders, 4*(1), 67–78.

Velleman, S. L. (2003). *Childhood apraxia of speech resource guide.* Delmar.

Velleman, S. L. (2016). *Speech sound disorders in children.* Wolters Kluwer Health.

Velleman, S. L., Currier, A., Caron, T., & Curley, A. (2006, May). *Phonological development in Williams syndrome* [Conference presentation]. International Clinical Phonetics and Linguistics Association.

Velleman, S. L., & Pearson, B. Z. (2010). Differentiating speech sound disorders from phonological dialect differences. *Topics in Language Disorders, 30*(3), 176–188.

Velleman, S. L., & Shriberg, L. D. (1999). Metrical analysis of the speech of children with suspected developmental apraxia of speech and inappropriate stress. *Journal of Speech Language and Hearing Research, 42*(6), 1444–1460.

Velleman, S. L., & Vihman, M. M. (2002). Whole-word phonology and templates: Trap, bootstrap, or some of each? *Language, Speech, and Hearing Services in the Schools, 33*, 9–23.

Vihman, M. M., & Croft, W. (2007). Phonological development: Toward a "radical" templatic phonology. *Linguistics, 45*(4), 683–725.

Vihman, M. M., Nakai, S., & DePaolis, R. A. (2006). Getting the rhythm right: A cross-linguistic study of segmental duration in babbling and first words. *Laboratory Phonology, 8*, 341–366.

Vihman, M. M., & Velleman, S. L. (2000). The construction of a first phonology. *Phonetica, 57*, 255–266.

Wells, B. (1994). Junction in developmental speech disorder: A case study. *Clinical Linguistics & Phonetics, 8*(1), 1–25. https://doi.org/10.1080/02699209408985572

Wetherby, A. M., Yonclas, D. G., & Bryan, A. A. (1989). Communicative profiles of preschool children with handicaps: Implications for early identification. *Journal of Speech and Hearing Disorders, 54*, 148–158.

Zampini, L., Fasolo, M., Spinelli, M., Zanchi, P., Suttora, C., & Salerni, N. (2016). Prosodic skills in children with Down syndrome and in typically developing children. *International Journal of Language & Communication Disorders, 51*(1), 74–83.

2 Morphosyntax

Using linguistic theory to frame
assessment and intervention of
morphosyntactic skills in English
speaking children

Stacy K. Betz

Abstract

This chapter explains key linguistic terminology and theory that apply
to clinical assessment and intervention of grammatical impairments in
children. Children with a wide range of language disorders, including developmental language disorder, Down syndrome, and Fragile X
syndrome, have difficulty with the morphologic and syntactic system.
Although they produce errors on a range of morphemes and syntactic structures, they tend to make a disproportionate number of errors
on verb morphology, specifically on morphemes that mark tense and
agreement properties. Together, the properties of tense and agreement are referred to as finiteness marking because they contrast the
marked form of the verb, such as *walked*, from the non-finite form of
the verb, as in *to walk*. Because the morpheme, such as past tense—*ed*,
is required to fulfill a syntactic requirement, that all verbs are marked
for tense, the term morphosyntax is also used to refer to these grammatical properties.

In English, the sounds that are used to indicate these morphemes are
quite different ranging from /d/ to mark past tense, /s/ to mark third
person singular present tense, to a free morpheme, /ɪz/, to indicate tense
and agreement on the verb "to be." However, research has shown that
children with language impairments make similar errors across these different sounding morphemes because their shared purpose is to mark
finiteness within a clause. Although much more limited than the evidence for using morphosyntactic skills to diagnose child language disorders, there is also some research demonstrating that this linguistic theory
applies to intervention as well. Children will generalize treatment gains
from one treated morpheme that marks finiteness to other, untreated
morphemes that mark finiteness.

DOI: 10.4324/9781003045519-3

Statement to the reader

Within the field of speech-language pathology, child language develop-ment classes often discuss Brown's morphemes as the foundational basis for understanding development of specific morphological and syntactic structures. Although this is a useful starting point, it can lead to a view that these structures should be assessed and treated as individual units without considering their underlying grammatical function. This chapter describes how speech-language pathologists can apply theoretical linguistics to interpret a child's grammatical errors in terms of underlying grammatical functions. Two areas of particular weakness for children with language impairments are used as an example—tense and agreement marking.

Introduction

In the field of pediatric speech-language pathology, it is second nature to evalu-ate a child's speech errors in terms of error patterns focused on the articulatory characteristics of place, manner, and voicing. That is, a child who substituted /t/ for /k/ and /d/ for /g/ would not be viewed as making two unrelated errors; rather, these errors would be described as a pattern of substituting alveolars for velars (i.e., velar fronting)—an error with place of articulation. This error pattern could then be used to guide treatment decisions. However, the field does not place as much emphasis on using morphosyntactic properties to inter-pret grammatical errors and plan treatment goals. In terms of morphosyn-tax, errors such as a child saying, *Him bounce it*, instead of *He bounced it* and *Me is sick* instead of *I was sick* are not as different as they might seem. Both of these incorrect utterances involve errors on case marking and verb tense. Using morphosyntactic properties to interpret errors such as these can guide more accurate classification of errors and more efficient treatment approaches. When determining whether a child's production is a morphosyntactic error, it is essential to have knowledge of the linguistic rules of the language and dialect the child is speaking. A child's production can only be considered an error if native speakers of that dialect would consider it ungrammatical. This chapter explains key linguistic terminology and theory that apply to clinical assessment and intervention of grammatical impairments in children that speak General American English (GAE). These general concepts can be applied to other lan-guages and other English dialects; however, the specific examples used might not be considered errors in all other English dialects. See Oetting, Berry, and Gregory-Martin (Chapter 4) for discussion of linguistic properties of other English dialects.

Morphosyntax

One straightforward way to define morphosyntax is the interaction of mor-phology and syntax. To understand this interaction, consider each of these domains of language separately. Morphology refers to how morphemes contribute to the structure of words. A morpheme is the smallest linguistic unit of meaning or function. For example, the word firehouse is composed of two morphemes that each has meaning: fire and house. The word teacher is also composed of two morphemes that each has meaning: *teach* and -*er*. In this case, -*er* changes the meaning of teach to mean someone who teaches. *Fire, house, teach,* and -*er* are all morphemes that have meaning but they do have one important difference in terms of structure. *Fire, house,* and *teach* can all be words on their own. Because of this, they are referred to as free morphemes. In contrast, the morpheme -*er* is not a word on its own. It is considered a bound morpheme because it must occur bound to another morpheme.

Other bound morphemes do not have a particular meaning but serve more of a grammatical function. For example, in the sentence, *The child talks*, the bound morpheme -*s* in the word talk does not have much meaning by itself. If the speaker would have instead said, *The child talk*, their listener probably would still understand their meaning but would also think that the sentence was ungrammatical. That is because the -*s* morpheme serves a grammatical purpose/function rather than contributing true meaning to the sentence. Grammar is the combination of morphology and syntax (although note that phonology is also considered to be part of a person's grammar).

Syntax refers to the structure of sentences. For example, in English, basic sentence construction occurs with the subject first, followed by the verb, and then the object. If a speaker said, *talk child the*, the sentence would be considered ungrammatical because it violates syntactic rules for how sentences are formed using the canonical subject-verb-object word order. Some grammatical structures need to follow both morphological and syntactic rules. Think back to the sentence, *The child talks*. The reason the -*s* morpheme is required on the verb is because of the properties of the subject of the sentence; if the subject would have been *children*, as in, *The children talk*, then the -*s* morpheme would not be needed. This is an example of morphosyntax because how a speaker uses morphology depends on other structures in the sentence.

One category of morphosyntactic forms is finiteness marking. Finiteness is a property that applies to verbs with all verbs being considered as either finite or non-finite. In English, finite verbs are those that indicate tense, person/number agreement with the subject, or mood (Quirk et al., 1985). The finiteness properties that have the largest impact on clinical practice with children with language impairments who speak GAE are tense and agreement. Therefore, mood (e.g., the selection of the forms *would* and *were* in utterances such as, *I would eat more if I were hungry*) will not be discussed in this chapter. Tense refers to the distinction between present and past. For example, the difference between *The boys play games* and *The boys played games* is that the first sentence is present tense and the second past tense. The -*ed* morpheme is referred to as a past tense marker because its use differentiates (i.e., marks) tense in those two examples.

Agreement refers to marking the verb so that it matches the subject in terms of person and number. For example, consider the sentence, *The girl plays games*.

Table 2.1 Auxiliary be verbs

Form of Agreement	Present Tense	Past Tense
1st person singular	I **am** playing	I **was** playing
1st person plural	We **are** playing	We **were** playing
2nd person singular	You **are** playing	You **were** playing
2nd person plural	You **are** playing	You **were** playing
3rd person singular	He/She/It **is** playing	He/She/It **was** playing
3rd person plural	They **are** playing	They **were** playing

Table 2.2 Copular be verbs

Form of Agreement	Present Tense	Past Tense
1st person singular	I **am** here	I **was** here
1st person plural	We **are** here	We **were** here
2nd person singular	You **are** here	You **were** here
2nd person plural	You **are** here	You **were** here
3rd person singular	He/She/It **is** here	He/She/It **was** here
3rd person plural	They **are** here	They **were** here

The subject of the sentence, *the girl*, is third person. Third person refers to a subject that is not the person speaking (that is first person) or the person the speaker is talking to (that is second person) but rather is someone/something being referred to during the conversation. The subject *the girl* is also singular. There is one girl being discussed not multiple (which would be plural). In the sentence *The girl plays games*, the verb *plays* contains the bound inflectional morpheme -*s*. The function of this morpheme is to indicate that the verb is present tense and that the subject of the sentence is third person singular. Therefore, the morpheme is referred to as third person singular present tense -*s*.

The past tense -*ed* and third person singular present tense -*s* are the only bound morphemes that mark finiteness in English. In addition, there are auxiliary and copular forms of the verb to-be that also mark both tense and agreement. These verbs are shown in bold in Tables 2.1 and 2.2. The forms of the verb are the same. The only difference is that copular verbs are the main verbs in the sentence, whereas auxiliary verbs occur with another main verb. For this reason, auxiliary verbs are often referred to as helping verbs.

At first glance, third person singular present tense morphemes, past tense morphemes, and auxiliary/copular forms of be might seem very different from each other. However, these grammatical structures are all similar because they all mark finiteness, either tense or tense and agreement. In contrast to other languages, English is considered to have a sparse inflectional system. In some languages, all verbs would be required to have a finiteness marker to indicate tense and agreement. However, in English, many verbs do not have any overt marking for finiteness. For example, a speaker knows that the sentence *They play games* is present tense even though there is no morphological marker on the verb *play* to indicate this.

When evaluating whether a child produces finiteness marking correctly, it is essential to accurately identify the instances where verbs must have an overt finiteness marker. These are referred to as obligatory contexts for finiteness because the sentence would not meet the grammatical rules of English if the finiteness marker was not used (i.e., that finiteness marker is obligatory). For example, the sentence *He eats candy* is grammatical but the sentence *He eat candy* is not grammatical. This is because the verb *eat* in conjunction with the third person singular subject *he* creates an obligatory context for using the third person singular present tense -*s*. That clause, *He eats candy*, is considered to be overtly marked for finiteness. If a child attempts to produce the sentence *He eats candy*, but makes a mistake marking finiteness, the error is almost always one of omission. In this case an omission error would be the child saying *He eat candy*. This error could be described as an attempt at producing the third person singular present tense -*s* but an attempt that was an omission of this morpheme. Young typically developing children and children with language impairments make this same pattern of errors in which they omit finiteness markers.

Morphosyntactic Errors in Children With Language Impairments

Assessment of finiteness marking in children is clinically important for two reasons. First, weaknesses in finiteness marking have been shown to have high diagnostic accuracy in identifying children who have language impairments but no known cause for the language weaknesses (e.g., no hearing loss or intellectual disability) (e.g., Conti-Ramsden et al., 2001; Guo et al., 2020; Rice & Wexler, 2001). The diagnosis given to this group of children is developmental language disorder (DLD) (also referred to as specific language impairment (SLI)). This does not mean that these children do not have difficulties with other domains of language, such as semantics, or other grammatical structures—only that the weaknesses in finiteness marking can differentiate children with DLD from children with typical language. However, measures of finiteness marking must be accurately collected to be used as a diagnostic indicator of DLD. The other reason finiteness marking is important during a clinical assessment is that in addition to children with DLD, children with other language impairments due to other etiologies have weaknesses with these grammatical forms. This includes children with Fragile X syndrome (Sterling et al., 2012) and children with Down syndrome (Eadie et al., 2002). Evaluating these children's accuracy in finiteness marking is important to then plan treatment. Therefore, being able to validly evaluate finiteness marking is essential for clinical practice with these populations.

The research documenting that children with language impairments have difficulties with finiteness marking is robust and a relative point of agreement within the field. However, the reason for these weaknesses is not as widely agreed on. The theory most directly linked to the identification of finiteness weaknesses as a hallmark feature of children with DLD is the extended optional infinitive hypothesis (Rice et al., 1995). This theory states that children with language impairments are likely to omit finiteness markers in obligatory contexts because their grammatical system treats these structures as optional even when the syntactic context requires tense and agreement marking. No direct cause for the optional nature of finiteness marking is suggested other than biological maturation; however, the search for genetic causes is ongoing (Rice, 2020).

Another theory for weak finiteness marking is the surface account (Leonard et al., 1992). This theory proposes that children with language impairments have difficulty with tense and agreement markers because they have less perceptual saliency than other grammatical structures. The procedural deficit hypothesis offers yet another possibility for these deficits (Ullman & Pierpont, 2005). This theory suggests that children with language impairments have deficits in more areas than just language. Weakness in finiteness marking occurs because children have difficulty with procedural memory which involves learning rules including grammatical rules. The debate over why children with language impairments have difficulty with finiteness marking is not likely to be resolved anytime soon. However, the fact that these children have deficits in this area means that effective assessment and treatment procedures are needed.

Assessment

Assessing Expressive Morphosyntactic Skills in Children

Because morphosyntactic deficits are common in children with language impairments, it is important to assess a child's skills in this area during initial diagnostic evaluations as well as ongoing assessment after a child begins receiving intervention. In terms of a child's skills in producing finiteness marking, the general concept behind evaluation is straightforward—have the child attempt to produce these structures and measure the accuracy of their productions. Similar to assessment procedures used for other areas of child language, there are two main ways to assess a child's productions: elicited production and spontaneous productions. Spontaneous productions can easily be collected during a language sample. Following the language sample, the clinician can then orthographically transcribe the sample and calculate a child's percent correct use of each finiteness marker. In addition to analyzing the accuracy of each individual finiteness marker, it is also useful to calculate an overall percentage correct use of finiteness marking. This overall percentage would include as the denominator all obligatory contexts for finiteness marking (i.e., third person singular present tense -s, past tense -ed, irregular past tense, copular *be* forms, and auxiliary forms). The numerator would be how many of those opportunities were produced correctly. Because all of these grammatical structures serve the linguistic function of marking tense and agreement, the overall percentage correct is a summary measure of the child's use of these grammatical features rather than specific forms of these features. This is similar to an analysis of a child's speech errors. If a child substituted /t/ for /k/ and /d/ for /g/, one measure of the child's accuracy would be the percent correct production of /k/ and the percent correct production of /g/. But because both of these errors can also be explained as instances of velar fronting, a clinician might also compute the percentage occurrence of velar fronting. Research suggests that clinicians approach treatment for tense and agreement as intervention on specific grammatical structures rather than the underlying grammatical function. For example, when asked in an open-ended format to list up to five grammatical forms they target most often with children, 60% of SLPs working with elementary school-aged children reported treating past tense, but only 6% mentioned third person singular, 12% auxiliary verbs, and 15% copula verbs (Finestack & Satterlund, 2018). No responses mentioned treating tense, agreement, or finiteness more broadly.

Elicited production tasks are ones in which the clinician creates a structured opportunity for the child to produce a specific linguistic structure. In general, elicitation methods use both visual and linguistic contexts to create a scenario that makes it extremely likely a child will attempt the grammatical structure that is being assessed. The Test of Early Grammatical Impairment (TEGI) is one formal assessment that uses two types of elicitation procedures to assess production of finiteness marking (Rice & Wexler, 2001). To elicit productions of third person singular present tense -*s*, the clinician shows the child a picture of one person actively engaged in an activity. The clinician then provides a prompt such as "Here is a teacher. Tell me what a teacher does?" The target response is for the child to produce a sentence that has a third person singular subject and a lexical verb. A grammatical response for speakers of GAE requires the child to use the third person singular present tense -*s* morpheme. Examples of responses that correctly use this finiteness marker include: *The teacher teaches*, *The teacher writes on the board*, and *She tells kids what to do*. Because this task is intended to measure finiteness marking, not semantics, a child's response would also be scored as correct if the third person singular present tense marker was used correctly but the content did not match the picture stimulus. For example, a response of *My teacher gives us candy* would be considered correct because the third person singular present tense marker is used correctly even though there is no candy in the picture. Similarly, if the child produces grammatical errors on structures other than the targeted third person singular present tense, those errors do not impact the child's score for that item. For example, if a child omits the determiner *the* and says, *The teacher writes on board*, the response would be scored as correct because the child correctly used the third person singular present tense marker.

Elicited production tasks aim to create a context in which a child will attempt to use a particular grammatical structure; however, children do not always respond in ways the clinician might expect. These responses can create difficulties for how to score and interpret the child's productions. For example, in an elicited production task targeting third person singular present tense, a child may produce a third person plural subject and say *The teachers write on the board*. Because the subject is not third person singular, there is not a linguistic context to use the third person singular present tense marker. Therefore, this type of response cannot be validly used to assess a child's ability to produce this morpheme. In these instances, the formal testing directions are to prompt the child for a second response by implicitly encouraging them to use a third person singular subject. For example, one suggested re-prompt is, "Tell me just what this teacher does" or to tell the child to "Start with he or she" (p. 14). If the child's second response uses a third person singular subject, then that response can be scored. If the clinician is ultimately not able to get the child to produce a response that includes the context for using the third person singular present tense morpheme, then the response is considered unscorable and is not used when calculating the child's percent correct use of the morpheme. If a child does not provide any response to the elicitation prompt, those responses are also considered unscorable. These formal testing procedures used in the Test of Early Grammatical Impairment lead to slightly more complicated scoring directions than are typically used in standardized tests of child language. According to the test directions, responses for the items that target third person singular present tense use can be classified in four ways:

- The child attempted the structure and the child's use was dialect appropriate: *The teacher teaches.*
- The child attempted the structure but the child's use was dialect inappropriate: *The teacher teach.*
- Unscorable attempt: *The teachers teach.*
- Unscorable no response: The child did not respond at all.

The administration and scoring procedures for this task ensure that the child is being assessed on their use of this one finiteness marker specifically. Other types of errors, both lexical and grammatical, do not impact how each item is scored. In this way it is a theoretically driven evaluation. The Test of Early Grammatical Impairment includes similar subtests to elicit productions of other finiteness markers. The procedures for this formal assessment can easily be used as the basis for creating informal assessments to use in diagnostic evaluations and to monitor treatment progress.

Assessment of Finiteness Marking Production Using Norm-Referenced Tests

The Test of Early Grammatical Impairment (Rice & Wexler, 2001) described earlier is designed specifically to assess a child's use of finiteness marking. Other formal tests including comprehensive standardized tests of child language include some test items focused on morphosyntax along with other domains of language. One common way these tests elicit production of specific finiteness markers is the use of a sentence completion task. In this type of task, the clinician begins saying a sentence and asks the child to fill in a word or phrase to complete the end of the sentence. For example, the clinician might show the child a picture of a dog jumping while saying *The dog likes to jump. Yesterday the dog. . .* Correct productions of the regular past tense marker would then be scored as correct. Similarly, third person singular present tense can be elicited by showing a child a picture of a dog jumping while saying, *The dog likes to jump. Every day the dog . . ..* In both of these examples, the linguistic context is intended to create an obligatory context for the child to produce a specific finiteness structure.

The way elicited production tasks are scored directly impacts the interpretation of a child's strengths and weaknesses in finiteness marking. In terms of scoring, most norm-referenced tests do not consider the same level of detail as the Test of Early Grammatical Impairment (TEGI; Rice & Wexler, 2001). One difference is how responses that would be considered as "unscorable" on the TEGI are interpreted. Some norm-referenced tests (e.g., Clinical Evaluation of Language Fundamentals—5th Edition [CELF-5]; Wiig et al., 2013) have similar administration procedures as the TEGI in which if the child initially produces a response that does not include an obligatory context for the intended finiteness marker, the clinician gives an additional prompt. These prompts are often generic with phrasing such as Try again, or, Say that another way. If a child gives a response that does not include the target finiteness marker but is still grammatically correct, the response is most frequently scored as incorrect. For example, *ate cookies*, in response to the question, *The boy likes to bake every day. Tell me what he did yesterday* would be considered an incorrect response. The justification for scoring this response as incorrect is that the purpose of the test item is to assess regular past tense *-ed* (i.e., *cooked*) but the child produced an irregular past tense instead. On the one hand, this response is not an example of the child correctly producing regular past tense. In that sense, scoring it as incorrect seems appropriate. However, the response is also not an incorrect production of past tense. From a linguistic point of view, this response is more accurately described as not being an obligatory context for producing this grammatical structure. This type of scoring system penalizes children not only for incorrect grammatical productions but also for responses that do not attempt the target structure.

One possible reason standardized tests often use a simplified scoring system for elicited production tasks is that the individual test items target a wide range of grammatical structures. For example, the Clinical Evaluation of Language Fundamentals Preschool—3rd Edition (CELF-P3; Wiig et al., 2006) Word Structure subtest focuses on production of grammatical structures such as past tense *-ed*, progressive *-ing*, plural *-s*, the derivational morpheme *-er* to indicate "one who," and the modal auxiliary *will*. Even the Structured Photographic Expressive Language Test (SPELT-3; Dawson et al., 2005), which evaluates only expressive morphology and syntax, includes a range of structures; finiteness marking is targeted but so are other grammatical forms such as plurals, negation, and prepositions. With so many different structures being assessed within the same test, it can be difficult to create administration and scoring guidelines for how to identify and re-prompt children's responses that do not provide obligatory contexts for the target grammatical structure. It certainly is possible to create such guidelines, but clinician reliability in administering the test might decrease due to the constantly changing nature of the task. Therefore, on tests like these, a child's score is influenced by their accuracy in producing finiteness markers but is not a direct measure of finiteness marking. If a child scores below age expectations on the CELF-P3 or SPELT-3, clinicians can interpret that as a weakness in expressive grammatical skills, but any conclusions about the child's ability to produce finiteness marking could only be made informally. In addition, those conclusions would be based on only a few opportunities for producing finiteness.

Assessing Comprehension of Finiteness Marking

In comparison to tasks assessing production of finiteness marking, comprehension of finiteness markers is less commonly included on formal assessments. From a theoretical perspective, the reason for this is that finiteness markers serve a grammatical function rather than a stand-alone meaning. This makes it difficult to assess those grammatical functions independent of other aspects of the sentence. As one example, think back to children who have deficits in finiteness marking and often omit copular be forms such as *is* or *are*. It is difficult to imagine a task that would assess whether a child understands the word *is* in isolation. Comprehension tasks at the sentence level are certainly possible. A child could be shown four pictures and asked to point to "She is happy." What the child's response tells you about their grammatical system would depend on the four picture options and which one the child selects. For example, the correct picture could be a girl with a large smile holding a bunch of balloons. One of the other pictures could be two children each with a large smile holding a bunch of balloons. A third picture could be a boy with a large smile holding a bunch of balloons. The final picture could be a girl with a cut on their leg crying. If a child points to the picture of the sad girl, that response does not provide any information on the child's understanding of finiteness marking. This is because the stimulus sentence used the form *is* and the picture could also be described with a sentence using the form *is*, such as *The girl is sad*. This incorrect response would most likely be due to a lexical error regarding the meaning of happy. Therefore, these types of comprehension tasks can evaluate a child's understanding of finiteness but only in tandem with their skills in other language domains.

Grammaticality Judgment Tasks

Although directly assessing comprehension of finiteness marking is difficult, clinicians should aim to collect information about a child's finiteness marking using more than only production tasks. Grammaticality judgment tasks are one way to do this. As the name implies, they involve having the child make a judgment about whether a linguistic structure is grammatical. For example, one task could assess a child's knowledge of copular -be forms. A grammaticality judgment task could involve the clinician saying *The girl is happy.* Does that sound right or wrong? Other items on the task would ask similar questions about ungrammatical structures. For example, the clinician might say *The girl happy.* Does that sound right or wrong? Throughout the task some items would be grammatical instances of the use of a finiteness marker. Other items would be ungrammatical examples. Because the most common error made by children with language impairments is omission of finiteness marking, the ungrammatical test items could involve omissions. Grammaticality judgment tasks are a type of meta-linguistic task. The term meta-linguistics refers to a person's ability to think about their own linguistic system. In a grammaticality judgment task, children are asked to do just that—reflect on whether a given structure is grammatical or ungrammatical. The task can be considered a measure of the child's linguistic competence, which is different than production (because they do not have to produce the finiteness marker being assessed) and also different than comprehension.

Interpreting a child's performance on grammaticality judgment tasks involves considering their performance on the task as a whole, not individual items. The clearest interpretation would be a child who demonstrated adult levels of linguistic competence. This would be a child who consistently responded by saying sentences with omitted finiteness markers were ungrammatical and items with correct uses of finiteness were grammatical.

Another fairly straightforward interpretation would be a child who inconsistently responded to both grammatical and ungrammatical items (i.e., if about 50% of the time they said grammatical sentences were grammatical but also about 50% of the time said that ungrammatical sentences were grammatical). This pattern of responses most likely indicates the child was guessing. In this case you could say that a child had difficulty with meta-linguistics but could not make clear conclusions about their finiteness marking system. The third pattern of responses is difficult to interpret. That is, children who consistently judge grammatical and ungrammatical items as being grammatical. If a child's production errors are such that they sometimes correctly mark finiteness but other times omit those same finiteness markers, it is reasonable to hypothesize that they could consider both of those forms to be grammatical. On the other hand, similar to the previous child, this child could also have difficulties with the meta-linguistic aspect of the task but instead of randomly guessing right or wrong as their judgment, they consistently rate all items as grammatical. Including other, earlier developing types of grammatical structures in the task can help determine whether a child understands how to make meta-linguistic judgments. For example, if a child accurately produces plural morphemes, ungrammatical test items that have errors in plural marking can be included. A child can be asked questions such as *A boy has three crayon.* Does that sound right or wrong? If a child consistently judged omitted plurals as wrong while consistently judging correct and omitted finiteness markers as correct, it would be evidence that the child understands the task and omissions of finiteness are considered grammatical for them.

A few formal child language tests include grammaticality judgment questions. Interspersed among other types of questions, the Preschool Language Scales—5th Edition (PLS-5; Zimmerman et al., 2011) has a few grammaticality judgment items. The Comprehensive Assessment of Spoken Language—2nd Edition (CASL-2; Carrow-Woolfolk, 2017) and the TEGI (Rice & Wexler, 2001) both have an entire grammaticality judgment subtest. The grammaticality judgment questions on the PLS-5 and CASL-2 also ask the child to fix any errors on items they judge to be ungrammatical. Similar to the fact that elicited imitation tasks on most norm-referenced tests assess a range of grammatical structures within the same subtest, grammaticality judgment tasks on many formal tests also include questions not only about finiteness marking but also about other structures such as derivational morphemes and pronoun case. The TEGI is one formal assessment that includes a grammaticality judgment task focused solely on finiteness marking. Grammaticality judgment tasks can be especially useful when working with children who use final consonant deletion. Because past tense *-ed* and third person singular present tense *-s* are marked with a final consonant added to the root word, if a child omits final consonants due to a speech error, the child would omit these bound morphemes. The reason for these omissions would be a speech error, not a morphological error. Because grammaticality judgment tasks do not require the child to produce the structure, they can be used to give some information about the child's linguistic competence of finiteness marking without interference from their speech system.

Treating Morphosyntactic Deficits

One of the primary ways linguistic theory relates to intervention for morphosyntactic impairments in children is how treatment goals are selected. Fey et al. (2003) suggested that clinicians identify intermediate goals when planning grammatical interventions. Intermediate goals are a middle ground between the broader aim for treatment to improve grammar overall and more specific basic goals that can be clearly targeted and measured within a therapy session. Intermediate goals can reflect linguistic categories. Fey and colleagues suggest that categories such as auxiliary use or nominative case pronouns could be intermediate goals. When treating a child who has deficits in finiteness marking, the property of tense marking or agreement marking could be considered an intermediate goal. If tense was selected as an intermediate goal, then basic goals could include increasing correct productions of specific forms that mark tense. This could include structures that differentiate past versus present tense such as regular past tense *-ed* and irregular past tense forms. Because third person singular present tense *-s* also marks tense, it could also be included as a basic goal that addresses this intermediate goal. Similarly, auxiliary and copula *be* verbs would also fit within this intermediate goal. Because these later forms, third person singular present tense -*s*, auxiliary *be* forms, and copular *be* forms, all mark both tense and agreement, a different intermediate goal focused on forms that mark both tense and agreement could be selected. Past tense -*ed* would not be an appropriate basic goal in that instance because the morpheme only marks tense, not agreement. Therefore, the exact intermediate goals a clinician selects can vary depending on how fine grained a linguistic distinction is made in terms of the function of grammatical forms.

For example, a child might consistently omit plural -*s*, third person singular -*s*, and the auxiliary *are*. The phonological forms of the first two of those structures are the same: /s z ɪz/. An initial conclusion someone might make is that focusing treatment on plural and third person singular present tense together makes sense because those structures sound the same. However, considering the grammatical function of those morphemes would lead to selecting third person singular present tense -*s* and auxiliary *are* as two related basic goals that both address the same intermediate goal of tense and agreement marking.

Similar to the use of linguistic theory when selecting intermediate goals in clinical practice, researchers who investigate grammatical interventions can use linguistic theory to select control and generalization targets related to their treatment targets. Many intervention studies primarily aim to improve one specific grammatical target, similar to the selection of a basic goal. For example, a researcher might hypothesize that their intervention will increase children's accuracy in producing auxiliary *be* forms. One of the primary variables for this type of study would likely be a measure of the percentage of correct productions of these auxiliaries pre- and post-treatment. An increase in children's accuracy pre- to post-treatment would be one way to document the intervention was beneficial. Because auxiliary *be* forms mark tense and agreement, the researchers might also hypothesize that the intervention might generalize to other grammatical forms that mark tense and agreement. To investigate this, they might select a generalization measure such as children's accuracy in producing copular *be* forms. If children's accuracy on copular *be* forms also increased pre- to post-treatment, that would be evidence that the intervention impacted not just the specific treatment forms, but also the marking of tense and agreement more broadly. However, in these cases, it could also be that the increased accuracy in auxiliary and copular *be* was due to maturational changes in the child and not the intervention. To verify this is not the reason for the treatment gains, researchers can measure a control variable that is a grammatical form that has a different linguistic function than the treatment and generalization measures. In this case, one possible control measure could be children's use of articles (i.e., *the*, *a*, and *an*). Articles, auxiliary *be* and copular *be* are all function words but articles do not mark tense and agreement. Therefore, if a child did not improve on their use of articles pre- and post-treatment it would add more evidence that the treatment targeted tense and agreement. Not all intervention research uses this design, but background in linguistic theory can make it easier to understand these designs and the type of progress that could be expected when using that treatment with a child in clinical practice. Clinicians can also select intervention targets using a similar strategy; one tense marker to treat, a different tense marker as to measure treatment generalization, and another morpheme the child produces incorrectly that is not related to tense as control data.

Treatment studies that include generalization and control measures help to document the degree to which the use of linguistic theory to structure the assessment of finiteness marking also relates to treatment. That is, linguistic theory provides a clear rationale for considering finiteness markers as a similar functional group despite the range of phonological forms. There is also strong evidence that children with language impairments often have more difficulties with finiteness markers than other grammatical structures. The question when interpreting intervention research is, do the currently available interventions also support the notion of finiteness marking as an important classification when planning treatment? Overall, the research in this area is mixed, partly because studies treating finiteness markers vary in what are considered generalization and control measures.

Leonard and colleagues (2004, 2006, 2008) conducted a longitudinal study focused on improving production of finiteness markers in children with SLI. There were three treatment groups: one group who received intervention focused on third person singular present tense *-s*; one group who received a similarly structured intervention but focused on use of auxiliary *be*; and a third control group who received general language stimulation not specific to finiteness marking. All three groups were assessed on their use of third person singular present tense forms, auxiliaries, and past tense *-ed*. The third person singular treatment group made the greatest improvement in production of the target structure, third person singular. They also improved in production of auxiliaries, which was considered a generalization measure, but they made less improvement than they did for the target structure. A similar pattern occurred for the auxiliary treatment group. They not only had the greatest gains in production of auxiliaries but also increased in production of third person singular *-s*. Production of past tense *-ed* was considered a control measure. There were no differences between the three groups in terms of past tense productions. The researchers hypothesized that gains in third person singular present tense and auxiliaries might generalize because they mark both tense and agreement. In contrast, past tense *ed* only marks tense. Overall, their results supported this pattern of generalization of treatment gains within the finiteness marking system.

Calder et al. (2021) also conducted a study that investigated whether treatment gains generalized across finiteness markers in children with DLD. Past tense *-ed* was the structure directly targeted in intervention. In contrast to the studies by Leonard and colleagues (2004, 2006, 2008), this study considered third person singular present tense *-s* to be a potential generalization measure and possessive *-s* a control measure. The children improved in their production of past tense *-ed* but accuracy of grammaticality judgments of past tense did not change. However, the gains in production of both third person singular present tense *-s* and possessive *-s* were not significant. These studies demonstrate that treatments are effective in treating finiteness marking, but how much generalization can be expected is an area where more research is needed.

Treatment Procedures Used to Improve Finiteness Marking

The interventions used in the Calder et al. (2021) and Leonard et al. (2004, 2006, 2008) studies differed in one primary way. Calder and colleagues used an explicit treatment approach whereas Leonard and colleagues used implicit intervention procedures. Explicit interventions involve direct instruction in grammatical rules. For example, the clinician may frequently state the grammatical rule that is being targeted and talk to the child about why their production does or does not follow that grammatical rule. Implicit treatments focus on providing opportunities for the child to hear correct productions of grammatical structures and to produce those structures, but the grammatical rule is not directly discussed. Historically, grammatical interventions primarily used implicit methods such as focused stimulation, elicited production, and recasting. Focused stimulation involves the clinician producing a large number of instances of the target grammatical structure for the child to hear. This usually occurs in naturalistic scenarios such as play or narratives. The use of elicited productions in treatment is similar to their use in assessment; the clinician creates contexts for the child to produce the grammatical structure that is being treated. The key feature of an implicit treatment is that if the child's production is incorrect, the clinician does not tell the child they were incorrect. Instead, many (but not all) implicit treatments then use another procedure, recasting. In recasting, the clinician will immediately restate the child's utterance but will correct their error on the treatment target. For example, if third person singular present tense -*s* was the treatment target, the clinician and child might be playing with a farm set that included one horse and one cow. An example of elicited production could be the clinician saying, *My horse eats hay. Tell me about your cow.* The child might then say, *The cow eat grass.* To recast the clinician could then say, *Oh the cow eats grass.* At that point, as an implicit intervention, nothing is expected of the child.

These implicit treatment techniques have been found to be successful in targeting finiteness marking in children with language impairments. The findings described earlier for Leonard and colleagues (2004, 2006, 2008) stemmed from the use of implicit intervention procedures including focused stimulation. However, Swanson et al. (2005) did not find improvements in grammar use after using a narrative-based treatment that combined recasting, focused stimulation, and multiple methods for elicited production including narrative retells and sentence imitation. A systematic review and meta-analysis (Cleave et al., 2015) found that at least for recasts as the implicit intervention procedure, overall, the evidence shows positive treatment benefits.

One formal method for providing explicit grammatical treatment is SHAPE CODING (Ebbels, 2007). Finiteness marking is directly treated through the use of visual markers to identify the tense and agreement properties of verbs.

The clinician writes a sentence or uses an app that presents written sentences to the child. Colors and shapes are then used to identify various grammatical properties of the sentence. Tense marking arrows are drawn underneath the verb that is marked for tense. An arrow drawn on the left side of the word indicates past tense, whereas an arrow drawn extending down from the middle of the verb indicates present tense. The position of the arrow can help children differentiate present from past tense. Perhaps more importantly for children who omit tense markers is that clinicians can use the arrows as a graphic reminder that all sentences need to be marked for tense. Subject-verb agreement is depicted by drawing a single line underneath singular subjects and underneath verbs that agree in number to singular subjects. A double line is used for plural subjects and agreement. Calder et al. (2021) reference the procedural deficit hypothesis as one theoretical motivation for SHAPE CODING. As described earlier, the procedural deficit hypothesis proposes that children with language impairments have difficulties with implicit learning (Ullman & Pierpont, 2005). SHAPE CODING then aims to use explicit teaching to help children overcome impairments related to difficulties with implicit learning. Numerous studies have found SHAPE CODING to improve children's production of finiteness marking including past tense *-ed*, auxiliary *be*, and copular *be* (Calder et al., 2021, 2020; Kulkarni et al., 2014; Tobin & Ebbels, 2019).

One difficulty documenting the benefits of explicit interventions is that (assuming typical hearing and vision) children with language impairments have heard correct productions of finiteness marking their whole lives. Hearing these correct productions can be considered a type of implicit teaching and learning. Therefore, studies that investigate explicit grammar treatments cannot definitively rule out the influence of that real-life exposure to hearing those forms produced and how adults respond to the child's incorrect productions outside the therapy sessions. To address this design weakness, Finestack (2018) conducted a study focused on the use of explicit interventions with children with DLD. Instead of using real English grammatical forms, three novel bound morphemes were used. All three structures were designed to mimic a real grammatical form. One structure was used on verbs to mark the gender of the subject. Another structure indicated habitual actions. The third structure was an agreement marker to agree with first person subjects. All of these novel forms share at least some properties with finiteness marking (e.g., subject-verb agreement) so results can be an indication of the usefulness of explicit treatments for children with DLD. Some children were taught these novel forms using an implicit approach and some with a combined explicit-implicit method. In general, the children with DLD made greater gains when explicit intervention was included along with implicit treatment. A similar result was found for children with autism spectrum disorder (ASD) although the intervention differences were only statistically significant for one of the grammatical markers they investigated (Bangert et al., 2019).

Because implicit intervention includes basic methods such as providing correct models of a treatment structure, the debate between explicit and implicit instruction should not be between these two methods but between the use of implicit-only methods and a combined use of explicit and implicit methods. A systematic review by Frizelle and colleagues (2021) concluded that the use of explicit interventions is beneficial including when they are used in morpho-syntactic treatment. This recent work on explicit interventions builds on years of research showing that implicit methods can also be beneficial, albeit perhaps not as effective as when explicit teaching is also included.

Conclusions

For someone with minimal linguistics training, a child's errors in omitting copular *be* verbs, past tense *-ed*, and third person singular *-s* may seem to be vastly different errors. However, when viewed within a theoretical linguistics framework, these are all instances of errors with finiteness marking. Because of their shared grammatical properties, they can be assessed and treated with similar methods. Finiteness marking errors are certainly not the only type of weakness that children with language impairment have. Additionally, of the errors children make, finiteness marking might not seem like the highest priority for treatment. However, a child who makes finiteness marking errors will clearly be identified by their conversational partners as being ungrammatical. This can have significant consequences for children. Therefore, accurate assessment of finiteness marking and implementation of appropriate treatment methods for these weaknesses will benefit children with developmental language disorders. Clinical work with these children can be more theoretically based when morphosyntactic errors are interpreted as patterns of errors and treatment focuses on the underlying grammatical functions of the morphosyntactic structures.

References

Bangert, K. J., Halverson, D. M., & Finestack, L. H. (2019). Evaluation of an explicit instructional approach to teach grammatical forms to children with low-symptom severity autism spectrum disorder. *American Journal of Speech-Language Pathology, 28*(2), 650–663. https://doi.org/10.1044/2018_AJSLP-18-0016

Calder, S. D., Claessen, M., Ebbels, S., & Leitão, S. (2020). Explicit grammar intervention in young school-aged children with developmental language disorder: An efficacy study using single-case experimental design. *Language, Speech, and Hearing Services in Schools, 51*(2), 298–316. https://doi.org/10.1044/2019_LSHSS-19-00060

Calder, S. D., Claessen, M., Ebbels, S., & Leitão, S. (2021). The efficacy of an explicit intervention approach to improve past tense marking for early school-age children with developmental language disorder. *Journal of Speech, Language, and Hearing Research, 64*(1), 91–104. https://doi.org/10.1044/2020_JSLHR-20-00132

Carrow-Woolfolk, E. (2017). *Comprehensive assessment of spoken language* (2nd ed.). Western Psychological Services.

Cleave, P. L., Becker, S. D., Curran, M. K., Van Horne, A. J. O., & Fey, M. E. (2015). The efficacy of recasts in language intervention: A systematic review and meta-analysis. *American Journal of Speech-Language Pathology, 24*(2), 237–255. https://doi.org/10.1044/2015_AJSLP-14-0105

Conti-Ramsden, G., Botting, N., & Faragher, B. (2001). Psycholinguistic markers for specific language impairment (SLI). *Journal of Child Psychology and Psychiatry, 42*(6), 741–748. https://doi.org/10.1111/1469-7610.00770

Dawson, J. I., Stout, C. E., & Eyer, J. A. (2005). *Structured photographic expressive language test* (3rd ed.). Janelle Publications.

Eadie, P. A., Fey, M. E., Douglas, J. M., & Parsons, C. L. (2002). Profiles of grammatical morphology and sentence imitation in children with specific language impairment and Down syndrome. *Journal of Speech, Language, and Hearing Research, 45*(4), 720–732. https://doi.org/10.1044/1092-4388(2002/058)

Ebbels, S. (2007). Teaching grammar to school-aged children with specific language impairment using shape coding. *Child Language Teaching and Therapy, 23*(1), 67–93. https://doi.org/10.1191/0265659007072143

Fey, M. E., Long, S. H., & Finestack, L. H. (2003). Ten principles of grammar facilitation for children with specific language impairments. *American Journal of Speech-Language Pathology, 12*(1), 3–15. https://doi.org/10.1044/1058-0360(2003/048)

Finestack, L. H. (2018). Evaluation of an explicit intervention to teach novel grammatical forms to children with developmental language disorder. *Journal of Speech, Language, and Hearing Research, 61*(8), 2062–2075. https://doi.org/10.1044/2018_JSLHR-L-17-0339

Finestack, L. H., & Satterlund, K. E. (2018). Current practice of child grammar intervention: A survey of speech-language pathologists. *American Journal of Speech-Language Pathology, 27*(4), 1329–1351. https://doi.org/10.1044/2018_AJSLP-17-0168

Frizelle, P., Tolonen, A., Tulip, J., Murphy, C., Saldana, D., & McKean, C. (2021). The impact of intervention dose form on oral language outcomes for children with developmental language disorder. *Journal of Speech, Language, and Hearing Research, 64*(8), 3253–3288. https://doi.org/10.1044/2021_JSLHR-20-00734

Guo, L. Y., Eisenberg, S., Schneider, P., & Spencer, L. (2020). Finite verb morphology composite between age 4 and age 9 for the Edmonton narrative norms instrument: Reference data and psychometric properties. *Language, Speech, and Hearing Services in Schools, 51*(1), 128–143. https://doi.org/10.1044/2019_LSHSS-19-0028

Kulkarni, A., Pring, T., & Ebbels, S. (2014). Evaluating the effectiveness of therapy based around shape coding to develop the use of regular past tense morphemes in two children with language impairments. *Child Language Teaching and Therapy, 30*(3), 245–254. https://doi.org/10.1177/0265659013514982

Leonard, L. B., Camarata, S. M., Brown, B., & Camarata, M. N. (2004). Tense and agreement in the speech of children with specific language impairment: Patterns of generalization through intervention. *Journal of Speech, Language, and Hearing Research, 47*(6), 1363–1379. https://doi.org/10.1044/1092-4388(2004/102)

Leonard, L. B., Camarata, S. M., Pawłowska, M., Brown, B., & Camarata, M. N. (2006). Tense and agreement morphemes in the speech of children with specific language impairment during intervention: Phase 2. *Journal of Speech, Language, and Hearing Research, 49*(4), 749–770. https://doi.org/10.1044/1092-4388(2006/054)

Leonard, L. B., Camarata, S. M., Pawtowska, M., Brown, B., & Camarata, M. N. (2008). The acquisition of tense and agreement morphemes by children with specific language impairment during intervention: Phase 3. *Journal of Speech, Language, and Hearing Research, 51*(1), 120–125. https://doi.org/10.1044/1092-4388(2008/008)

Leonard, L. B., McGregor, K. K., & Allen, G. D. (1992). Grammatical morphology and speech perception in children with specific language impairment. *Journal of Speech & Hearing Research, 35*(5), 1076–1085. https://doi.org/10.1044/jshr.3505.1076

Quirk, R., Greenbaum, S., Leech, G., & Svartvik, J. (1985). *A comprehensive grammar of the English language.* Longman.

Rice, M. L. (2020). Causal pathways for specific language impairment: Lessons from studies of twins. *Journal of Speech, Language, and Hearing Research, 63*(10), 3224–3235. https://doi.org/10.1044/2020_JSLHR-20-00169

Rice, M. L., & Wexler, K. (2001). *Rice/Wexler test of early grammatical impairment*. The Psychological Corporation.

Rice, M. L., Wexler, K., & Cleave, P. L. (1995). Specific language impairment as a period of extended optional infinitive. *Journal of Speech & Hearing Research, 38*(4), 850–863. https://doi.org/10.1044/jshr.3804.850

Sterling, A. M., Rice, M. L., & Warren, S. F. (2012). Finiteness marking in boys with fragile X syndrome. *Journal of Speech, Language, and Hearing Research, 55*(6), 1704–1715. https://doi.org/10.1044/1092-4388(2012/10-0106)

Swanson, L. A., Fey, M. E., Mills, C. E., & Hood, L. S. (2005). Use of narrative-based language intervention with children who have specific language impairment. *American Journal of Speech-Language Pathology, 14*(2), 131–143. https://doi.org/10.1044/1058-0360(2005/014)

Tobin, L. M., & Ebbels, S. H. (2019). Effectiveness of intervention with visual templates targeting tense and plural agreement in copula and auxiliary structures in school-aged children with complex needs: A pilot study. *Clinical Linguistics & Phonetics, 33*(1–2), 175–190. https://doi.org/10.1080/02699206.2018.1501608

Ullman, M. T., & Pierpont, E. I. (2005). Specific language impairment is not specific to language: The procedural deficit hypothesis. *Cortex: A Journal Devoted to the Study of the Nervous System and Behavior, 41*(3), 399–433. https://doi.org/10.1016/S0010-9452(08)70276-4

Wiig, E. H., Secord, W. A., & Semel, E. (2006). *Clinical evaluation of language fundamentals—preschool* (3rd ed.). Pearson.

Wiig, E. H., Semel, E., & Secord, W. A. (2013). *Clinical evaluation of language fundamentals* (5th ed.). PsychCorp.

Zimmerman, I. L., Steiner, V. G., & Pond, R. E. (2011). *Preschool language scales* (5th ed.). PsychCorp.

Appendix 2.1

Individual grammatical forms that comprise finiteness marking in GAE.

During assessment each of these forms can be evaluated individually and those measures combined for an overall measure of the child's production of finiteness marking.

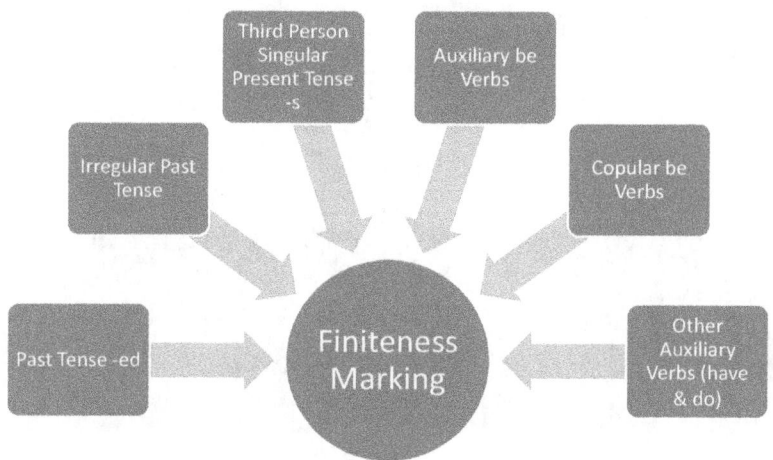

Appendix 2.2

Example of using multiple measures to assess finiteness marking.

Assess a child's production: Spontaneous or elicited production

Examples of Omitted Finiteness Marking Across Structures

- Past tense -ed: He bake a cake
- Third person singular -s: He bake a cake
- Copular be: He here
- Auxiliary be: He eating

Examples of Correct Productions

- Past tense -ed: He baked a cake
- Third person singular -s: He bakes a cake
- Copular be: He is here
- Auxiliary be: He is eating

If the child omits finiteness markers in production tasks, conduct additional assessments using grammaticality judgments.

Assess a Child's Grammaticality Judgments

Examples of Correct Finiteness Marking

- Past tense -ed: He bake a cake
- Third person singular -s: He bake a cake
- Copular be: He here
- Auxiliary be: He eating

Examples of Correct Productions

- Past tense -ed: He baked a cake
- Third person singular -s: He bakes a cake
- Copular be: He is here
- Auxiliary be: He is eating

Examples of Non-Finiteness Markers to Include to Rule out Metalinguistic Difficulties

- Incorrect use of plural -s: I have two cat.
- Correct use of plural -s: I have two dogs.

3 Prosody

Child prosody and approaches to assessment and intervention

Jill Thorson

Abstract

Prosody refers to the melodic and rhythmic variation of speech, and encompasses suprasegmental aspects such as lexical stress, accentuation, speech melody, and phrasing. By varying the primary acoustic correlates of prosody, one can relay a wide range of information about syntactic structure, semantic and pragmatic meaning, dialect, and affective states. Due to its interaction with linguistic and communicative function, prosody is an essential component of language development. The perception of prosody begins before birth and plays a critical role during the acquisition of a first language by aiding in early word segmentation and word learning. Additionally, child-directed speech patterns (i.e., motherese/parentese), which include exaggerated prosodic features, have been shown to aid in these early processes. As speech emerges, children have been shown to successfully produce a range of prosodic contours. The first aim of this chapter is to review the literature on prosodic development in typically developing children.

Prosodic impairment in children is often seen as one part of a speech and/or language disorder. Limited assessments are available, not widely used, and are typically targeted in their approach or more comprehensive in nature. Most evidence-based interventions for children with prosodic impairment use a motor programming approach. The second aim of this chapter is to review approaches to assessment and intervention for children with prosodic impairments and discuss the need for additional evidence-based options. On the basis of research, suggestions for how to approach assessment and intervention are also provided.

DOI: 10.4324/9781003045519-4

Statement to the reader

As a clinician, you have most likely learned more generally about prosody. However, you may not have had exposure to the diversity of components that all fall under the umbrella of prosody or how they interact with different types of disorders. In this chapter, a theory for how to hierarchically organize prosody is presented along with an overview of child prosody across these different levels. Additionally, prosodic approaches for assessment and intervention that are appropriate for children are discussed. Recommendations for clinicians are provided in how to approach assessment and intervention when an evidence-based option is not available.

Introduction

As children acquire speech and language, they must learn that it is not only *what* they say, but also *how* they say it. By varying the melodic and rhythmic components of speech (prosody), we express a wide range of critical linguistic and affective information. As listeners, children also need to process and comprehend prosodic information to effectively communicate with others. Thus, prosodic development plays a robust role in communication and is used to express both linguistic information and speaker affect.

Linguistically, prosody aids in structuring information as well as conveying semantic and pragmatic meaning. Organizing information by manipulating the placement of prosodic phrasal boundaries helps create meaningful syntactic units and signal turns in conversation. The placement of boundaries at the appropriate location signals meaning and helps resolve ambiguity. For example, changing the location of these boundaries can indicate meaningful differences between the following two sentences (marked with commas): *Jules loves chocolate muffins, and cookies* [she loves two things] versus *Jules loves chocolate, muffins, and cookies* [she loves three things]. Prosody also relays pragmatic information that is essential for a successful interaction by encoding speech acts (e.g., question, request) and information status (given versus new information) (Ladd, 2008; Nespor & Vogel, 2007; Prieto, 2015). In some languages, like English, phrasal prosody is also used to express lexical stress (e.g., through the assignment of a pitch accent to the syllable with primary word stress; *REcord* versus *reCORD*) and focus or prominence distinctions (e.g., *Who ate the cookie? JULIE ate the cookie.*). A pitch accent in English serves as a cue to prominence (e.g., a stressed syllable in a word or an acoustically highlighted word in a sentence) and is made through the manipulation of pitch, duration, and loudness. Pitch accents consist of targets that are high (H), low (L), or a combination of the two (L and H, or H and L). In tonal languages such as Mandarin and Cantonese, prosody is used to express lexical tone (e.g., rising, falling, high rising), where different pitch patterns on a word are used to signal different meanings.

Prosody also expresses speaker affect and emotion, such as being happy, angry, or sad, as well as how we communicate irony and sarcasm. In child language acquisition, prosody plays a critical role in learning and has been shown to aid in guiding infant attention, segmenting the speech stream, acquiring syntactic information, and supporting early word learning (see de Carvalho et al., 2018; Teixidó et al., 2018; and Thorson, 2018, for reviews). Thus, an impairment in prosodic perception or production can lead to breakdowns in learning and/or communication.

Children learn to perceive and produce the correct association between pro-sodic form and its function in relaying syntactic, semantic, pragmatic, affec-tive, and, in some languages, phonological information. Prosodically encoded meaning is realized through modulations in prosodic prominence and phrasal grouping (Prieto & Esteve-Gibert, 2018). Marking prominence highlights information in an utterance. A prominent word stands out, relative to other words in the same phrase, by virtue of pitch accent, and increased duration and/or intensity. For example, by accenting and deaccenting information in an utterance, a speaker can relay which part of a sentence is new or in focus to their listener (i.e., information/words that receive a pitch accent and are more acoustically prominent; an example of a word in focus would be the name *Paul* in response to the question *Who is running?* → *PAUL is running*). At the same time, modulations in prosody over the course of an utterance can provide cues as to whether a sentence is a statement or a question (e.g., rising for yes-no questions versus falling for a statement or a wh-question). A speaker also uses prosodic phrasal markers to break up syntactic units and provide cues to where a word or phrase begins and ends. The primary acoustic correlates manipulated to provide these cues are fundamental frequency (F_0, ~pitch), intensity (~loud-ness), duration (relating to timing), and spectral information (~voice quality), with the majority of work focusing on differences in pitch, loudness, and dura-tion (Bolinger, 1989; Lehiste, 1970, 1976; Shattuck-Hufnagel & Turk, 1996).

How we approach the study of prosody is important to provide a linguisti-cally and theoretically grounded foundation for analyses that are consistent across researchers and clinicians. For example, prosodic phonology has proven to be a useful way to discuss prosody and its acquisition. This theory hypoth-esizes that prosody is structured in a hierarchical manner from the syllable (or mora, which is a timing unit that is equal to or shorter than the syllable) at the bottom of the hierarchy up to intonational phrases and utterances at the top (see Figure 3.1, Nespor & Vogel, 2007). This framework for conceptualizing prosody as a hierarchy is widely referred to in the field of prosody and provides a foundation for thinking about the multiple levels of prosody. In this hierarchy, an intonational phrase consists of one prosodic contour (i.e., the melodic and rhythmic contour) over a stretch of spoken material. While there is discussion around which levels are present in this hierarchy, Figure 3.1 shows an adap-tation of Nespor and Vogel's (2007) version by Kehoe (2018) (see Demuth, 2018; Kehoe, 2018, for reviews on prosodic phonology and word production in development, and Vihman, 2018, for an alternative usage-based approach to prosodic structure). At each level, crucial prosodic information is transmitted. Syntactic and semantic form is often tied to the higher levels, such as the into-national and phonological phrases. The phonological phrase is an intermediate

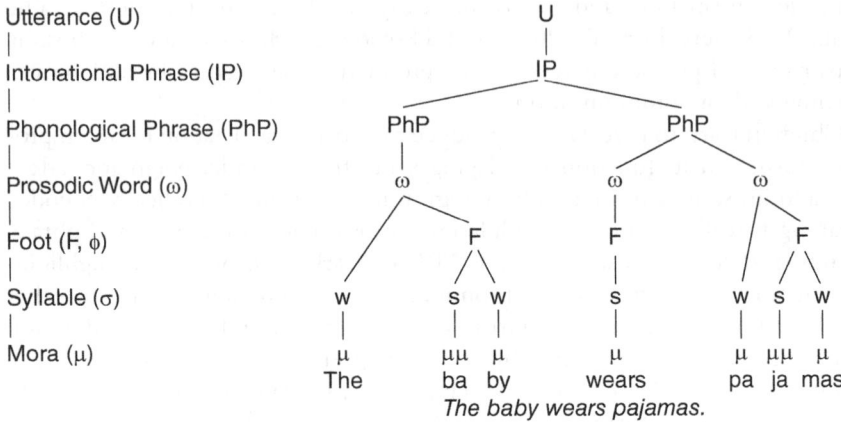

Figure 3.1 Prosodic hierarchy proposed by Kehoe (2018) and adapted from Nespor and Vogel (2007). Example utterance showing levels; w = weak syllable, s = strong syllable.

phrase that consists of multiple prosodic words and at least one stressed element. It may be shorter than the full prosodic contour reflected in the intonational phrase. On the lower end, stress assignment is most often tied to the foot and syllable levels. Typically, in English, a foot is made up of a strong and a weak syllable. These terms are commonly used in the discussion of prosodic abilities and prosodic development.

On the basis of relative lengths of timing units in this hierarchy, languages are considered to fall into one of three broad rhythmic classes: stress-timed, syllable-timed, and mora-timed. Stress-timed languages demonstrate more variation in the length of syllables, but show equal intervals between two stressed syllables. This variation in syllable length can be due to intrinsic vowel length differences and the variability in the number of consonants in onset or coda position. Generally, weak syllables are shorter and strong syllables are longer. English, Thai, and Swedish are examples of stress-timed languages. Syllable-timed languages are considered to have relatively similar syllable durations due to consistent segmental patterns across the syllable. Mandarin, French, and Tagalog are examples of syllable-timed languages. Comparatively, vowel reduction is less common in syllable-timed languages and is more common in unstressed syllables in stress-timed languages. Finally, mora-timed languages such as Japanese and Ganda base their timing on the mora (versus the syllable), where each one has relatively equal duration. In addition to these three groups, it has been proposed that stress- and syllable-timed languages can be better described as fitting along a continuum of relative syllable length. These rhythmic groupings can be helpful in considering differences between languages.

The ability to perceive, comprehend, and produce prosodic distinctions is essential for both language learning and communicating effectively with others. If an individual has an impairment in prosody, this can lead to difficulties with the intelligibility and naturalness of speech as well as the perception and learning of language. For children, directly addressing prosodic challenges is important to perceive others' intentions and emotions, be understood themselves, learn language, and successfully engage with others.

The goal of this chapter is twofold: (1) to provide an overview of the perception and production of prosody for typically developing children and (2) to review the literature regarding the assessment and intervention of prosodic impairment in children (for more information on prosody and the role in adult speech and language, see Chapter 10; for more information on the interaction between phonotactics and prosody, see Chapter 1).

Child prosody: perception and production

Perception

Infants use prosodic information in the speech signal to guide their language learning. This process begins before an infant is born, when they are exposed to the prosodic signal *in utero*. Beginning around 20 weeks of gestational age, the fetus can begin to detect and eventually, at birth, distinguish among speech sounds that are transmitted from the mother as well as others (Fifer & Moon, 1988; Hepper & Shahidullah, 1994; Querleu et al., 1988). For speech, the information that reaches the fetus is primarily prosodic, with pitch, loudness, and rhythmic variation being some of the first aspects that the fetus will hear. Studies of infants only a few days old show that they can discriminate speech between their native versus non-native language, different rhythmic classes, their mother's voice versus an unfamiliar woman's voice, and even a familiar versus an unfamiliar story read to them in the womb (DeCasper & Fifer, 1980; DeCasper & Spence, 1986; Mehler et al., 1978, 1988; Nazzi, Bertoncini, et al., 1998). These early discriminative abilities have been suggested to stem from the experience of the fetus in the womb, where they hear a low-passed filtered version of the speech signal, and thus receive melodic and rhythmic input before they are born (DeCasper & Spence, 1986).

Early sensitivity to prosody begins before birth and continues to play an important role throughout development, particularly in the first year of life. One of the first tasks that an infant faces is breaking up the speech stream into smaller chunks, from the larger clausal levels all the way down to the word level (see the levels shown in Fig. 3.1). Taking the analogy of hearing a foreign language for the first time as an adult, it is very difficult to decipher where the beginning and end of a unit or word is located. To do so, you may use some prosodic information to break up the speech stream and begin to figure out where these boundaries are occurring, such as using the edge of a phrase, a pause, or other rhythmic markers. For infants, exploiting their language's prosodic information is essential to begin to segment continuous speech into these smaller units (i.e., word segmentation). Studies have shown that infants as young as 7 months are sensitive to clausal units indicated by prosody. Hirsh-Pasek et al. (1987) showed that infants 7 to 10 months old demonstrate a preference for listening to speech where pauses are at clause boundaries versus within clauses. Additional cross-linguistic work has shown that infants can use a combination of silent pauses, phrase final lengthening, and the more extreme pitch excursions found at the ends of utterances to discover clausal boundaries from an early age (Johnson & Seidl, 2008; Seidl, 2007). Language-specific prosodic cues that signal smaller units take longer to acquire as more experience with the native language is necessary (Soderstrom et al., 2003; Wellmann et al., 2012).

Infants must tune in to subtle prosodic information during the earliest phases of lexical development. Infants and young children need to learn to segment individual words from the speech stream, identify a referent/object or action, and then map the linguistic form to meaning (Thorson, 2018). In a continuous stream of speech, there are no pauses between most words. How then does an infant learn where these utterance-internal word boundaries are located? The role of rhythm has been shown to aid in this process. Rhythmic patterns are closely linked with the placement of weak and strong syllables (or feet). For the two primary rhythmic patterns, weak–strong disyllables are called iambs (e.g., *baLLOON*, *reLAX*), while strong–weak disyllables are called trochees (e.g., *BUnny*, *SNUggle*). Stress-timed languages differ in the relative ratio of iambic to trochaic words, with English having 90% of multisyllabic words as trochees (Cutler & Carter, 1987).

Using this rhythmic information, English-acquiring infants between 6 and 9 months can perceptually group pairs of syllables, and by 9 months old, infants demonstrate a rhythmic bias for trochees (Jusczyk et al., 1993; Morgan, 1994, 1996; Morgan & Saffran, 1995). Jusczyk et al. (1999) showed that English-acquiring infants can segment trochaic words from the speech stream at 7.5 months old, and then segment iambic words by 10.5 months old. Prosody alone is not sufficient to fully explain how infants segment words, with other aspects interacting in this process including the phonotactics (i.e., permissible sound sequences of a language), adjacent familiar words, and the statistical regularities of speech (i.e., transitional probabilities between syllables; Bortfeld et al., 2005; Jusczyk & Aslin, 1995; Mattys et al., 1999; Mattys & Jusczyk, 2001; Saffran et al., 1996). Like rhythm, infants display early sensitivities to intonation (Nazzi, Floccia, et al., 1998; Papoušek et al., 1990; Trehub et al., 1984). Work in European Portuguese shows infants as young as 5 to 9 months can discriminate words with a falling declarative pattern (i.e., statement) from those with a falling–rising interrogative pattern (Frota et al., 2014), although the discrimination of other prosodic contrasts in pitch timing may not develop until a year old (Butler et al., 2016).

Another important feature that interacts with word segmentation is the speech that is typically used by caregivers known as infant- or child-directed speech (IDS/CDS; also known as motherese or parentese). CDS exhibits unique prosodic properties in comparison to adult-directed speech (ADS) and is preferred by young children over ADS. It has been characterized prosodically as having increased overall pitch, wider variations in pitch range, longer durations of segments leading to a slower speaking rate, and increased intensity (Fernald, 1985, 1989; Fernald & Simon, 1984). Thiessen et al. (2005) showed that 7-month-olds more readily segmented whole words from the speech stream if produced in CDS versus ADS. In general, CDS is a prosodically distinct register and has been shown not only to aid word segmentation, but also to direct attention, help with word recognition, and facilitate speech processing (Cooper & Aslin, 1994; Fernald & Mazzie, 1991; Song et al., 2010).

Prosody continues to play a key role in early word learning as infants progress from segmenting the linguistic label in the speech stream to mapping it to a real-word referent or action. Children rely on cues from pitch accent placement to interpret the referent of a word. In German, Grassmann and Tomasello (2010) looked at how accentuation and newness of an object in a discourse affected referent identification by 2-year-old toddlers. They found that the child needed the referent to be new and to receive an accent in order for the child to attend to that referent. In American English, research has shown that 18-month-olds use discourse newness and/or the presence of a pitch movement on the target word to guide their attention to the referent (Thorson & Morgan, 2014). By 4 and 5 years of age, children additionally use the deaccented status of a word as identifying a previously established referent in the discourse (Arnold, 2008). Tuning into these language-specific patterns of accentuation helps young children identify objects and actions in their surroundings, paving the way to map linguistic form to meaning.

Making a lasting connection between a word and its intended meaning is the goal of a young word learner in order to meet necessary language milestones. Social interactions have been argued to be the optimal environment for word learning to occur, with the social pragmatics of the environment playing a role in whether or not a child interprets a novel word as a verb or a noun (Akhtar et al., 1996; Tomasello & Akhtar, 1995). Beyond the context alone, prosodic highlighting (i.e., accentuation) of new information interacts with word learning to aid in mapping a novel word to a new referent (Grassmann & Tomasello, 2007; Thorson, 2015). Prosodic phrasal boundaries and lexical stress patterns also support early word learning. Infants as young as 6 months can link a word with its referent when the word form is at a prosodic phrase boundary (Shukla et al., 2011), and by 16 months old, toddlers show a bias to map trochaic words to nouns and iambic words to verbs (the general pattern found in English; Curtin et al., 2012). Finally, specific pitch accents and CDS have been shown to facilitate both word segmentation and the mapping of linguistic labels to meaning (Graf Estes & Hurley, 2013; Ma et al., 2011; Thiessen et al., 2005; Thorson, 2015). Overall, word learning is an integrative and evolving process, where language-specific lexical stress patterns, prominent accentuation forms, and prosodic characteristics of CDS interact to aid in the learning process.

Beyond word learning, the structural organizational aspects of prosody facilitate learning about syntax as well. Phrasal prosody has also been argued to play a role in constraining syntactic class assignment and determining syntactic structure. Prosodic bootstrapping hypothesizes that early sensitivities to prosodic cues such as pitch, tempo, and intensity guide the learner in figuring out syntactic classes (Gleitman & Wanner, 1982; Morgan, 1996; Morgan & Demuth, 2014), with other researchers adding that this process evolves over development and works alongside other non-prosodic information in the speech signal (Jusczyk, 1997). Research shows that by 18 months infants can use the prosodic structure to figure out the syntactic structure of a sentence as well as infer a likely meaning of the referent (de Carvalho et al., 2015). Still, young children continue to demonstrate difficulties using prosody to resolve syntactic ambiguities in English into the preschool years (e.g., *You can feel [the frog with the feather]* (the frog is holding the feather) versus *You can feel the frog [with the feather]* (you feel the frog using the feather) (Snedeker & Trueswell, 2001; Snedeker & Yuan, 2008). In summary, the crucial role of prosody in development stems from early sensitivities to prosody in the womb to making use of lexical stress and intonation patterns to help access lexical and syntactic information in the native language. Overall, prosody plays an essential role in early language learning.

Production

In comparison to the perception of prosody, infants are initially more limited in production. While sensitivities to prosody begin *in utero*, expressive prosodic abilities develop over the first year of life and continue to be refined through adolescence. It is well known that vocal development progresses over the first year of life, with repeated consonant-vowel (CV) productions as the hallmark sign of the canonical babbling phase between 6 and 10 months of age. On average, children produce their first word at 12 months old, which is around the same time they are able to produce a range of language-specific intonational and rhythmic patterns. Even before the production of their first word, newborns will cry in a rising or falling pitch pattern based on the most frequent pattern of phrase-level pitch prosody found in their native language (Mampe et al., 2009).

As language emerges, children learn to encode a wide range of linguistic and affective information. When word production takes off in the second year of life, we see rapid advances in prosodic abilities and the mapping of prosodic contours onto pragmatic meanings. At the same time, the link between prosody and gesture (referring to manual movements) develops in parallel and continues to strengthen, with implications for those with speech disorders (see Rusiewicz & Esteve-Gibert, 2018 for a review on the relationship between gesture and prosody). Acquiring all these varying characteristics of prosody is essential for the child to become a competent communicative partner.

As noted, children display early sensitivities to rhythmic patterns between languages (Nazzi, Bertoncini, et al., 1998). It is not until the second year of life that they gradually acquire the ability to produce rhythmic differences in their own language. As discussed previously, languages have been classified into one of three rhythmic groups: syllable-timed (e.g., French), stress-timed (e.g., English), or mora-timed (e.g., Japanese). While this approach has been criticized for not accurately capturing the full range of rhythmic patterns found in languages, it did spark the creation of a set of metrics that are useful for analyzing rhythm, and which have proven to be beneficial in the analysis of particular communication disorders that show impairments in rhythm and timing (e.g., apraxia of speech; Prieto, Vanrell et al., 2012).

Common rhythmic metrics measure relative length of syllables based on the length of vowels and consonants, such as vocalic and consonantal interval measures (Ramus et al., 1999), and the Pairwise Variability Index (PVI' Grabe & Low, 2002; Low et al., 2000). Cross-linguistically, a pattern emerges where children tend to begin with more even-timed rhythm with more vowels than consonants in their utterances (DePaolis et al., 2008; Payne et al., 2012; Vihman et al., 2006). Then, by 1 year old, children begin to narrow in on their native language rhythm patterns in their own productions. Relatedly, syllables containing more consonants take longer to develop and begin as more unevenly timed. Thus, rhythmic production abilities in languages that are syllable-timed are learned earlier than in languages that are stress-timed like English, in which it can take up to age 6 to become more target-like in their rhythm (Payne et al., 2012; see Post & Payne, 2018, for a review on the development of speech rhythm).

At the level of the intonational phrase, the Autosegmental-Metrical framework is commonly used to analyze intonation cross-linguistically (Ladd, 2008; Pierrehumbert, 1980). This framework uses a series of high (H) and low (L) targets that are assigned to stressed syllables (pitch accents: H*, L*, etc.) and to the ends of phrases (boundary tones: L%, H%, etc.) to describe the intonational contour. For example, a rising yes-no question would end with a high (H%) boundary tone, while a falling statement or wh-question would end in a low (L%) boundary tone. Research shows that this approach captures differences in child intonation (Prieto, Estrella et al., 2012; Thorson & Morgan, 2021).

Relatively early in development, children show near adult-like inventories for the final portion of an intonational phrase—the part of the intonational contour consisting of the final pitch accent and the boundary tone (at about 24 months for Dutch, Chen & Fikkert, 2007; at the onset of speech for European Portuguese, Frota et al., 2016, Frota & Vigário, 2008, and Spanish and Catalan, Prieto et al., 2012, Prieto & Vanrell, 2007). Figure 3.2 shows an example of an English-acquiring 2.5-year-old producing a low to high (L+H) pitch accent on the word *sun* in the sentence *no, that sun* with a final low boundary tone (L%) (adapted from Thorson & Morgan, 2021). By the second year of life, the use of other pitch accent targets in the utterance advances rapidly in addition to form-to-meaning mappings (Chen & Fikkert, 2007; Jun, 2014; Thorson

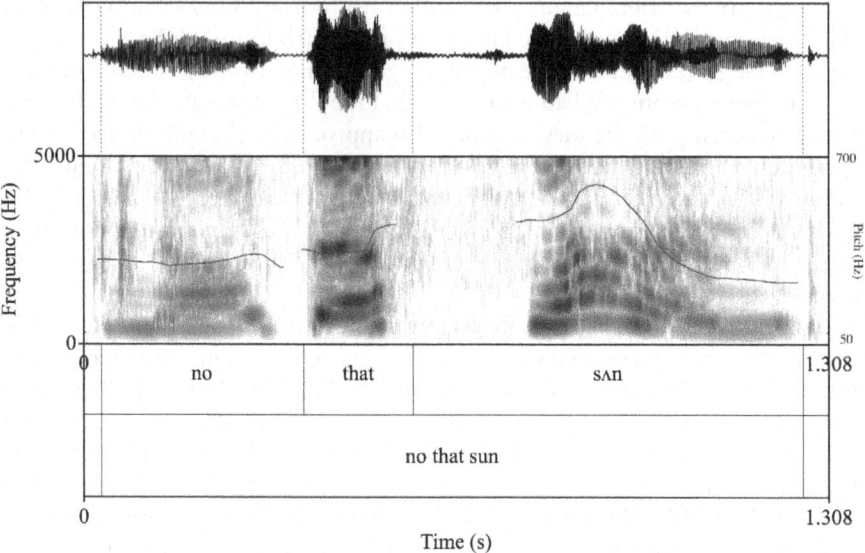

Figure 3.2 Waveform and spectrogram with overlaid pitch contour showing a pitch accent on the word *sun* in the child utterance *No that sun* from Thorson and Morgan (2021).

et al., 2015, among others). While children become proficient in producing the phonological categories of intonation very early in development, the phonetics continue to refine over several years (Chen & Fikkert, 2007; Frota et al., 2016; Prieto, Estrella et al., 2012). Some research has also shown that prior to age 2, children may place a pitch accent on individual words before making them part of the same phrase (e.g., accenting both *red* and *cat* in a two-word utterance like *'red cat'*; Behrens & Gut, 2005 for English; Chen & Fikkert, 2007 for Dutch; Frota et al., 2016 for European Portuguese). Children also express focus and information status (e.g., new versus given information) through the use of pitch accents, with abilities reflecting adult input patterns that continue to refine over the first years of life (Chen, 2011 for Dutch; Grünloh et al., 2015 for German; Thorson & Morgan, 2021 for English). More work is required to fully understand the full range of intonational abilities in children and how these develop over the first years of life.

Approaches to assessment and intervention

Atypical prosody can impact one's ability to converse successfully with others, whether due to receptive or expressive difficulties. Atypical prosody characteristics vary depending on the disorder, with deficits affecting phonology and/or phonetics. Considering the prosodic hierarchy presented in Figure 3.1, there may be impairment along any one or more of the levels: atypical or misplaced stress patterns at the syllable or foot level, unusual patterns at the phonological or intonational level, and/or segmental or pause duration irregularities at the syllable or prosodic word level leading to overall speech rhythm and timing issues. An example of a segment or pause duration irregularity includes inappropriate segmental lengthening and pauses between segments (e.g., *The cat loves* [pause] *wa..*[pause]*..ter*, where a pause would not be expected between *loves* and *water* in fluent speech or between the two syllables in *water*). The acoustic correlates of prosody may also be impacted, including disorders in which pitch, loudness, and/or duration, are affected. There are a variety of conditions in which we see prosodic impairment, and it is crucial that we assess children early and provide a reliable measure of their prosodic ability. In turn, there is a need for evidence-based interventions that target specific prosodic abilities. This section will focus on assessments and interventions that are grounded in a linguistic approach.

First, it is important to highlight some of the characteristics that define prosodic impairment in particular conditions. Two groups of disorders that may give rise to prosodic impairment in childhood include the motor speech disorders (childhood apraxia of speech (CAS); dysarthria) and autism spectrum disorder (ASD). CAS is a neurodevelopmental communication disorder with a core impairment in the programming and/or planning of motor movements. No validated assessment procedure exists for CAS, and it is identified by three diagnostic characteristics. Alongside the distortion of speech sounds, the other two core characteristics of CAS are prosodic in nature: lengthened transitions between segments (i.e., segmentation), and inappropriate or equal phrasal or lexical stress patterns (ASHA, 2007; McNeil et al., 1997). Dysarthria is a set of neurologic speech disorders defined by impairments in neuromuscular control including changes in muscle strength, condition, and movement that result in paralysis, incoordination, hyperkinesis (involuntary movements), hypokinesis, flaccidity, or spasticity involving one or more of the speech subsystems or their coordination, which can lead to reduced intelligibility (Yorkston et al., 2007). Dysarthria in childhood is commonly caused by cerebral palsy (CP), a traumatic brain injury (TBI), or other neurological impairment. It has been shown that symptoms of dysarthria in children are more perceptually ambiguous in comparison to adults due to the co-presence of other developmental phenomena (Schölderle et al., 2020). Prosodic research in children with congenital dysarthria due to CP shows slower speech and overall increased fundamental frequency (F_0; ~pitch) patterns that decrease overall intelligibility (Patel et al., 2012).

There have been mixed findings on how to describe the prosodic characteristics found in ASD. ASD is a neurodevelopmental disorder characterized by impairments in social communication and the presence of restricted or repetitive behaviors, interests, or activities. While prosody is not part of its diagnostic criteria, many of the social areas affected in ASD have a prosodic link, such as difficulties with making inferences and understanding non-literal or ambiguous meaning—both marked by suprasegmental prosodic elements. Prosody in ASD may be disrupted during prosodic imitation, the acoustic realization of expressive prosody, the prosody-to-meaning mapping, and/or the perception of prosody (see McCann & Peppé, 2003 for a review). Perceptually, the prosody of children with ASD is distinct and often immediately recognizable (Tager-Flusberg et al., 2005). It has been described as exaggerated or monotonous, with these differences possibly due what aspect of prosody is analyzed (i.e., pitch versus rhythm; Peppé, 2018). Many of the terms used to describe prosody in ASD are opposites (e.g., exaggerated/flat pitch; fast/slow speech; loud/soft), reflecting the need for continued research as well as the fact that not all individuals will necessarily present with distinct prosodic patterns (Diehl et al., 2009). Acoustically, findings show wider pitch ranges and longer duration of vowels and words than typically developing (TD) peers (Bonneh et al., 2011; Diehl et al., 2009; Grossman et al., 2010; Van Santen et al., 2010). At the syllable and intonational levels, studies have found difficulties with stress placement, intonation patterns, and expressing affect (Peppé et al., 2007).

Approaches to assessment

The assessment of prosody can be challenging as prosody relays a vast amount of linguistic and affective information. It can be difficult to find an assessment that will evaluate all these unique factors (e.g., lexical stress, intonation, affect) perceptually and expressively. In comparison to other standardized language assessments, prosodic assessment is far behind in part due to less overall knowledge of the general prosodic milestones. There are relatively few assessments available to examine prosody and those that do exist are not commonplace in a clinical setting, as many lack standardization, normative comparison samples, and ecological validity (Diehl & Paul, 2009). Without a standardized and norm-based prosodic assessment available, clinicians are often left to create their own manner of assessing prosody or prosody may not be addressed at all.

The first impression of a prosodic impairment is often perceptual, with the atypical expressive prosody of a child drawing attention first. Due to these outward expressive difficulties, prosodic assessments initially focused on expressive abilities only. There are four main assessments that have been created and used with children:

1) Prosody Profile (PROP; Crystal, 1982)
2) Prosody-Voice Screening Profile (PVSP; Shriberg et al., 1990)
3) Perception of Prosody Assessment Tool (PPAT; Klieve, 1998)
4) Profiling Elements of Prosody in Speech-Communication (PEPS-C; Peppé & McCann, 2003)

The PROP employs a linguistic approach to prosodic assessment and was designed for adults and children (Crystal, 1982). The basis of PROP rose out of

Halliday's work on intonation, which analyzed different aspects of the intonational contour (Halliday, 1967). The goal of the tool was to analyze expressive patterns in clinical populations (e.g., intonation, tempo, stress). The procedure for PROP consisted of collecting a spontaneous speech sample that was later transcribed and prosodically judged to be typical or atypical along these three variables.

Similarly, the PVSP was established to assess spontaneous conversational speech in 3- to 19-year-olds (Shriberg et al., 1990, 1992). A speech sample was recorded, analyzed for both prosody (phrasing, speech rate, stress) and voice (pitch, loudness, laryngeal quality, resonance), and then analyzed for appropriateness along a rating scale. For example, rate could be marked as appropriate, slow articulation/pause time, slow/pause time, fast, or fast/acceleration. Like PROP, the PVSP requires the clinician or researcher to transcribe and analyze the data along a set of prescribed criteria. The natural speech samples in both approaches are advantageous as they increase ecological validity. The disadvantage of natural speech is that the variability introduced due to its uncontrolled nature impacts the ability to conduct a more detailed acoustic analysis. Further, there is less ability to compare results across individuals.

The PPAT assesses prosodic perception in older children aged 7- to 12-years old who use cochlear implants (Klieve, 1998; Klieve & Jeanes, 2001). It includes six receptive subtests, five of which are embedded in linguistic contexts such as question/statement/command forms, tone and affect, and new-given utterance-level focus (where elements that have not been mentioned before are considered new and are acoustically stronger than ones that are given or have been mentioned before—what the authors call stress). The PPAT was made for research use and has a limited normative sample of six children with cochlear implants. Overall, the PROP, PVSP, and the PPAT are not well known across the field of speech-language pathology and have been used sparingly in a clinical or research setting.

The most comprehensive and widely used prosodic assessment is the PEPS-C (Peppé & McCann, 2003). Unlike the prior three assessments, the PEPS-C focuses on both expressive and receptive prosodic abilities. It includes 14 subtests that look at both prosodic function and form. The function tasks evaluate both the expressive and receptive skills across six tasks: turn-end (question/statement distinction), affect, lexical stress, phrase stress, boundary, and contrastive stress. For example, a receptive boundary task asks which picture aligns with *chocolate, cookies, and cake* versus *chocolate cookies, and cake*, which differ in the placement of prosodic phrasal boundaries. Similarly, the expressive version of this task asks the participant to describe a picture where the ambiguity is resolved by prosodic boundary placement. The form tasks include an auditory discrimination task and an imitation task. For example, the auditory discrimination task asks whether two stimuli are the same or different. Meanwhile, the imitation task is a function task that relates prosodic skills to meaning while the two form tasks probe more basic prosodic differences related to perception and imitation. By having specific words used in the expressive tasks, the assessment more easily allows for post-hoc acoustic analyses to compare within and across individuals.

The PEPS-C was originally designed for typically developing and language-impaired children but has been broadened over the years for both adults and children over age 4 (Peppé & McCann, 2003). It has additionally been used with children with ASD (Peppé et al., 2007). Advantages of the PEPS-C are that it assesses both perception and production, it is designed for use across the age span, and it is available in five English dialects as well as several other languages including Spanish. Disadvantages of the test are that it takes 40–60 minutes to administer all 14 subtests (though subtests can also be given separately), it is not standardized, and there are limited normative data available for only particular populations (Peppé et al., 2007; Wells et al., 2004; Wells & Peppé, 2003). For ASD, no specific prosodic assessments are available, but the PEPS-C has been used with individuals who can complete this type of protocol. Questions still remain about the most effective way to assess prosody in individuals who are minimally verbal and/or have difficulty in completing standardized assessments (Thorson et al., 2016). Understanding perceptual and expressive prosodic abilities in this population would provide valuable insight into their language development path as well as aid intervention approaches.

Other assessments have been created to assess prosody in specific disorders, such as CAS. One example is a speech recognition technology to automatically detect symptoms consistent with CAS, including prosodic errors due to lexical stress difficulties (Tabby Talks; Shahin et al., 2015). The classification rates for lexical stress are 83.3% for 4- to 16-year-olds. A diagnostic marker has also been proposed, which plays an important role for the assessment of CAS. A Pause Marker (PM) measure aims to differentiate CAS from speech delay based on the number and type of between-word pauses in continuous speech (Shriberg et al., 2017). Generally, the methods for assessing prosody can be considered either instrumental approaches, like using an acoustic analysis, or ones that measure prosodic function, as seen with the PEPS-C (Kalathottukaren et al., 2015).

If none of these assessments are available for use or if they are inappropriate to use with a specific population, a clinician can take an instrumental and/or a prosodic function approach to prosodic assessment. First, it is helpful to assess the different aspects of prosody separately and in a naturalistic manner. Areas to assess expressively might include lexical stress, phrasal stress, intonation, and affect. It is important to elicit these differences in as naturalistic manner as possible since prosody is very sensitive to the pragmatics of an interaction, which can inadvertently affect an individual's performance. Subsequent analyses can be performed both perceptually and acoustically. Training one's ear to distinguish prosodic output (e.g., unequal or excess lexical stress, inappropriate pauses, high or low boundaries) is invaluable and will aid in providing a measure of intelligibility and naturalness. Acoustic analyses using an acoustic software program such as Praat (freely available online) are also helpful for the clinician to use when they would like to systematically and objectively examine the acoustic correlates of prosody (fundamental frequency, duration, and intensity) between or within individuals (Boersma & Weenink, 2018).

Approaches to intervention

The ultimate goal of prosodic intervention is to aid in communication. Expressive aims for prosody may be to relay the intended message more clearly such as by matching a specific target, and/or to convey the appropriate linguistic, pragmatic, or social meaning. Receptive aims may include being able to process prosodic cues for learning or for understanding linguistic, pragmatic, or social cues. Few prosody-specific interventions exist, with most focusing on the production of prosody. For the motor speech disorders, many of the interventions that exist are grounded in a motoric approach that then impacts linguistic skills (Maas et al., 2014; for a linguistic approach to intervention in CAS, see Chapter 1). Fewer yet have been specifically designed to be conducted with children.

Interventions such as the Treatment to Establish Motor Program Organization (TEMPO^SM; Ballard et al., 2010; Miller et al., 2021), formerly known as Rapid Syllable Transition (ReST; Murray et al., 2015), are founded in the principles of motor learning (PML) and use the repetition of certain types of syllable sequences to improve the core deficits of CAS. As two of the core diagnostic criteria for CAS are prosodic in nature, segmentation and lexical/phrasal stress difficulties are the focus for these interventions. For example, with TEMPO^SM, the focus is on the underlying impairment of CAS in order to make changes in prosody at the syllable level (i.e., lexical stress distinctions). Similarly, Dynamic Temporal and Tactile Cueing (DTTC) indirectly targets prosody by targeting the efficiency of neural processing to address underlying motor impairments in disorders such as CAS, which is characterized by impairments in motor programming (Strand, 2020). DTTC is individualized for each child and works on overall movements versus individual sounds. Overall prosody including phrasing, pauses, intonation, speech rate, and stress is a focus during treatment. Cues are provided as needed and faded to encourage independence (e.g., saying a target word in unison with the child, saying a word slowly, modeling mouth movements, and tactile cues). These two interventions are based on the PML, using those principles to guide intervention in aspects such as stimuli creation (increasing complexity) and intensity of treatment (high).

In Hargrove et al. (2009), 14 interventions were identified as targeting one of the primary aspects of prosody including pitch, loudness, rate, stress, or affect, and only four of those included children 12 or younger. The four interventions discussed include (1) Rosenbek et al.'s (2004) six steps for treating affective prosody, which uses a cognitive-linguistic approach, (2) Samuelsson's (2011) focus on various prosodic issues at the word, phrasal, and discourse level, (3) the aforementioned TEMPO^SM protocol that targets, in addition to sound accuracy and segmentation, lexical stress (Ballard et al., 2010; Miller et al., 2021), and the Lee Silverman Voice Treatment (LSVT) that targets loudness (e.g., Ramig et al., 1995). The last three of these have been used with young children. Grounded in intonational linguistic theory, Samuelsson (2011) was conducted in Swedish and focused on a 5-year-old boy with language impairment. LSVT focuses on increasing loudness in various populations. For children, LSVT has shown to be effective in increasing loudness and speech intelligibility in children with CP and dysarthria, but beyond intensity no other aspects of prosody are addressed (Fox et al., 2005, 2008; Fox & Boliek, 2012).

Hargrove (2013) discusses why there is a dearth of prosodic interventions, citing reasons such as how prosodic impairments occur across a wide range of conditions and are therefore not tied to one clinical condition, and how prosody is not often seen as the primary concern for intervention. She argues that by increasing interest in prosody and including it in clinical goals, the field will respond in kind with increased intervention options. Hargrove (2013) concludes with a call for more evidence-based measures, the monitoring of trade-offs between prosodic and non-prosodic targets, clearer descriptions of intervention protocols, better understanding of when intervention should be started in development, and for clinicians to work together to support implementing prosodically focused interventions in a clinical setting.

For ASD specifically, the main types of intervention styles used include antecedent-based, behavioral, in vivo modeling, parent-implemented,

Table 3.1 Summary of specific interventions discussed in this chapter (not an exhaustive list of all prosodic interventions and approaches), the child population(s) they target, the prosody targets that they aim to address, and their primary resources.

Intervention	Target Population	Prosody Targets	Resources
Treatment to Establish Motor Program Organization TEMPO^SM (formerly known as ReST)	CAS	Segmentation of syllables/segments; lexical & phrasal stress	Miller et al. (2021)
Dynamic Temporal and Tactile Cueing (DTTC)	CAS	None direct. *Targets movements that indirectly affect prosodic impairment with a focus on overall prosody*	Strand (2020)
Lee Silverman Voice Treatment (LSVT)	childhood dysarthria	Loudness	Fox et al. (2005, 2008), Fox and Boliek (2012), Ramig et al. (1995)
Auditory Motor Mapping Training (AMMT)	Minimally verbal/vocal children with ASD	None direct. *Uses prosody as the medium to promote functional speech production*	Chenausky et al. (2016), Wong et al. (2013)

peer-mediated, reinforcement, scripting, social narratives, and video modeling, with many employing a combination of these types. Most of these showed moderate to significant gains when targeting prosody directly, but minimal to no effect when targeting it indirectly, and many were considered weak in terms of meeting evidence-based criteria (Holbrook & Israelsen, 2020). The target areas that improved the most were global intonation patterns and intensity measures. Beyond expressive aims, a large portion of the prosodic research in ASD has focused on affect and the processing of emotions. For example, Matsuda and Yamamoto (2013) showed improvements for young autistic children in processing affective prosody by matching emotions with different facial expressions. An important takeaway is that the most effective interventions for ASD seem to directly target prosody over a longer period of time. Importantly, the interventions have been designed for individuals who are verbal.

Another line of interventions uses prosody as the primary medium to improve functional speech production. Auditory motor mapping training (AMMT; Chenausky et al., 2016; Wan et al., 2011) rose out of melodic intonation therapy, a treatment that uses intonation to target language abilities in individuals with neurological trauma (Albert et al., 1973; Sparks & Holland, 1976). AMMT was designed for use with minimally verbal/vocal children with ASD to increase expressive speech output. This approach uses entoned (i.e., sung) speech along with rhythmic tapping of tuned drums to train participants on particular words (e.g., *that is a **ba-by***). The goal is for these skills to generalize to new stimuli. Critics of this approach claim that generalization is difficult with this type of model and that it can impact the way in which children produce words, making them sound sung instead of like a typical prosodic speech contour. Overall, the interventions discussed target different aspects of prosody, with some designed for specific populations (see Table 3.1 for a summary). There is a need for more linguistically based approaches to be researched and used clinically.

Like assessment, the clinician has at their disposal both instrumental and function-based approaches to intervention. For disorders with underlying motor impairments, interventions that are founded in the PML can provide frameworks for how to create stimuli, structure intervention, provide feedback, and plan intensity and duration of treatment. Generally, working on prosodic skills that are measurable and natural is important to affect meaningful change. For aspects that are not perceptually salient, the clinician may additionally employ objective acoustic measures as a method to monitor and track change over time.

Conclusion

Prosody is a rich and complex system that involves all the different aspects of speech and language from phonology to pragmatics. Understanding the different levels of the prosodic hierarchy will aid clinicians in better assessing and treating prosodic impairment. Knowing which level is impacted and teasing apart what prosodic skills are intact or impaired will lead to more effective and targeted approaches. Finally, employing both instrumental and prosodic function approaches to assessment and intervention is helpful to affect both objective and functional change. Since prosody interacts with aspects of speech and language, it is important to consider its role during all clinical settings. Disregarding prosody when working on other skills may lead to a decrease in naturalness. Importantly, prosody will be present no matter the context and taking it into consideration will be critical for natural and effective communication.

Acknowledgments

I thank Amy Ramage, Don Robin, Meg Morgan, and Paul Robertson for their invaluable feedback and edits on earlier versions of this chapter. Special thanks to the reviewers and the editors for their helpful comments.

References

Akhtar, N., Carpenter, M., & Tomasello, M. (1996). The role of discourse novelty in early word learning. *Child Development, 67*(2), 635–645.

Albert, M. L., Sparks, R. W., & Helm, N. A. (1973). Melodic intonation therapy for aphasia. *Archives of Neurology, 29*(2), 130–131.

Arnold, J. E. (2008). THE BACON not the bacon: How children and adults understand accented and unaccented noun phrases. *Cognition, 108*(1), 69–99. https://doi.org/10.1016/j.cognition.2008.01.001

ASHA. (2007). *Childhood apraxia of speech* [Technical report]. American Speech-Language-Hearing Association. www.practice-portal/clinical-topics/childhood-apraxia-of-speech/

Ballard, K. J., Robin, D. A., McCabe, P., & McDonald, J. (2010). A treatment for dysprosody in childhood apraxia of speech. *Journal of Speech, Language, and Hearing Research: JSLHR, 53*(5), 1227–1245. https://doi.org/10.1044/1092-4388(2010/09-0130)

Behrens, H., & Gut, U. (2005). The relationship between prosodic and syntactic organization in early multiword speech. *Journal of Child Language, 32*(1), 1–34.

Boersma, P., & Weenink, D. (2018). *Praat: Doing phonetics by computer (6.0.40)* [Computer software]. www.praat.org/

Bolinger, D. (1989). *Intonation and its uses: Melody in grammar and discourse.* Stanford University Press.

Bonneh, Y. S., Levanon, Y., Dean-Pardo, O., Lossos, L., & Adini, Y. (2011). Abnormal speech spectrum and increased pitch variability in young autistic children. *Frontiers in Human Neuroscience, 4.* https://doi.org/10.3389/fnhum.2010.00237

Bortfeld, H., Morgan, J. L., Golinkoff, R. M., & Rathbun, K. (2005). Mommy and me: Familiar names help launch babies into speech-stream segmentation. *Psychological Science, 16*(4), 298–304.

Butler, J., Vigário, M., & Frota, S. (2016). Infants' perception of the intonation of broad and narrow focus. *Language Learning and Development, 12*(1), 1–13.

Chen, A. (2011). Tuning information packaging: Intonational realization of topic and focus in child Dutch. *Journal of Child Language, 38*(5), 1055–1083. https://doi.org/10.1017/S0305000910000541

Chen, A., & Fikkert, P. (2007). Intonation of early two-word utterances in Dutch. *Proceedings of the 16th International Congress on Phonetic Sciences,* 315–320.

Chenausky, K., Norton, A., Tager-Flusberg, H., & Schlaug, G. (2016). Auditory-motor mapping training: Comparing the effects of a novel speech treatment to a control treatment for minimally verbal children with autism. *PLoS One, 11*(11), e0164930. https://doi.org/10.1371/journal.pone.0164930

Cole, J., Hilger, A., & Patel, S. (this volume). Adult prosody. In C. Grindrod & N. Gurevich (Eds.), *Clinical applications of linguistics to speech-language pathology: A guide for clinicians.*

Cooper, R. P., & Aslin, R. N. (1994). Developmental differences in infant attention to the spectral properties of infant-directed speech. *Child Development, 65*(6), 1663–1677.

Crystal, D. (1982). *Profiling linguistic disability.* Arnold.

Curtin, S., Campbell, J., & Hufnagle, D. (2012). Mapping novel labels to actions: How the rhythm of words guides infants' learning. *Journal of Experimental Child Psychology, 112*(2), 127–140. https://doi.org/10.1016/j.jecp.2012.02.007

Cutler, A., & Carter, D. M. (1987). The predominance of strong initial syllables in the English vocabulary. *Computer Speech & Language, 2*(3–4), 133–142.

de Carvalho, A., Dautriche, I., Millotte, S., & Christophe, A. (2018). Early perception of phrasal prosody and its role in syntactic and lexical acquisition. *The Development of Prosody in First Language Acquisition, 23*, 17.

de Carvalho, A., He, A., Lidz, J., & Christophe, A. (2015). *18-month-olds use the relationship between prosodic and syntactic structures to constrain the meaning of novel words.* 40th Boston University Conference on Language Development.

DeCasper, A. J., & Fifer, W. P. (1980). Of human bonding: Newborns prefer their mothers' voices. *Science, 208*(4448), 1174–1176.

DeCasper, A. J., & Spence, M. J. (1986). Prenatal maternal speech influences newborns' perception of speech sounds. *Infant Behavior and Development, 9*(2), 133–150.

Demuth, K. (2018). Understanding the development of prosodic words. *The Development of Prosody in First Language Acquisition,* 207–224.

DePaolis, R. A., Vihman, M. M., & Kunnari, S. (2008). Prosody in production at the onset of word use: A cross-linguistic study. *Journal of Phonetics, 36*(2), 406–422.

Diehl, J. J., & Paul, R. (2009). The assessment and treatment of prosodic disorders and neurological theories of prosody. *International Journal of Speech-Language Pathology, 11*(4), 287–292. https://doi.org/10.1080/17549500902971887

Diehl, J. J., Watson, D. G., Bennetto, L., McDonough, J., & Gunlogson, C. (2009). An acoustic analysis of prosody in high-functioning autism. *Applied Psycholinguistics, 30*(3), 385. https://doi.org/10.1017/S0142716409090201

Fernald, A. (1985). Four-month-old infants prefer to listen to motherese. *Infant Behavior and Development, 8*(2), 181–195.

Fernald, A. (1989). Intonation and communicative intent in mothers' speech to infants: Is the melody the message? *Child Development,* 1497–1510.

Fernald, A., & Mazzie, C. (1991). Prosody and focus in speech to infants and adults. *Developmental Psychology, 27*(2), 209–221.

Fernald, A., & Simon, T. (1984). Expanded intonation contours in mothers' speech to newborns. *Developmental Psychology, 20*(1), 104.

Fifer, W. P., & Moon, C. (1988). Auditory experience in the fetus. *Behavior of the Fetus,* 175–188.

Fox, C. M., & Boliek, C. A. (2012). Intensive voice treatment (LSVT LOUD) for children with spastic cerebral palsy and dysarthria. *Journal of Speech, Language, and Hearing Research, 55*, 930–945.

Fox, C., Bolieck, C. A., Namdaran, N., Nickerson, C., Gardner, B., Piccott, C., Hilstad, J., & Archibald, E. (2008). Intensive voice treatment (LSVT® LOUD) for children with spastic cerebral palsy: 1160. *Movement Disorders, 23.*

Fox, C., Boliek, C. A., & Ramig, L. (2005). The impact of intensive voice treatment (LSVT) on speech intelligibility in children with spastic cerebral palsy: P504. *Movement Disorders, 20.*

Frota, S., Butler, J., & Vigário, M. (2014). Infants' perception of intonation: Is it a statement or a question? *Infancy, 19*(2), 194–213.

Frota, S., Cruz, M., Matos, N., & Vigário, M. (2016). Early prosodic development. *Intonational Grammar in Ibero-Romance: Approaches Across Linguistic Subfields, 6,* 295.

Frota, S., & Vigário, M. (2008). The intonation of one-word and first two-word utterances in European Portuguese. *XI International Conference for the Study of Child Language,* 1–4.

Gleitman, L. R., & Wanner, E. (1982). *Language acquisition: The state of the art.* Cambridge University Press.

Grabe, E., & Low, E. L. (2002). Durational variability in speech and the rhythm class hypothesis. In C. Gussenhoven & N. Warner (Eds.), *Papers in laboratory phonology 7* (pp. 515–546). Cambridge University Press.

Graf Estes, K., & Hurley, K. (2013). Infant-directed prosody helps infants map sounds to meanings. *Infancy, 18*(5), 797–824.

Grassmann, S., & Tomasello, M. (2007). Two-year-olds use primary sentence accent to learn new words. *Journal of Child Language, 34*(3), 677. https://doi.org/10.1017/S0305000907008021

Grassmann, S., & Tomasello, M. (2010). Prosodic stress on a word directs 24-month-olds' attention to a contextually new referent. *Journal of Pragmatics, 42*(11), 3098–3105. https://doi.org/10.1016/j.pragma.2010.04.019

Grossman, R. B., Bemis, R. H., Plesa Skwerer, D., & Tager-Flusberg, H. (2010). Lexical and affective prosody in children with high-functioning Autism. *Journal of Speech, Language, and Hearing Research, 53*(3), 778–793. https://doi.org/10.1044/1092-4388(2009/08-0127)

Grünloh, T., Lieven, E., & Tomasello, M. (2015). Young children's intonational marking of new, given and contrastive referents. *Language Learning and Development, 11*(2), 95–127. https://doi.org/10.1080/15475441.2014.889530

Halliday, M. A. K. (1967). *Intonation and grammar in British English.* Mouton.

Hargrove, P. M. (2013). Pursuing prosody interventions. *Clinical Linguistics & Phonetics, 27*(8), 647–660.

Hargrove, P. M., Anderson, A., & Jones, J. (2009). A critical review of interventions targeting prosody. *International Journal of Speech-Language Pathology, 11*(4), 298–304.

Hepper, P. G., & Shahidullah, B. S. (1994). Development of fetal hearing. *Archives of Disease in Childhood—Fetal and Neonatal Edition, 71*(2), F81–F87. https://doi.org/10.1136/fn.71.2.F81

Hirsh-Pasek, K., Nelson, D. G. K., Jusczyk, P. W., Cassidy, K. W., Druss, B., & Kennedy, L. (1987). Clauses are perceptual units for young infants. *Cognition, 26*(3), 269–286.

Holbrook, S., & Israelsen, M. (2020). Speech prosody interventions for persons with autism spectrum disorders: A systematic review. *American Journal of Speech-Language Pathology, 29*(4), 2189–2205. https://doi.org.unh.idm.oclc.org/10.1044/2020_AJSLP-19-00127

Johnson, E. K., & Seidl, A. (2008). Clause segmentation by 6-month-old infants: A cross-linguistic perspective. *Infancy, 13*(5), 440–455.

Jun, S. A. (2014). Prosodic typology: By prominence type, word prosody, and macro-rhythm. *Prosodic Typology II: The Phonology of Intonation and Phrasing, 520,* 539.

Jusczyk, P. W. (1997). *The discovery of spoken language—a Bradford book.* The MIT Press.

Jusczyk, P. W., & Aslin, R. N. (1995). Infants' detection of the sound patterns of words in fluent speech. *Cognitive Psychology, 29,* 1–23.

Jusczyk, P. W., Cutler, A., & Redanz, N. J. (1993). Infants' preference for the predominant stress patterns of English words. *Child Development, 64*(3), 675–687.

Jusczyk, P. W., Houston, D. M., & Newsome, M. (1999). The beginnings of word segmentation in English-learning infants. *Cognitive Psychology, 39*(3), 159–207.

Kalathottukaren, R. T., Purdy, R., McCormick, S. C., & Ballard, E. (2015, Spring). Behavioral measures to evaluate prosodic skills: A review of assessment tools for children and adults. *Contemporary Issues in Communication Science and Disorders, 42*, 138–154.

Kehoe, M. (2018). Prosodic phonology in acquisition. *The Development of Prosody in First Language Acquisition, 23*, 165.

Klieve, S. A. (1998). *Perception of prosodic features by children with cochlear implants. Is it sufficient for understanding meaning differences in language?* [Unpublished master's thesis, University of Melbourne].

Klieve, S. A., & Jeanes, R. C. (2001). Perception of prosodic features by children with cochlear implants: Is it sufficient for understanding meaning differences in language? *Deafness & Education International, 3*(1), 15–37.

Ladd, D. R. (2008). *Intonational phonology.* Cambridge University Press. https://doi.org/10.1017/CBO9780511808814

Lehiste, I. (1970). *Suprasegmentals.* MIT Press.

Lehiste, I. (1976). Suprasegmental features of speech. In N. J. Lass (Ed.), *Contemporary issues in experimental phonetics* (pp. 225–454). Academic Press.

Low, E. L., Grabe, E., & Nolan, F. (2000). Quantitative characterisations of speech rhythm: "Syllable-timing" in Singapore English. *Language and Speech, 43*(1), 377–401.

Ma, W., Golinkoff, R. M., Houston, D. M., & Hirsh-Pasek, K. (2011). Word learning in infant-and adult-directed speech. *Language Learning and Development, 7*(3), 185–201.

Maas, E., Gildersleeve-Neumann, C., Jakielski, K. J., & Stoeckel, R. (2014). Motor-based intervention protocols in treatment of childhood apraxia of speech (CAS). *Current Developmental Disorders Reports, 1*(3), 197–206.

Mampe, B., Friederici, A. D., Christophe, A., & Wermke, K. (2009). Newborns' cry melody is shaped by their native language. *Current Biology, 19*(23), 1994–1997.

Matsuda, S., & Yamamoto, J. (2013). Intervention for increasing the comprehension of affective prosody in children with autism spectrum disorders. *Research in Autism Spectrum Disorders, 7*(8), 938–946.

Mattys, S. L., & Jusczyk, P. W. (2001). Phonotactic cues for segmentation of fluent speech by infants. *Cognition, 78*(2), 91–121.

Mattys, S. L., Jusczyk, P. W., Luce, P. A., & Morgan, J. L. (1999). Phonotactic and prosodic effects on word segmentation in infants. *Cognitive Psychology, 38*(4), 465–494.

McCann, J., & Peppé, S. (2003). Prosody in autism spectrum disorders: A critical review. *International Journal of Language & Communication Disorders, 38*(4), 325–350. https://doi.org/10.1080/1368282031000154204

McNeil, M. R., Robin, D. A., & Schmidt, R. A. (1997). Apraxia of speech: Definition, differentiation, and treatment. In M. R. McNeil (Ed.), *Clinical management of sensorimotor speech disorders* (pp. 311–344). Thieme.

Mehler, J., Bertoncini, J., Barriere, M., & Jassik-Gerschenfeld, D. (1978). Infant recognition of mother's voice. *Perception, 7*, 491–497.

Mehler, J., Jusczyk, P., Lambertz, G., Halsted, N., Bertoncini, J., & Amiel-Tison, C. (1988). A precursor of language acquisition in young infants. *Cognition, 29*(2), 143–178.

Miller, H. E., Ballard, K. J., Campbell, J., Smith, M., Plante, A. S., Aytur, S. A., & Robin, D. A. (2021). Improvements in speech of children with apraxia: The efficacy of treatment for establishing motor program organization (TEMPOSM). *Developmental Neurorehabilitation, 24*(7), 494–509.

Morgan, J. L. (1994). Converging measures of speech segmentation in preverbal infants. *Infant Behavior and Development, 17*(4), 389–403.

Morgan, J. L. (1996). A rhythmic bias in preverbal speech segmentation. *Journal of Memory and Language*, *35*(5), 666–688.

Morgan, J. L., & Demuth, K. (2014). *Signal to syntax: Bootstrapping from speech to grammar in early acquisition*. Psychology Press.

Morgan, J. L., & Saffran, J. R. (1995). Emerging integration of sequential and suprasegmental information in preverbal speech segmentation. *Child Development*, *66*(4), 911–936.

Murray, E., McCabe, P., & Ballard, K. J. (2015). A randomized controlled trial for children with childhood apraxia of speech comparing rapid syllable transition treatment and the Nuffield dyspraxia programme—third edition. *Journal of Speech, Language, and Hearing Research*, *58*(3), 669–686.

Nazzi, T., Bertoncini, J., & Mehler, J. (1998). Language discrimination by newborns: Toward an understanding of the role of rhythm. *Journal of Experimental Psychology: Human Perception and Performance*, *24*(3), 756.

Nazzi, T., Floccia, C., & Bertoncini, J. (1998). Discrimination of pitch contours by neonates. *Infant Behavior and Development*, *21*(4), 779–784.

Nespor, M., & Vogel, I. (2007). *Prosodic phonology: With a new foreword*. Walter de Gruyter.

Papoušek, M., Bornstein, M. H., Nuzzo, C., Papoušek, H., & Symmes, D. (1990). Infant responses to prototypical melodic contours in parental speech. *Infant Behavior and Development*, *13*(4), 539–545.

Patel, R., Hustad, K. C., Connaghan, K. P., & Furr, W. (2012). Relationship between prosody and intelligibility in children with dysarthria. *Journal of Medical Speech-Language Pathology*, *20*(4).

Payne, E., Post, B., Astruc, L., Prieto, P., & Vanrell, M. del M. (2012). Measuring child rhythm. *Language and Speech*, *55*(2), 203–229.

Peppé, S. (2018). Prosodic development in atypical populations. *The Development of Prosody in First Language Acquisition*, *23*, 343.

Peppé, S., & McCann, J. (2003). Assessing intonation and prosody in children with atypical language development: The PEPS-C test and the revised version. *Clinical Linguistics & Phonetics*, *17*(4–5), 345–354. https://doi.org/10.1080/0269920031000079994

Peppé, S., McCann, J., Gibbon, F., O'Hare, A., & Rutherford, M. (2007). Receptive and expressive prosodic ability in children with high-functioning autism. *Journal of Speech, Language, and Hearing Research*, *50*(4), 1015–1028.

Pierrehumbert, J. (1980). *The phonetics and phonology of English intonation* [Doctoral dissertation, University of Massachusetts].

Post, B., & Payne, E. (2018). Speech rhythm in development. *The Development of Prosody in First Language Acquisition*, *23*, 125.

Prieto, P. (2015). Intonational meaning. *Wiley Interdisciplinary Reviews: Cognitive Science*, *6*(4), 371–381.

Prieto, P., Vanrell, M. del M., Astruc, L., Payne, E., & Post, B. (2012). Phonotactic and phrasal properties of speech rhythm: Evidence from Catalan, English, and Spanish. *Speech Communication*, *54*(6), 681–702.

Prieto, P., & Esteve-Gibert, N. (2018). *The development of prosody in first language acquisition* (Vol. 23). John Benjamins Publishing Company.

Prieto, P., Estrella, A., Thorson, J. C., & Vanrell, M. D. M. (2012). Is prosodic development correlated with grammatical and lexical development? Evidence from emerging intonation in Catalan and Spanish. *Journal of Child Language*, *39*(2), 221–257. https://doi.org/10.1017/S030500091100002X

Prieto, P., & Vanrell, M. del M. (2007). Early intonational development in Catalan. *Proceedings of the 16th International Congress of Phonetic Sciences*, 309–314.

Querleu, D., Renard, X., Versyp, F., Paris-Delrue, L., & Crèpin, G. (1988). Fetal hearing. *European Journal of Obstetrics & Gynecology and Reproductive Biology, 28*(3), 191–212.

Ramig, L. O., Countryman, S., Thompson, L. L., & Horii, Y. (1995). Comparison of two forms of intensive speech treatment for Parkinson disease. *Journal of Speech, Language, and Hearing Research, 38*(6), 1232–1251.

Ramus, F., Nespor, M., & Mehler, J. (1999). Correlates of linguistic rhythm in the speech signal. *Cognition, 73*(3), 265–292.

Rosenbek, J. C., Crucian, G. P., Leon, S. A., Hieber, B., Rodriguez, A. D., Holiway, B., Ketterson, T. U., Ciampitti, M., Heilman, K., & Gonzalez-Rothi, L. (2004). Novel treatments for expressive aprosodia: A phase I investigation of cognitive linguistic and imitative interventions. *Journal of the International Neuropsychological Society: JINS, 10*(5), 786.

Rusiewicz, H. L., & Esteve-Gibert, N. (2018). Set in time: Temporal coordination of prosody and gesture in the development of spoken language production. *The Development of Prosody in First Language Acquisition, 23*, 103.

Saffran, J. R., Newport, E. L., & Aslin, R. N. (1996). Word segmentation: The role of distributional cues. *Journal of Memory and Language, 35*(4), 606–621.

Samuelsson, C. (2011). Prosody intervention: A single subject study of a Swedish boy with prosodic problems. *Child Language Teaching and Therapy, 27*(1), 56–67. http://doi.org. unh.idm.oclc.org/10.1177/0265659010372185

Schölderle, T., Haas, E., & Ziegler, W. (2020). Age norms for auditory-perceptual neurophonetic parameters: A prerequisite for the assessment of childhood dysarthria. *Journal of Speech, Language, and Hearing Research, 63*(4), 1071–1082.

Seidl, A. (2007). Infants' use and weighting of prosodic cues in clause segmentation. *Journal of Memory and Language, 57*(1), 24–48.

Shahin, M., Ahmed, B., Parnandi, A., Karappa, V., McKechnie, J., Ballard, K. J., & Gutierrez-Osuna, R. (2015). Tabby talks: An automated tool for the assessment of childhood apraxia of speech. *Speech Communication, 70*, 49–64. https://doi.org/10.1016/j. specom.2015.04.002

Shattuck-Hufnagel, S., & Turk, A. E. (1996). A prosody tutorial for investigators of auditory sentence processing. *Journal of Psycholinguistic Research, 25*(2), 193–247. https://doi. org/10.1007/BF01708572

Shriberg, L. D., Kwiatkowski, J., & Rasmussen, C. (1990). *Prosody-voice screening profile (PVSP): Scoring forms and training materials.* Communication Skill Builders.

Shriberg, L. D., Kwiatkowski, J., Rasmussen, C., Lof, G. L., & Miller, J. F. (1992). *The prosody-voice screening profile (PVSP): Psychometric data and reference information for children.* Citeseer.

Shriberg, L. D., Strand, E. A., Fourakis, M., Jakielski, K. J., Hall, S. D., Karlsson, H. B., Mabie, H. L., McSweeny, J. L., Tilkens, C. M., & Wilson, D. L. (2017). A diagnostic marker to discriminate childhood apraxia of speech from speech delay: Introduction. *Journal of Speech, Language & Hearing Research, 60*(4), S1094–S1095. https://doi. org/10.1044/2016_JSLHR-S-16-0148

Shukla, M., White, K. S., & Aslin, R. N. (2011). Prosody guides the rapid mapping of auditory word forms onto visual objects in 6-mo-old infants. *Proceedings of the National Academy of Sciences, 108*(15), 6038–6043. https://doi.org/10.1073/pnas.10176 17108

Snedeker, J., & Trueswell, J. (2001). *Unheeded cues: Prosody and syntactic ambiguity in mother-child communication.* 26th Boston University Conference on Language Development.

Snedeker, J., & Yuan, S. (2008). Effects of prosodic and lexical constraints on parsing in young children (and adults). *Journal of Memory and Language, 58*(2), 574–608.

Soderstrom, M., Seidl, A., Nelson, D. G. K., & Jusczyk, P. W. (2003). The prosodic boot-strapping of phrases: Evidence from prelinguistic infants. *Journal of Memory and Language, 49*(2), 249–267.

Song, J. Y., Demuth, K., & Morgan, J. (2010). Effects of the acoustic properties of infant-directed speech on infant word recognition. *The Journal of the Acoustical Society of America, 128*(1), 389–400. https://doi.org/10.1121/1.3419786

Sparks, R. W., & Holland, A. L. (1976). Method: Melodic intonation therapy for aphasia. *Journal of Speech and Hearing Disorders, 41*(3), 287–297.

Strand, E. A. (2020). Dynamic temporal and tactile cueing: A treatment strategy for childhood apraxia of speech. *American Journal of Speech-Language Pathology, 29*(1), 30–48.

Tager-Flusberg, H., Paul, R., & Lord, C. (2005). Language and communication in autism. In F. R. Volkmar, A. Klin, & D. Cohen (Eds.), *Handbook of autism and pervasive developmental disorders* (Vol. 1, pp. 335–364). Wiley.

Teixidó, M., François, C., Bosch, L., & Männel, C. (2018). The role of prosody in early speech segmentation and word-referent mapping. *The Development of Prosody in First Language Acquisition, 23*, 79.

Thiessen, E. D., Hill, E. A., & Saffran, J. R. (2005). Infant-directed speech facilitates word segmentation. *Infancy, 7*(1), 53–71.

Thorson, J. C. (2015). *The development of intonation and information structure: Perceptual and productive investigations* [Doctoral dissertation, Brown University].

Thorson, J. C. (2018). The role of prosody in early word learning: Behavioral evidence. In P. Prieto & N. Esteve-Gibert (Eds.), *The development of prosody in first language acquisition* (Vol. 23, p. 59). John Benjamins.

Thorson, J. C., Borras-Comes, J., Crespo-Sendra, V., del Mar Vanrell, M., & Prieto, P. (2015). The acquisition of melodic form and meaning in yes-no interrogatives by Catalan and Spanish speaking children. *Probus, 27*(1), 73–99.

Thorson, J. C., Meyer, S., Plesa-Skwerer, D., Patel, R., & Tager-Flusberg, H. (2016). Assessing prosody in minimally to nonverbal children with autism. *Proceedings of Speech Prosody 8, an International Conference*, 1206–1210.

Thorson, J. C., & Morgan, J. L. (2014). *Directing toddler attention: Intonation and information structure.* Supplement to the Proceedings of the 38th Annual Boston University Conference on Language Development (BUCLD). Boston University Conference on Language Development (BUCLD).

Thorson, J. C., & Morgan, J. L. (2021). Prosodic realizations of new, given, and corrective referents in the spontaneous speech of toddlers. *Journal of Child Language, 48*, 541–568.

Tomasello, M., & Akhtar, N. (1995). Two-year-olds use pragmatic cues to differentiate reference to objects and actions. *Cognitive Development, 10*(2), 201–224.

Trehub, S. E., Bull, D., & Thorpe, L. A. (1984). Infants' perception of melodies: The role of melodic contour. *Child Development*, 821–830.

Van Santen, J. P., Prud'Hommeaux, E. T., Black, L. M., & Mitchell, M. (2010). Computational prosodic markers for autism. *Autism, 14*(3), 215–236.

Vihman, M. M. (2018). The development of prosodic structure. *The Development of Prosody in First Language Acquisition*, 185–206.

Vihman, M. M., Nakai, S., & DePaolis, R. A. (2006). Getting the rhythm right: A cross-linguistic study of segmental duration in babbling and first words. In D. H. Whalen & C. Best (Eds.), *Laboratory phonology 8: Phonology and phonetics* (pp. 341–366). Mouton de Gruyter.

Wan, C. Y., Bazen, L., Baars, R., Libenson, A., Zipse, L., Zuk, J., Norton, A., & Schlaug, G. (2011). Auditory-motor mapping training as an intervention to facilitate speech output in non-verbal children with autism: A proof of concept study. *PLoS One*, *6*(9), e25505. https://doi.org/10.1371/journal.pone.0025505

Wellmann, C., Holzgrefe, J., Truckenbrodt, H., Wartenburger, I., & Höhle, B. (2012). How each prosodic boundary cue matters: Evidence from German infants. *Frontiers in Psychology*, *3*, 580.

Wells, B., & Peppé, S. (2003). Intonation abilities of children with speech and language impairments. *Journal of Speech, Language, and Hearing Research*, *46*(1), 5–20. https://doi.org/10.1044/1092-4388(2003/001)

Wells, B., Peppé, S., & Goulandris, N. (2004). Intonation development from five to thirteen. *Journal of Child Language*, *31*(4), 749–778. https://doi.org/10.1017/S030500090400652X

Wong, C., Odom, S. L., Hume, K. A., Cox, A. W., Fettig, A., Kucharczyk, S., Brock, M. E., Plavnick, J. B., Fleury, V. P., & Schultz, T. R. (2013). *Evidence-based practices for children, youth, and young adults with autism spectrum disorder*. The University of North Carolina, Frank Porter Graham Development Institute, Autism Evidence-Based Practice Review Group.

Yorkston, K. M., Hakel, M., Beukelman, D. R., & Fager, S. (2007). Evidence for effectiveness of treatment of loudness, rate, or prosody in dysarthria: A systematic review. *Journal of Medical Speech-Language Pathology*, *15*(2), xi.

4 Sociolinguistics

Use of linguistic theory to inform
clinical practice for children with
Developmental Language Disorder
within African American English

*Janna B. Oetting, Jessica R. Berry,
and Kyomi D. Gregory-Martin*

Abstract

Linguistic theory provides a roadmap to identify a child's system-level strengths and weaknesses not readily observed with traditional measures of language, such as mean length of utterance. In this chapter, we demonstrate how use of linguistic theory has helped us learn about the system-level strengths and weaknesses of childhood Developmental Language Disorder (DLD) within African American English (AAE). Focusing on finite markers (i.e., forms of auxiliary BE such as *is, are, was,* and *were,* past tense such as *walked* and *fell,* and verbal -s, such as *runs*) and recognizing AAE as a dialect with variable form use (i.e., use of alternative forms to express the same meaning), we show that children with DLD demonstrate limited productivity of overt finite forms (weakness), while also producing patterns of finite form use that align with those of their typically developing (TD), AAE-speaking peers (strength). The chapter ends by introducing dialect discovery worksheets to help clinicians learn about variable finite form use within AAE when serving children with DLD.

Statement to reader

As a clinician, you understand the importance of considering dialectal differences when serving children with Developmental Language Disorder (DLD). However, you may not have realized how linguistic theory can help you do this by focusing on system-level strengths and weaknesses within a child's dialect. In this chapter, we demonstrate how use of linguistic theory has helped us learn about childhood DLD within African American English (AAE). The chapter ends by introducing dialect discovery worksheets to help clinicians learn about a child's use of AAE when serving children with DLD.

DOI: 10.4324/9781003045519-5

Introduction

We write this chapter as scientists who use various linguistic theories to guide clinical practice for children with developmental language disorder (DLD).[1] Use of linguistic theory provides a roadmap to identify a child's system-level strengths and weaknesses[2] not readily observed with traditional measures of language, such as mean length of utterance. Although we are interested in all forms of linguistic diversity, this chapter focuses on the grammatical profile of DLD within AAE (AAE; see Chapter 2 for studies of DLD within General American English, GAE).

The study of childhood DLD within AAE has not always been driven by theory. The American Speech-Language-Hearing Association's (1983) dialect versus disorder framework asks professionals to differentiate language behaviors reflecting a dialect difference (from GAE) from behaviors reflecting a "true" language disorder. This approach has led to classifying AAE grammar structures as either non-contrastive or contrastive (Seymour et al., 1998; Seymour & Pearson, 2004). Non-contrastive structures are expressed in similar ways across dialects, whereas contrastive structures are expressed differently across dialects. Examples of non-contrastive structures include progressive -*ing*/-*in*,[3] conjunction *and*, and preposition *in*. In both AAE and GAE, these morphemes can be produced in the same way to create the utterance, *We were helping Jade and Teriana in the lab*. Auxiliary BE is an example of a contrastive structure. Whereas GAE is limited in the BE forms that can be used with plural subjects, allowing only *are* and *were* (e.g., *we are, we were*), AAE and other dialects of English allow plural subjects to be combined with five different auxiliaries, including *is, are, was, were* and zero in some contexts (e.g., *we's, we are, we was, we were, we Ø*).

Once categorized as noncontrastive and contrastive, clinicians are then encouraged to exclude the contrastive structures (e.g., auxiliary BE) from clinical practice when a child speaks AAE. There are two ways to do this. A clinician can select a test, such as the *Diagnostic Evaluation of Language Variation: Norm-Referenced* (DELV-NR; Seymour et al., 2005), that does not target the contrastive structures. Alternatively, for tests that include contrastive structures, such as the *Clinical Evaluation of Language Fundamentals—5th edition* (Wiig et al., 2013), scoring can be modified so that a child is not penalized for producing a dialect-specific form that differs from GAE (for a similar approach with language samples, see McGregor et al., 1997). Excluding the contrastive structures within clinical practice allows the clinician to measure a child's language abilities without the fear of misinterpreting a dialect-specific form (e.g., *we's, we was, we Ø*) as a disorder.

1. We adopt the term DLD to recognize changes in terminology preferences within the field (Ebbels, 2014; see also Bishop et al., 2016, 2017; Green, 2020; McGregor, 2020; Volkers, 2018).
2. Within clinical practice, we would refer to a child's weaknesses as needs and/or skills in need of treatment to avoid deficit terminology.
3. The progressive inflection here excludes the verb *going* and the clause, *I'm going to,* as this verb and clause can be reduced to *gon* and *I'ma* in AAE (Green, 2002).

Unfortunately, excluding the contrastive structures, such as auxiliary forms of BE, within clinical practice leads to a lack of information about how a child acquires and uses these structures. Exclusionary practices also lead to disparities if the contrastive structures are examined and treated in one dialect but not in another (Oetting et al., 2021). Moreover, modified scoring systems intended to "accommodate" dialect-specific forms within children's responses have not increased the diagnostic accuracy of assessments for AAE-speaking children (Hendricks & Adlof, 2017; Oetting et al., 2019, 2021). Finally, from a linguistic perspective, the exclusion of contrastive grammar structures when serving AAE-speaking children is untenable. Linguistic theories, because they are focused on the organization and representation of language, treat the non-contrastive and contrastive structures of AAE as theoretically related to each other and to other grammatical elements within a child's utterance.

To demonstrate the use of linguistic theory to learn about childhood DLD, we highlight findings from a study of 70 kindergartners who spoke AAE (Oetting et al., 2021). The children's ages averaged 66 months (SD = 3.68), and their primary caregiver's highest level of education averaged 12 years (SD = 2.57; 12 = high school). The children earned standard scores that were within or above the normative range (≥ −1.2 SD) on the *Primary Test of nonverbal intelligence* (Ehrler & McGhee, 2008) and *Goldman-Fristoe Test of Articulation-2* (Goldman & Fristoe, 2000). Using the syntax subtest of the DELV-NR (Seymour et al., 2005), 35 were classified as presenting DLD, and 35 were classified as TD. As expected, the proportion of children in the DLD group whose caregivers reported a positive family history of a speech or language disorder was significantly higher than the proportion in the TD group (46% versus 12%; for a review of other family history studies, see Leonard, 2014).

The study was based on the children's language samples, which were elicited by examiners in the children's schools. The samples totaled 16,599 complete and intelligible utterances (per sample: M = 237.13, SD = 56.43), and analyses focused on auxiliary *is*, *are*, and *was/were*,[4] regular and irregular past tense, and regular verbal -s. The samples contained 5,949 (per sample: M = 84.99, SD = 31.10) of these structures. In this chapter, these structures are referred to as markers of finiteness (see Chapter 2 for further explanation of this term).

As background, we describe the term *finite form* from a linguistic framework and the term *variable form use* from a sociolinguistic variationist framework. Then, we use data to draw three conclusions: (1) Children with DLD produce overt finite forms at lower percentages than their TD peers (weakness); (2) Despite differences, children with DLD produce patterns of finite form use that parallel those produced by their TD peers (strength); and (3) Children with DLD, like their TD peers, do not produce overt finite forms in AAE-inappropriate contexts in conversational speech (strength).

---

4. *Was* and *were* auxiliaries were combined as each had too few tokens to analyze separately.

Table 4.1 Finite and Nonfinite Past Tense Forms with Main Verbs in GAE and AAE[†]

Main Verbs	GAE	AAE
a. *Yesterday, they cook<u>ed</u>.*	Finite	Finite
b. *Today, she cook<u>s</u>.*	Finite	Finite
c. *Today, I, we, you, they cookØz.*	Finite[††]	Finite
d. *Yesterday, he cookØ.*	Nonfinite	Nonfinite
e. *Yesterday, he cookØz.*	NA	Finite
f. *Yesterday, he <u>fount</u>, <u>brung</u>, <u>brang</u> it.*	NA	Finite

Note:
†   NA indicates that the dialect does not include the form type.
†† GAE contains some past tense zero forms that carry finiteness (e.g., *cut, hit, put, quit*) but these forms are limited in number, and AAE also contains these forms.

Finite marking in AAE

In most linguistic theories, English tense (e.g., past tense as in *jump<u>ed</u>*) and agreement (e.g., verbal -s as in *run<u>s</u>* and auxiliaries as *he <u>was</u> running*) are viewed together and described as marking finiteness (e.g., Chomsky, 1995; Hegarty, 2005; Radford, 1997; Wexler, 1994). Main verbs carry the marking of finiteness when the main clause does not contain an auxiliary. As shown in Table 4.1, (1a) *cook<u>ed</u>* and (1b) *cook<u>s</u>* are both considered main verbs with overt forms of finite marking. They are considered overt forms because listeners can perceive them. In example (1c) *today they cookØz*, *cookØz* is also finite, but the features of finiteness are phonetically silent (i.e., not perceived by the listener; Guasti, 2002). We have notated the finite form in (1c) as *Øz* to distinguish it from (1d) *yesterday he cookØ*, which is not marked for finiteness, reflects a bare form, and is considered inappropriate in both AAE and GAE once TD children pass the age of 5 or 6 years.

However, AAE speakers can also produce (1e) *yesterday he cookØz* as a zero form that is marked for finiteness. In other words, the finite form *cookØz* in (1e) is phonetically silent just as it is in (1c) *today they cookØz*. We know that (1e) in AAE marks finiteness, because when this main clause is followed by a tag question (which is generated from the main clause), auxiliary DO must be added to carry the finite marking of the main clause (i.e., *he cookØz, <u>didn't</u> he?*). In this example, if the finite marker was omitted in the main clause (i.e., *he cookØ*), then a grammatical tag couldn't be created. In addition to zero finite forms, AAE contains several overt finite forms that are not found in GAE. A few of these are listed in (1f).

Next, consider the case of auxiliaries. When auxiliary BE (i.e., *am, is, are, was, were*), HAVE (i.e., *have, has, had*), or DO (i.e., *do, did, does*) is present within a clause, it carries the finiteness of the clause (see Table 4.2). The auxiliary in (2a) *they <u>are</u> cooking* is an example of an overt finite form that can be produced in AAE and GAE, and (2b) *they Ø cooking* is an example of a nonfinite bare form that cannot occur after the age of 5 or 6 years. Like main verbs, however,

Table 4.2 Finite and nonfinite auxiliary be forms in GAE and AAE[†].

Auxiliaries	GAE	AAE
a. *They are cooking.*	Finite	Finite
b. *They Ø cooking.*	Nonfinite	Nonfinite
c. *They Øz cooking.*	NA	Finite
d. *They's cooking.*	NA	Finite
e. *They was cooking.*	NA	Finite

† NA indicates that the dialect does not include the form type.

AAE also allows a zero auxiliary finite form as shown in (2c) *they Øz cooking*, and as mentioned earlier, overt auxiliary finite forms that are not produced in GAE as shown in (2d) *they's cooking* and (2e) *they was cooking*. Together, the examples in (1) and (2) illustrate the larger inventory of form types that carry finiteness within AAE clauses as compared to GAE clauses.

A question arises as to how one knows when an AAE-speaking child is producing a finite zero form (e.g., *cookØz*) or a nonfinite bare form (e.g., *cookØ*). On the surface, both are perceived by the listener as the same form (i.e., *cook*). Interpreting various types of zero forms is not a new problem for linguists, child language researchers, or sociolinguists. Givón (2017) has written an entire book titled *The Story of Zero* to highlight the naturalness and importance of various types of phonetically silent forms across languages for speaking, listening, reading, and writing. Hoekstra and Hyams (1998) also recognize different types of zero forms, such as bare forms and root infinitives in child studies of English as compared to Dutch, French, and German. Finally, Green (2019) makes a distinction between AAE zero forms that are produced for verbal -s as compared to past tense.

Our position is that we don't always know which form a child has produced; however, we assume that TD children learning AAE produce close to adult AAE levels of finite forms by the age of 5 or 6 years, because this is the age children learning GAE produce finite forms at levels close to adult GAE levels. For the 5- and 6-year-old TD kindergartners studied here, our working hypothesis is that the children have moved beyond immature nonfinite bare forms (e.g., *cookØ*) and are producing overt finite forms and zero finite forms (e.g., *cooked* and *cookØz*) at frequency distributions that align relatively well with adult AAE.

Our hypothesis is supported by data. As shown in Figure 4.1, AAE-speaking TD kindergartners produced percentages of overt finite forms at varying rates, with high percentages for auxiliary *was/were*, lower percentages for auxiliary *is*, and even lower percentages for auxiliary *are*. The TD children also produced higher percentages of overt finite forms for past tense than for verbal -s. Similar patterns of overt form use by other groups of AAE-speaking children have been documented for auxiliary BE using language samples (Roy et al., 2013) and for past tense and verbal -s using a recall task (Green, 2019; Newkirk-Turner & Green, 2016). For comparison, we have plotted the percentages of overt marking from these three other studies in Figure 4.2. Additional AAE child studies that have documented a similar pattern of overt marking by type

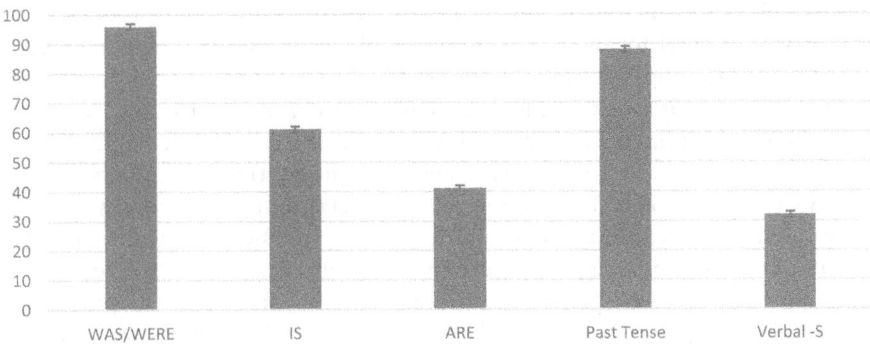

Figure 4.1 Percentage of overt finite forms by TD children within AAE (Oetting et al.,
2021). Percentages calculated by dividing the sum of each child's dialect-general
and dialect-specific overt finite forms by the sum of these and the child's zero
forms.

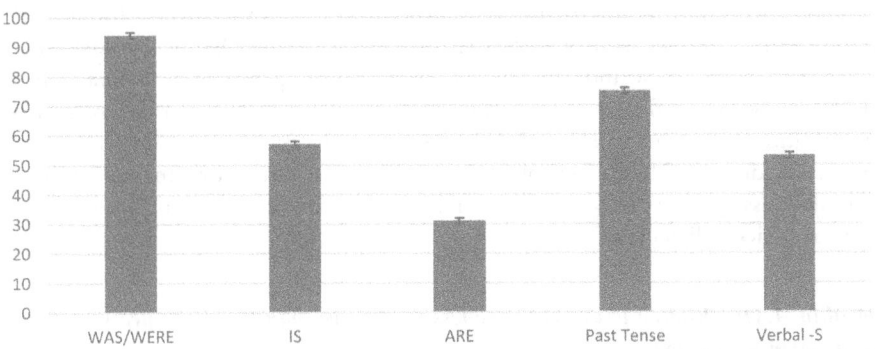

Figure 4.2 Percentage of overt finite forms as reported in Roy et al. (2013) for auxiliaries,
Green (2019) for past tense, and Newkirk-Turner and Green (2016) for verbal -s.

of structure include Wyatt (1991) who studied *is* and *are*, Burns et al. (2000),
who studied *am, is, are, was,* and *were*, and Garrity and Oetting (2010) who
studied *am, is,* and *are*.

Importantly, the AAE-speaking TD children's patterning of overt finite
forms aligns well with the adult AAE literature (Blake, 1997; Rickford, 1998,
1999; Rickford et al., 1991). Rickford (1999) provides data from three groups
of AAE speakers, labeled as teen, middle-aged, and old. For each group, the
speakers produced overt forms for *is* at higher percentages than for *are*, and
overt forms for past tense at higher percentages than for verbal -s.[5] This pattern

5. Reported as percentages of zero forms in original study; these were converted to percentages of overt
forms for comparison purposes.

is identical to the AAE child data reported in Figures 4.1 and 4.2. Furthermore, Blake (1997) provides convincing data that AAE-speaking adults produce high percentages of overt forms for *was* and *were*, which match the high percentages of the AAE-speaking TD kindergartners.

The presence of overt forms (e.g., *cooked*) and zero forms (e.g., *cookØz*) within adult AAE has been studied for over 50 years (e.g., Labov, 1972, 1984). This work is referred to as variationist sociolinguistics (Chambers, 2009; Chambers et al., 2004; Tagliamonte, 2012). Variationist frameworks seek to understand the internal and external linguistic processes involved in *variable form use*, or the choosing among alternatives within a grammar (Paolillo, 2002). This approach involves quantifying the percentages (and often the probabilities) at which a speaker selects one linguistic variant (e.g., *cooked*) over another (e.g., *cookØz*).

A focus on *variable form use* and the application of a variationist framework have helped demonstrate the systematicity and complexity of a wide range of languages, creoles, and dialects (e.g., Lightfoot & Havenhill, 2019). Variationist studies have also revealed differences between speakers of various dialects when studied at the same time and changes within speakers of the same dialect across time. For example, Wolfram and Thomas (2002) used a variationist framework to examine three generations of African American and White speakers who resided in Pamlico Sound, an enclave community in North Carolina. Their findings revealed differences between the African American and White speakers within each generation, and differences within each group across generations. Weldon (2021) also employed a variationist framework in her study of middle-class speakers in South Carolina to help draw distinctions between and within various dialects of AAE.

Within AAE, children with DLD are less productive than their TD peers in overt finite form production

We now turn to AAE-speaking children with DLD. Recognizing that children with DLD experience linguistic weaknesses within their dialects rather than outside their dialects, we assess and treat children from a disorder within dialects framework (Oetting, 2018; Oetting et al., 2013; 2016, 2019, 2021). This cross-linguistic approach allows us to assess and treat the entire linguistic system of AAE-speaking children with DLD and requires the use of AAE-speaking TD peers as the normative benchmark (for similar studies with bilingual children, see Bedore et al., 2018; Castilla-Earls et al., 2021; Gatlin-Nash et al., 2021).

As reported in Oetting et al. (2021), the most striking difference between children with and without DLD within AAE relates to their percentages of overt finite forms. Percentages are calculated by summing the children's dialect-general overt forms (e.g., *ate, fell, she jumps, they are, they were*) and dialect-specific overt forms (e.g., *ated, had fall, had falled, drunk, fount, I jumps, they was, they's*), and dividing the total by the sum of these and the zero forms. This coding system recognizes the many ways finiteness can be marked in AAE rather than relying on the finite marking system of a different dialect, such as GAE. As we have mentioned elsewhere, this system also distinguishes between the overt finite forms and zero finite forms of AAE, just as one distinguishes between a child's use of nouns (e.g., *girl, women, lady*) and pronouns (e.g., *she*). All dialects of English include nouns and pronouns, and children need both to communicate effectively. We apply this same logic to the overt and zero finite forms of AAE; both are part of AAE, and children who speak this dialect need both forms to communicate effectively both inside and outside of a school setting.

Strategic scoring of the children's 5,949 tense and agreement structures revealed clinical group differences in percentages of overt finite forms, with the DLD group averaging 56% (SD = 14%) compared to the TD group's 70% (SD = 13%). The effect size of the difference was large (partial eta squared = .19). Others who have identified reliable differences between AAE-speaking children with and without DLD include Seymour et al. (1998) for past tense and Hendricks and Adlof (2020) for past tense and verbal -s (for other studies from our lab, see Oetting, 2019). We interpret these group differences as showing the AAE-speaking children with DLD to be delayed in their use of adult levels of overt finite forms relative to their TD peers. We also interpret the DLD group's higher percentage of zero forms as reflecting a combination of adult finite zero forms (e.g., *cookØz*) and immature non-finite, bare forms (e.g., *cookØ*). In support of this interpretation, the DLD group produced an overt finite form for 51% of their auxiliary BE structures (combining *is, are, was, were*), and this percentage is very similar to the 55% (SD = 25%) reported for 48 AAE-speaking, TD three-year-olds studied by Newkirk-Turner et al. (2014).[6] A two-year delay (5 years compared to 3 years) in overt finite marking is consistent with studies of childhood DLD that have been conducted in other English dialects (Oetting & Horohov, 1997; Rice, 2003; Rice & Wexler, 1996; Rice et al., 1995; see also, Leonard, 2014).

Within AAE, children with DLD produce patterns of overt finite forms in ways that parallel their TD peers

Despite AAE-speaking children with DLD producing lower percentages of overt finite forms than expected for their age and dialect, the patterning of their overt finite form use matches that of their TD peers. To illustrate, we have re-presented in Figure 4.3 the TD children's percentages of overt forms along with the DLD group's parallel percentages.

Figure 4.4 demonstrates an additional parallel between the two groups. This figure shows the proportion of each structure (combining the overt and zero forms) found within the language samples. As shown, both groups produced similar proportions of structures to talk about the past and present. Although

---

6. Percentages include forms for *am*.

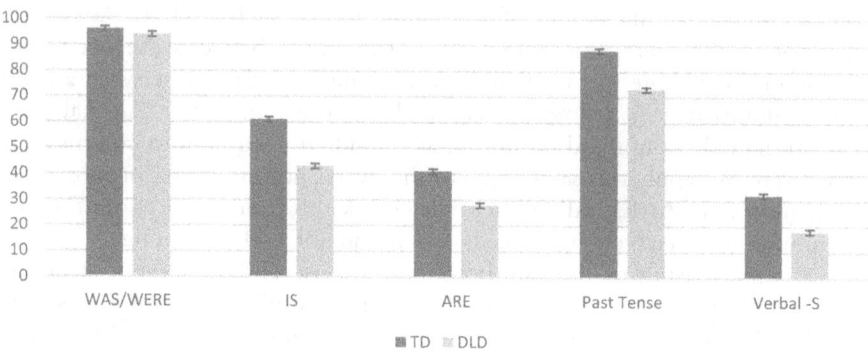

Figure 4.3 Percentage of overt finite forms by group (Oetting et al., 2021). Percentages calculated by dividing the sum of each child's dialect-general and dialect-specific overt finite forms by the sum of these and their zero forms.

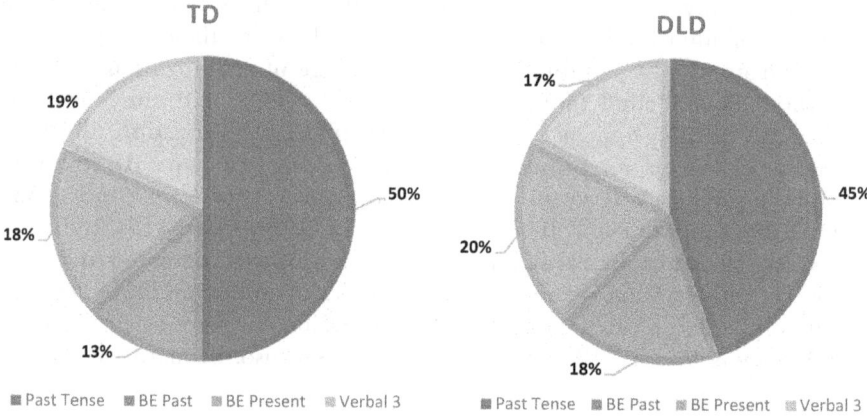

Figure 4.4 Proportion of each type of structure by group.

the TD group produced 5% more main verbs with past tense and the DLD group produced 5% more auxiliaries with past tense, the overall percentages of past versus present tense forms are practically identical for the two groups. This finding demonstrates considerable uniformity in the groups' use of grammatical structure, despite the DLD group producing lower percentages of overt finite forms for these structures relative to their TD peers.

Within AAE, children with DLD do not produce overt finite forms in AAE-inappropriate contexts

Another strength of the DLD grammar system within AAE relates to the dialect-appropriateness of the children's overt finite forms. Here we draw a

Table 4.3 Mean (SD) percentage of dialect-inappropriate overt finite forms in language samples by group.

	TD	DLD
All Structures Combined	.08 (1.0)	1.4 (1.9)
Is	1.0 (4.4)	.80 (4.2)
Are	.00 (.00)	.74 (4.3)
Was/Were	.00 (.00)	1.5 (.87)
Past Tense	1.1 (1.5)	2.3 (3.7)
Verbal–s	.90 (2.9)	2.1 (4.3)

distinction between dialect-appropriate use of an overt form (e.g., *She wanted to walk home*) and dialect-inappropriate use (e.g., *She wanted to walked home*). For the past tense marker on *walked*, we use the term dialect-inappropriate rather than error of commission in recognition that dialects differ in what is viewed as an error. From a linguistic perspective, the second regular past tense marker within the clause *wanted to walked* is dialect inappropriate in AAE as well as in GAE (Guasti, 2002; Hegarty, 2005; Radford, 1997; Rice & Wexler, 1996).

Of the 5,949 tense and agreement structures produced by the two groups (DLD = 2,808, TD = 3,141), only 1% (n = 64, DLD = 40, TD = 24) reflected a dialect-inappropriate overt form. Even when the various tense and agreement structures are examined separately, dialect-inappropriate forms are rare and never greater than 3% of the children's total forms (see Table 4.3). Green and White-Sustaíta (2015) report a similar finding in a study of TD children, aged 5 to 7 years. They studied the children's productions of three types of questions: inverted (e.g., *What did he say?*), noninverted (e.g., *What this is?*), and zero auxiliary (e.g., *What he say?*). Although all three question types are produced in adult AAE, use of the various types is dependent on context. Consistent with adult AAE, the TD children produced all three types of questions, and none produced a non-inverted question or zero auxiliary question in a dialect-inappropriate context. On the basis of the findings of the current study, we predict that AAE-speaking children with DLD, like their TD peers, would also not produce significant numbers of non-inverted questions or zero questions in dialect-inappropriate contexts.

Clinical implications

Many of the findings reported here for children with DLD within AAE have been attested within GAE (Leonard, 2014; Rice, 2003; Rice & Wexler, 1996; Rice et al., 1995). Given this, we can use the findings to begin crafting assessments and treatments that can be applied across dialects. For example, the findings suggest that we should look across dialects for immaturity of finite marking relative to same dialect-speaking TD peers. For AAE, this would mean calculating structure-specific percentages and plotting these percentages as was done in Figures 4.1, 4.2 and 4.3 to identify immature finite marking relative to normative expectations based on TD children. The findings also suggest that clinical efforts should be focused on increasing a child's overt finite form use when use is lower (and only when it is lower) than normative AAE expectations. Given that dialect-inappropriate use of finite forms is not a feature of DLD across dialects, it is also not necessary to ask children with DLD to stop producing dialect-specific overt finite forms (e.g., *they was, had fall*); these forms are part of AAE, and they are needed for successful communication with others who speak the child's dialect.

The across-dialect findings for childhood DLD have led us to develop dialect discovery worksheets to catalogue a child's dialect-general and dialect-specific overt and zero forms by structure, verb, and context (see Appendix 4.1 for an example for past tense). This type of worksheet helps a clinician learn how a child produces tense and agreement structures within AAE. In Table 4.4, we offer one example using the overt forms and zero forms for regular past tense for one child with DLD. In the table, we have listed the forms by phonetic context. As shown, the child produced overt forms of past tense 30% (i.e., 3/10) of the time, which is lower than the percentages presented in Figures 4.1 and 4.2 for TD children; however, he was most likely to produce an overt form when the verb ended with a vowel, liquid, or glide (e.g., *sigh, pull*), and when the past tense form was either at the end of the utterance, which leads to a pause (e.g., *Then I sighed*), or when the word following the past tense form began with a vowel (e.g., *I pulled a truck*). By comparison, the child produced zero forms most often when an overt form for past tense would have created a consonant cluster. The influence of phonetic context on overt marking for regular past tense is well documented for TD children and adults who speak AAE (for a review of studies and data, see Pruitt & Oetting, 2009). Note also that the child's inventory of verbs produced within past tense is relatively limited with the same five verbs used repeatedly.

With this information, a clinician can characterize the child's past tense system as immature for his age and dialect, but also linguistically like the systems of his TD peers. A clinician can then target increased use of past tense overt forms

Table 4.4 Example of regular past tense forms produced by children with DLD.

Type of Form	Verb	Consonant + Consonant	Consonant + Vowel, Pause	Vowel/liquid/guide + Consonant	Vowel/liquid/glide + Vowel or Pause
Dialect General Overt	Pull Yell				*Pull/ed an* *Yell/ed (pause)*
Dialect Specific Overt	Pull				*Had pull/ed a*
Zero	Jump Walk Jump Jump Go	*JumpØ to* *WalkØ down* *JumpØ two* *JumpØ there* *GoØ very*	*JumpØ up* *WalkØ on*		

at an AAE-appropriate level (e.g., 60–80%) while also expecting (and support-ing) the role of phonetic context in the child's variable use of his past tense overt forms and zero forms. Therapy goals focused on increasing a child's use of finite forms (both overt and zero) with a diverse set of verbs and subjects, and within a diverse set of clausal structures and discourse contexts also naturally flow from these worksheets. Helping children with DLD produce dialect-appropriate markers of finiteness when engaged in conversations, narratives, and expositions (both orally and in print) should be the end goal for all dialects of a language, as this level of proficiency is needed to be an effective communicator.

Appendix 4.1

Child Name: _____ Date of sample: _____Clinician: _____

Dialect Discovery Worksheet: A Focus on Past Tense within AAE
Source: Oetting et al. (2021; D4 Lab, Louisiana State University)[7]

Code switching pedagogy uses a child's dialect-specific forms (e.g., *walkØ*) as **springboards** to talk about dialect variation and the use of dialect-general English forms (e.g., *walked*) when completing school-based tasks (see figure 4.5). Dialect-specific and dialect-general forms may be referred to as nonmainstream and mainstream, respectively. Dialect-general forms may also be referred to as GAE, although they are as much a part of AAE as they are GAE.

With **Dialect Discovery Worksheets,** clinicians use a child's dialect-specific and dialect-general forms as **springboards** to learn about the child's dialect (see figure 4.6).

Use the attached worksheet to catalogue the child's past tense forms. Include dialect-specific and dialect-general forms because both may be part of the child's dialect. For cells in the table not filled out, work with the child to see if she can produce an utterance for that cell.

Types of Past Tense Forms to Record on the Worksheet

Dialect-General Overt Forms: These forms mark finiteness in AAE, GAE, and many other dialects of English. Examples: *She cooked; She fell*.

Dialect-Specific Overt Forms: These forms mark finiteness in AAE and other dialects of English but not in GAE. Examples: *She cookeded; She felled; She falled; She had cook; She had cooked;, She had fall; She had fell, brung, seen, fount*.

Zero Forms: Zero forms are produced in AAE and many other dialects of English; they are also produced in GAE, but are limited to a small set of verbs (e.g., *cut, put, hit*). Zero finite forms (*Øz*) and zero nonfinite forms (*Ø*)

7. Permission granted by authors for reproduction of this form for teaching and clinical use.

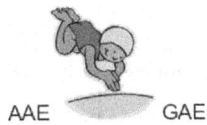

Figure 4.5 Approach asks clinician to dive toward GAE, focusing activity on child's use of GAE.

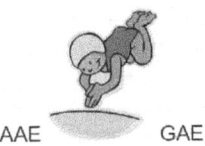

Figure 4.6 Approach asks clinician to dive toward AAE to learn about child's use of AAE.

are indistinguishable when produced in a single utterance, but we expect the nonfinite zero forms (Ø) to disappear across dialects as TD children reach the age of 5 or 6 years (and we infer this when a child's overt form use reaches AAE adult levels). For this worksheet, include all zero forms produced. Examples: *She cookØz, She fallØz, She cookØ, She fallØ.*

Dialect–Inappropriate Overt Forms: These are rare in conversational speech across dialects (<3%) and are not felicitous in AAE of GAE. They are so rare we have not added a row for them in the tables to keep our focus on children's dialect-appropriate forms. Dialect-inappropriate examples include clauses with more than one overt finite form (*wanted to cooked*) and misplaced forms (*She want to cooked*).

VERBS AND SUBJECTS PRODUCED WITH PAST TENSE (see Appendix Table 4.1). List the child's verbs produced with regular and irregular past tense. Also record the child's subjects (nouns, pronouns) within the clauses marked for past tense. Are there any patterns in the child's past tense forms? Does the child produce higher percentages of overt forms for regular verbs versus irregular verbs or for verbs with noun versus pronoun subjects? How many different types of verbs and subjects does the child produce with the various types of past tense forms?

Appendix Table 4.1

	Regular Past Tense	Irregular Past Tense
Number of Different Verbs Produced with Past Tense		
Dialect-General Overt		
Dialect-Specific Overt		
Zero		

(*Continued*)

Appendix Table 4.1 (Continued)

	Regular Past Tense	Irregular Past Tense
Number of Different Pronoun Subjects Produced with a Verb in Past Tense		
Dialect-General Overt		
Dialect-Specific Overt		
Zero		
Number of Different Noun Subjects Produced with a Verb in Past Tense		
Dialect-General Overt		
Dialect-Specific Overt		
Zero		

PHONETIC CHARACTERISTICS PRECEDING THE PAST TENSE FORM (see Appendix Table 4.2). Studies have shown that child and adult AAE speakers are more likely to produce overt past tense regular forms when the verb ends in a vowel, liquid, or glide as compared to other phonemes. List the child's past tense forms by type of regular verb ending. Does the child's past tense forms show this AAE pattern?

Appendix Table 4.2

	Regular Past Tense
Verbs Ending in Vowels, Liquids, or Glides	
Dialect-General Overt	
Dialect-Specific Overt	
Zero	
Verbs Ending in Other Phonemes	
Dialect-General Overt	
Dialect-Specific Overt	
Zero	

PHONETIC CHARACTERISTICS FOLLOWING THE PAST TENSE FORM (see Appendix Table 4.3). Studies have shown that AAE adult speakers are more likely to produce overt past tense regular forms when the phonetic context following the morpheme begins with a vowel or involves an utterance final pause (e.g., *walked on* a board; *he walked*) rather than other consonants. List the child's past tense forms by type of following context. Does the child's use of various types of past tense forms show this AAE pattern?

Appendix Table 4.3

	Regular Past Tense
Vowel	
Dialect-General Overt	
Dialect-Specific Overt	
Zero	
Utterance Final Pause	
Dialect-General Overt	
Dialect-Specific Overt	
Zero	
Consonant	
Dialect-General Overt	
Dialect-Specific Overt	
Zero	

SYNTACTIC CONTEXT OF THE PAST TENSE FORM (see Appendix Table 4.4). Children need to be able to produce past tense forms in simple and complex sentences. List the child's past tense forms by the complexity of the clause. Does the child's produce various types of past tense forms in a variety of syntactic contexts?

Appendix Table 4.4

	Regular Past Tense	Irregular Past Tense
Simple Independent Clause		
Dialect-General Overt		
Dialect-Specific Overt		
Zero		
Conjoined Independent Clause		
Dialect-General Overt		
Dialect-Specific Overt		
Zero		
Embedded Clause		
Dialect-General Overt		
Dialect-Specific Overt		
Zero		

DISCOURSE CONTEXT OF THE PAST TENSE FORM (see Appendix Table 4.5). Children need to be able to produce past tense forms in a variety of discourse contexts. List the child's past tense forms by type of discourse. Does the child's produce various types of past tense forms in a variety of discourse contexts?

Appendix Table 4.5

	Regular Past Tense	Irregular Past Tense
Conversation		
Dialect-General Overt		
Dialect-Specific Overt		
Zero		
Narrative		
Dialect-General Overt		
Dialect-Specific Overt		
Zero		
Exposition		
Dialect-General Overt		
Dialect-Specific Overt		
Zero		

References

American Speech-Language-Hearing Association. (1983). *Social dialects* [Position Statement]. www.asha.org/policy

Bedore, L. M., Peña, E. D., Anaya, J. B., Nieto, R., Lugo-Neris, M. J., & Baron, A. (2018). Understanding disorder within variation: Production of English grammatical forms by English language learners. *Language, Speech, and Hearing Services in Schools, 49*(2), 277–291.

Bishop, D. V. M., Snowling, M. J., Thompson, P. A., Greenhalgh, T., & CATALISE Consortium. (2016). CATALISE: A multinational and multidisciplinary Delphi consensus study: Identifying language impairments in children. *PLoS One, 11*(7), e0158753.

Bishop, D. V. M., Snowling, M. J., Thompson, P. A., Greenhalgh, T., & the CATALISE-2 consortium. (2017). Phase 2 of CATALISE: A multinational and multidisciplinary Delphi consensus study of problems with language development: Terminology. *Journal of Child Psychology and Psychiatry, 58*(10), 1068–1080.

Blake, R. (1997). Defining the envelope of linguistic variation: The case of don't count forms in the copula analysis of African American English. *Language Variation and Change, 9*(1), 57–79.

Burns, F., Paulk, C., Seymour, H., & Pearson, B. (2000, November). *Copula/auxiliary comparisons in African American and impaired standard American English* [Paper presentation]. Presentation at the annual convention of the American Speech-Language-Hearing Association.

Castilla-Earls, A., Pérez-Leroux, A. T., Fulcher-Rood, K., & Barr, C. (2021). Morphological errors in Spanish-speaking bilingual children with and without developmental language disorders. *Language, Speech, Hearing Services in Schools, 52*(2), 497–511.

Chambers, J. K. (2009). *Sociolinguistic theory.* Wiley-Blackwell.

Chambers, J. K., Trudgill, P., & Schilling-Estes, N. (2004). *The handbook of language variation and change.* Blackwell.

Chomsky, N. (1995). *A minimalist program.* MIT Press.

Ebbels, S. (2014). Introducing the SLI debate. *International Journal of Language and Communication Disorders, 49*(4), 377–380.

Ehrler, D. J., & McGhee, R. L. (2008). *Primary test of nonverbal intelligence.* Pro-Ed.

Garrity, A., & Oetting, J. (2010). Auxiliary BE production by African American English-speaking children with and without specific language impairment. *Journal of Speech, Language, and Hearing Research, 53*(5), 1307–1320.

Gatlin-Nash, B., Peña, E. D., Bedore, L. M., Simon-Cereijido, G., & Iglesias, A. (2021). English BESA morphosyntax performance among Spanish-English bilinguals who use African American English. *Journal of Speech, Language, Hearing Research, 57*(1), 143–157.

Givón, T. (2017). *The story of zero*. John Benjamins Publishing Company.

Goldman, R., & Fristoe, M. (2000). *Goldman-Fristoe test of articulation* (2nd ed.). AGS.

Green, L. (2020). The specific language impairment/developmental language disorders forum: Fostering a discussion of terminology. *Perspectives of the ASHA Special Interest Groups (SIG 1), 5*, 3–5.

Green, L. J. (2002). *African American English: A linguistic introduction*. Cambridge University Press.

Green, L. J. (2019). All zeros are not equal in African American English. In D. W. Lightfoot & J. Havenhill (Eds.), *Variable properties in language: Their nature and acquisition* (pp. 183–194). Georgetown University Press.

Green, L. J., & White-Sustaíta, J. (2015). Development of variation in child African American English. In S. Lanehart (Ed.), *The Oxford handbook of African American language* (pp. 475–511). Oxford University Press.

Guasti, M. T. (2002). *Language acquisition: The growth of grammar*. MIT Press.

Hendricks, A. E., & Adlof, S. M. (2017). Language assessment with children who speak non-mainstream dialects: Examining the effects of scoring modifications in norm-referenced assessment. *Language, Speech, Hearing Services in Schools, 48*(3), 218–231.

Hendricks, A. E., & Adlof, S. M. (2020). Production of morphosyntax within and across different dialects of American English. *Journal of Speech, Language, and Hearing Research, 63*(7), 2322–2333.

Hegarty, M. (2005). *A feature-based syntax of functional categories: The structure, acquisition and specific impairment of functional systems*. Mouton de Gruyter.

Hoekstra, T., & Hyams, N. (1998). Aspects of root infinitives. *Lingua, 106*, 81–112.

Labov, W. (1972). *Sociolinguistic patterns*. University of Pennsylvania Press.

Labov, W. (1984). Field methods of the project on linguistic change and variation. In J. Baugh & J. Sherzer (Eds.), *Language in use* (pp. 28–53). Prentice Hall.

Leonard, L. (2014). *Children with specific language impairment* (2nd ed.). MIT Press.

Lightfoot, D. W., & Havenhill, J. (Eds.). (2019). *Variable properties in language: Their nature and acquisition* (pp. 183–194). Georgetown University Press.

McGregor, K. K. (2020). How we fail children with developmental language disorder. *Language, Speech, and Hearing Services in Schools, 51*(4), 981–992.

McGregor, K. K., Williams, D., Hearst, S., & Johnson, A. C. (1997). The use of contrastive analysis in distinguishing difference from disorder: A tutorial. *American Journal of Speech-Language Pathology, 6*(3), 45–56.

Newkirk-Turner, B. L., & Green, L. J. (2016). Third person singular –s and event marking in child African American English. *Linguistic Variation, 16*(1), 103–130.

Newkirk-Turner, B. L., Oetting, J. B., & Stockman, I. J. (2014). BE, DO, and modal auxiliaries of three-year-old African American English speakers. *Journal of Speech, Language, and Hearing Research, 57*(4), 1383–1393.

Oetting, J. B. (2018). Prologue: Toward accurate identification of children with developmental language disorder in linguistically diverse schools. *Language, Speech, Hearing Services in Schools, 49*(2), 213–217.

Oetting, J. B. (2019). Variability within varieties of language: Profiles of typicality and impairment. In T. Ionin & M. Rispoli (Eds.), *Selected proceedings of the 7th generative approaches to language acquisition—North America conference* (pp. 59–82). John Benjamins.

Oetting, J., B., Berry, J. R., Gregory, K. D., Rivière, A. M., & McDonald, J. (2019). Specific language impairment in African American English and SWE: Measures of tense and agreement with dialect-informed probes and strategic scoring. *Journal of Speech, Language, and Hearing Research, 62*(9), 3443–3461.

Oetting, J. B., Gregory, K. D., & Rivière, A. M. (2016). Changing how speech-language pathologists think and talk about dialect variation. *Perspectives of the ASHA Special Interest Groups (SIG 16)*, *1*, 28–37.

Oetting, J. B., & Horohov, J. (1997). Past tense marking by children with and without specific language impairment. *Journal of Speech, Language, and Hearing Research*, *40*(1), 62–74.

Oetting, J. B., Lee, R., & Porter, K. (2013). Evaluating the grammars of children who speak nonmainstream dialects of English. *Topics in Language Disorders*, *33*(2), 140–151.

Oetting, J., B., Rivière, A. M., Berry, J. R., Gregory, K. D., Villa, T. M., & McDonald, J. (2021). Marking of tense and agreement in language samples by children with and without SLI in African American English and SWE: Evaluation of scoring approaches and cut scores across structures. *Journal of Speech, Language, and Hearing Research*, *64*(2), 491–509.

Paolillo, J. C. (2002). *Analyzing linguistic variation: Statistical models and methods*. Center for the Study of Language and Information.

Pruitt, S. L., & Oetting, J. B. (2009). Past tense marking by African American English-speaking children reared in poverty. *Journal of Speech, Language, and Hearing Research*, *52*(1), 2–15. https://doi.org/10.1044/1092-4388(2008/07-0176)

Radford, A. (1997). *Syntactic theory and the structure of English*. Cambridge University Press.

Rice, M. L. (2003). A unified model of specific and general language delay: Grammatical tense as a clinical marker of unexpected variation. In Y. Levy & J. Schaeffer (Eds.), *Language competence across populations: Toward a definition of specific language impairment* (pp. 63–95). Lawrence Erlbaum.

Rice, M. L., & Wexler, K. (1996). Toward tense as a clinical marker of specific language impairment in English-speaking children. *Journal of Speech, Language, and Hearing Research*, *39*(6), 1239–1257.

Rice, M. L., Wexler, K., & Cleave, P. (1995). Specific language impairment as an period of extended optional infinitive. *Journal of Speech, Language, Hearing Research*, *38*(4), 850–863.

Rickford, J. R. (1998). The creole origins of African American vernacular English: Evidence from copula absence. In S. S. Mufwene, J. R. Rickford, G. Bailey, & J. Baugh (Eds.), *African American English: Structure, history, and use* (pp. 154–200). Routledge.

Rickford, J. R. (1999). Grammatical variation and divergence in vernacular Black English. In J. R. Rickford (Ed.), *African American vernacular English* (pp. 261–277). Blackwell.

Rickford, J. R., Ball, A., Blake, R., Jackson, R., & Martin, N. (1991). Rappin on the copula coffin: Theoretical and methodological issues in the analysis of copula variation in African American vernacular English. *Language Variation and Change*, *3*(1), 103–132.

Roy, J., Oetting, J., & Moland, C. (2013). Linguistic constraints on children's overt marking of BE by dialect and age. *Journal of Speech, Language, and Hearing Research*, *56*(3), 933–944.

Seymour, H. N., Bland-Stewart, L., & Green, L. J. (1998). Difference vs. deficit in child African American English. *Language, Speech, and Hearing Services in the Schools*, *29*(2), 96–108.

Seymour, H. N., & Pearson, B. Z. (Eds.). (2004). Evaluating language variation: Distinguishing developmental and dialect from disorder. In *Special issue of seminars in speech and language*. Thieme Medical Publishers.

Seymour, H. N., Roeper, T., & de Villiers, J. (2005). *Diagnostic evaluation of language variation—norm referenced*. Ventris Publishing.

Tagliamonte, S. (2012). *Variationist sociolinguistics*. Wiley-Blackwell.

Volkers, N. (2018). Diverging views on language disorders. Part one of two: SLI vs. DLD. *The ASHA Leader*, *23*(12), 44–53. https://doi.org/10.1044/leader.FTR1.23122018.44

Weldon, T. L. (2021). *Middle-class African American English*. Cambridge University Press.

Wexler, K. (1994). Optional infinitives, verb movement and the economy of derivation in child grammar. In D. Lightfoot & N. Hornstein (Eds). *Verb movement*. Cambridge University Press.

Wiig, E., Semel, E., & Secord, W. (2013). *Clinical evaluation of language fundamentals* (5th ed.). Pearson.

Wolfram, W., & Thomas, E. (2002). *The development of African American English*. Blackwell.

Wyatt, T. (1991). *Linguistic constraints on copula production in Black English child speech* [Unpublished doctoral dissertation, University of Massachusetts].

5 Sign language

Signed language structure and considerations for language intervention with deaf children

James McCann, Lauren E. Kelley, and David Quinto-Pozos

Abstract

Deaf and hard-of-hearing (D/HH) children may present with a language disorder in the signed modality that is unrelated to their hearing levels. Often speech-language pathologists (SLPs) do not have a background in signed languages but need to make decisions regarding assessment and intervention in the child's signed language. Developmental Signed Language Disorder (DSILD), similar to unexplained language disorder in hearing children acquiring spoken language, could include deficits with phonology, morphology, syntax, and/or narrative production. While there may exist overlap in specific areas of deficits (e.g., morphological/syntactic agreement), how such deficits are encoded in the visual modality differs from how they are encoded in spoken language. In this chapter, a basic overview of American Sign Language (ASL) linguistics is provided to inform selection of treatment targets and stimuli for intervention.

Statement to the reader

As a clinician, you know that some deaf and hard of hearing (D/HH) children who use signed language as a primary mode of communication may struggle with language acquisition. However, you might not be familiar with the linguistic features of a signed language, like American Sign Language (ASL). Such features are important to consider when planning language intervention with D/HH signing children, since intervention might be focused on the signed language of the child. In this chapter, we provide a basic overview of some linguistic features of ASL such as verb inflection, use of space, and grammatical non-manual markers; comparable features can also be found in other signed languages, and we encourage clinicians to examine linguistic descriptions of the ambient sign language of their area. We discuss various aspects of ASL and provide the clinician with a resource that can be used to examine

DOI: 10.4324/9781003045519-6

language samples to help identify signed language treatment targets for D/HH children with developmental signed language disorders (DSILD).

The authors of this chapter are two hearing speech-language pathologists (SLPs) and a hearing ASL linguist, all of whom are fluent in ASL. Collectively, the authors have worked with Deaf ASL users for approximately 60 years. We believe that assessment and intervention with children with DSILD requires a collaborative approach that includes members of the Deaf community. We regret that Deaf educational specialists are not represented among the chapter's authors, and we support the inclusion of such experts in the assessment and intervention work with deaf signing children. Unfortunately, over the years few Deaf educational specialists have been given the opportunity to participate in formal language intervention with deaf signing children, and we hope that this state of affairs changes in the future.

Introduction

Over the past 15 years, questions about DSILD have been addressed by researchers who work on distinct signed languages. Pioneers in this area of research described various aspects of the language comprehension and production of D/HH children who sign British Sign Language (BSL), which were the first examples of specific language impairment (SLI) in the signed modality (Morgan et al., 2007; Mason et al., 2010; Woll & Morgan, 2012). Later, researchers in the United States added to the literature by including studies of American Sign Language (ASL), both with reports from school specialists and with various case study reports of D/HH children with typical cognition who were exposed to ASL from birth, but who appeared to present with a DSILD (Quinto-Pozos, 2011; Quinto-Pozos et al., 2013, 2017; Quinto-Pozos & Cooley, 2020). Among the areas discovered were deficits in morphology (Morgan et al., 2007; Mason et al., 2010), phonology and articulation (Quinto-Pozos & Cooley, 2020), sequential processing of fingerspelling (Quinto-Pozos et al., 2017), and visual–spatial processing (Quinto-Pozos et al., 2013). To date, previous work on DSILD has generally not addressed language intervention with the deaf children identified in the studies.

For D/HH children who present with DSILD in the context of early exposure to fluent ASL input, hearing levels and the underlying language disorder are generally unrelated. However, early sign exposure is not available to many D/HH children (Lillo-Martin & Henner, 2021). Separating the effects of language deprivation from effects of an unrelated language learning disorder for children with late language access is difficult (Henner et al., 2018). Children who go through a period of language deprivation may experience persistent delays with language acquisition that have implications for academic and behavioral outcomes (Hall et al., 2017; Scott & Dostal, 2019). Language disorders secondary to a period of deprivation may include difficulty with grammar, limited vocabulary, and difficulty with spatial organization (Hall et al., 2017). These difficulties appear to have some overlap with those present in children with DSILD so the tools and strategies provided in this chapter may be useful.

In this chapter we provide the SLP practitioner (and student) with a brief sketch of some of the linguistic features of signed languages that are relevant for the treatment of DSILD. We begin with an overview of signed language structure and its general features and possible areas of concern. A brief review of documented approaches to therapy and suggestions for the SLP are discussed last.

Overview of select signed language features and development

Since signed languages are produced with the hands and non-manual articulators (e.g., the mouth, eyebrows, and torso), they seem notably different from spoken languages. However, various aspects of linguistic structure are similar across modalities. For example, some syntactic constructions (such as word order, existence of null subjects or objects, and subject-verb-object agreement) can be readily compared to similar constructions in spoken languages. Signed languages tend to be null-subject languages (i.e., subjects are not obligatory in all contexts), they exhibit a variety of basic word orders cross-linguistically, and they have verbs that exhibit agreement patterns by using locations in the signing space. The use of signing space provides a mechanism for signed languages to have relatively flexible word order, even though basic word orders may be fixed. Signed languages, however, do differ from each other in other specific aspects of grammar (e.g., relative clause constructions and the use of auxiliary verbs for agreement).

Phonology

The phonology of signed languages consists of handshapes and their orientations, locations, both major and minor, where the hand(s) is placed, and movements (originating from engaging joints of the shoulder, elbow, and hand/wrist). These *parameters* of sign formation co-occur simultaneously, resulting in phonological structure that is notably different from spoken languages that use sequential patterns of phonemes and syllables. It takes about twice as long, on average, to produce a sign in comparison to the production of a spoken language word (Klima & Bellugi, 1979). However, the comparably slower rate of production (of signs) might be helpful for children (and adults) who would otherwise exhibit processing challenges due to rapid sequences of phonemes, syllables, and words in spoken languages (Quinto-Pozos, 2014).

Handshape is often cited as the most difficult phonological parameter to acquire based on production errors in young children (Cheek et al., 2001; Siedlecki & Bonvillian, 1993). Adult-like production of the handshapes of a signed language generally follows a developmental trajectory, which may be influenced by motoric and anatomical factors. According to Boyes-Braem

(1990), the earliest handshapes in ASL correspond with the manual alphabet letters A, C, S, and the numbers 1, and 5. These are followed by the handshapes for B, F, and O. Later in the developmental trajectory is adult-like production of W, D, H, typically followed by handshapes for R, T, and the number 8, which are seemingly among the most difficult for children to produce in adult-like form. While these handshapes do not represent the full inventory of handshapes of ASL (or most signed languages), they are among the handshapes represented in many lexical signs. Simms et al. (2013) also take into account developmental trajectories for handshapes within the Visual Communication and Sign Language Checklist (VCSL), with some handshapes being categorized on a continuum between simple and complex. See https://en.wiktionary.org/wiki/Appendix:Sign_language_handshapes for images of signed language handshapes.

An example of a phonological/articulatory error is described here. A five-year-old native-signing child demonstrated an error in producing the ASL sign FRIEND (see https://asl-lex.org/visualization/?sign=friend for a video-example of this sign). Instead of achieving contact between the palm side of his index fingers, as is typical in the sign FRIEND, the child failed to achieve contact between fingers. The resulting sign CHANGE (see https://asl-lex.org/visualization/?sign=change for a video example of this sign) was produced instead, even though the child intended to sign FRIEND (which was contextually accurate for the interaction). Both CHANGE and FRIEND have similar phonological locations and movements, but they differ in the articulatory contact and details about the index-finger extension. While there are no known published reports of phonological production abilities for children in their early school years, at 5 years old, we might expect a native signing child to have mastered the majority of his basic phonological system, so this error could be said to be atypical (see Quinto-Pozos & Cooley, 2020 for the case of an older native signer who exhibits articulatory problems). One possibility, however, is that this child might have been experiencing an issue with lexical access, and he produced a sign that was phonologically related, but not semantically correct.

Non-manual markers

In addition to the manual component of signed languages, there also exist non-manual features that serve syntactic, prosodic, and discourse functions. For example, facial features (e.g., brow raises and furrows, mouth openings of various forms, and eye gaze) are important parts of the grammars of signed languages, and specific non-manual signals might differ across signed languages (e.g., brow furrow for content questions in ASL versus backward head tilt for the same in Mexican Sign Language; Quinto-Pozos, 2002). These non-manual signals often share the same facial real estate as displays of emotion and affect.

Some of these non-manual markers/signals are grammatical in nature (e.g., for indicating topicalization, content questions, yes/no questions), but the same articulators can also be used for affective/emotional information. Reilly and colleagues (summarized in Reilly, 2006) investigated acquisition of non-manual markers in children exposed to ASL, with a focus on those of the face and head. Affective use of non-manual markers has been reported to appear earlier than grammatical use of non-manuals. Reilly reported D/HH children use a communicative head shake as a gesture around age one. From 18 to 26 months, they observed that when a new negative sign emerged (e.g., NO, CAN'T), a head shake did not accompany the sign. Their interpretation of this pattern is that early non-manual signals might appear separately from manual material, which is followed by a combination of the two as the child's grammar continues to develop. Use of non-manual markers associated with wh-questions also suggests that acquisition of the non-manual features happens after the lexical use of the question signs with no co-occurring non-manual signal. They use this evidence to suggest that it takes time for typically developing children to coordinate both manual and non-manual structures. When a construction is marked by both types of signals, children maintain the manual sign and drop the non-manual marker early on. Reilly described this phenomenon as developing "hands before face." This acquisition pattern has implications for assessment and target selection. It may not be until later in childhood development (e.g., the early years of formal schooling) where some children integrate both manual and non-manual features, whereas yes/no question non-manual markers, where there is no lexical question sign, often appear much earlier.

ASL, like various signed languages, demonstrates flexibility in word order. Even though the basic word order of ASL is subject-verb-object (SVO), one typical order is object-subject-verb (OSV), where the object is accompanied by one or more non-manual markers (brow raise, head tilt, and/or a pause) to indicate a topicalized constituent. When the markers are absent, agent/theme (subject/object) roles can be ambiguous, particularly with sentences that contain two animate noun phrases that are reversible (i.e., they could serve either role). Anecdotally, SLPs working with children who acquired ASL later have reported word order variation that does not incorporate adult-like grammatical markers resulting in ambiguity of agent and theme roles.

Verb inflection

Signed languages also differ in how they inflect verbs using handshape and space. For example, signed languages generally have verbs that fall into three main classes (plain, agreement, and locative), which are typically, but not always, distinguished by whether the verbs can incorporate morphemes for person, number, or aspect (Padden, 1983). Some signs are directed toward particular locations that are referenced in the signing space (known as agreement verbs/signs or indicating signs, depending on the theoretical approach that one adopts). Signed languages also leverage signs for daily communication that are only partially specified in the lexicon. That is, the handshape of the sign may be a fixed part of the lexeme, but aspects of movement and location (i.e., where the handshape is placed in the signing space) are more variable.

Such constructions have been referred to as classifiers in the signed language literature, even though they differ notably from spoken language classifiers (Schembri, 2003).

Some common ways that the signing space is used include indicating subject and/or object within a sentence, referencing present or imagined referents, and providing information about the motion/location, handling, or geometric features of an object (i.e., so-called classifier constructions, Schembri, 2003). The indication of subject and/or object of a verb (which does not occur with all verbs in a signed language) is commonly considered the representation of grammatical agreement.

With respect to children with DSILD, multiple studies have reported issues with aspects of the use of space (Morgan et al., 2007; Quinto-Pozos et al., 2013; Woll & Morgan, 2012). For example, Morgan and colleagues (2007) note that "Paul," a five-year-old deaf native signer, struggled with grammatical inflections in BSL, among other things. He also failed to produce necessary grammatical inflections on signs for a story-retelling task. Notably, Paul's morphological and syntactic abilities were impaired despite exhibiting age-appropriate phonological skills.

Another aspect worth noting for the consideration of DSILD is how the signing space is used for referencing present versus imaged (i.e., absent) referents. Agreement marking is a frequently reported difficulty for children with language disorders. In ASL, "agreement verbs" include information about the person and number of the agent and theme based on how the sign is carried out in space. Reports of agreement acquisition for native signers have varied from as early as 2;0 (Quadros & Lillo-Martin, 2007) to 3;0–3;6 (Meier, 1982) for present referents. Loew (1984) reported more difficulty with absent referents and noted "stacking errors" where a child sometimes placed several referents into the same space.

Classifiers

Classifiers are a group of morphosyntactic constructions (they involve both morphological and syntactic properties) that may include information on movement, size and shape characteristics, semantic class, or handling (Schembri, 2003). While the label "classifier" has been debated, we use the term because it is the label that most SLPs are likely to be familiar with. Classifiers are polymorphemic and require sentence structure knowledge, handshape selection, and representation of objects in space. Classifiers might be mastered relatively late. Beal-Alvarez and Easterbrooks (2013) summarized the research on the course of classifier development. Deaf children with early exposure typically produce and comprehend classifiers by 2–3-years-old, and continue to refine production to more adultlike through age 12 (or older). There is an early preference for handling classifiers that appears to be motivated by iconicity, the relationship between a linguistic form (here the shape and movement of the hand) and its referent. Children produce location and movement in classifiers more accurately and earlier than handshape. From 3- to 5-years old, children often show increased frequency of classifier production, but continue to have errors in handshape and use of figure/ground aspects. While handshapes and movements are conventionalized in ASL, learners may use the iconic elements to support their early acquisition (Slobin et al., 2003). The protracted course of acquisition may be due to the need to control multiple aspects of meaning when using these constructions. These meaningful parts include establishing referents, choosing how to represent the referents, coordinating figure ground relationships, using space, and using perspective. Individually some of these skills may be difficult for a child with DSILD, so necessitating the integration of them suggests that classifiers would be a potential area of difficulty. The length of time from emergence to mastery also suggests that detailed information on the child's use would direct target selection.

Quinto-Pozos and colleagues (2013) described the case of an adolescent native signer of ASL who presented with visual–spatial deficits that affected her use of classifiers within topographical space. That is, this young deaf signer had an underlying deficit of visual–spatial processing (specifically, perspective taking), which appeared in her use of the signing space in producing classifier constructions. Notably, she was not impaired with respect to the use of grammatical space for indicating arguments of verbs and pronominal forms. Additionally, she had typical comprehension skills, other than for the processing of classifiers that required perspective taking. This case study indicates the importance of differentiating visual–spatial processing difficulties from language disorders.

Role/referential-shift

Both spoken and signed languages have methods for quoting another's words. In signed languages, these quotative constructions are commonly known as role shift, which engages shifts in indexicals and agreement patterns in space (Steinbach, 2021). Role shift leverages non-manual markers, such as eye gaze, head, and torso shifts. Signers also use enactment strategies (known as constructed action), which are integrated into the grammars of those languages.

The use of role shift begins early but typically takes time to master. This protracted period of development also suggests that it may be an area of difficulty for children with DSLID or late language access. Children begin using non-manual features of role shift/constructed action from 3 to 4 years of age but have been reported to experience difficulty with adult-like productions until six or seven (Reilly, 2006) or even later (Emmorey & Reilly, 1998). Other reports indicate earlier observations of constructed action (Lillo-Martin & Quadros, 2011) but the productions are lacking key features, such as identifying referents of the shifts.

Documented approaches to therapy

Few studies have examined interventions targeting signed language outcomes despite language and communication being among the most studied areas in deaf education (Cripps et al., 2016; Scott & Dostal, 2019). Studies have focused on how different languages of instruction (e.g., ASL, spoken English, both combined) have been used to deliver print literacy instruction with outcome measures addressing print literacy rather than signed language. The few studies examining intervention effects on signed language outcomes are promising.

An ASL-English shared book reading intervention for a group of Kindergarten to second grade children improved receptive ASL syntax more than children in a conventional instruction control group (Wolsey et al., 2018). Dostal and Wolbers (2014) reported increased ASL mean length of utterance and decreased unintelligible utterances in a group of middle schoolers following Strategic and Interactive Writing Instruction (SIWI). The modality of the participants' school was identified as simultaneous communication. The SIWI intervention was provided to separate ASL and English to support linguistic competence in both languages. Beal-Alvarez and Easterbrooks (2013) examined the effects of a 6-week intervention consisting of repeated viewings of ASL stories paired with scripted teacher mediation on second to fourth-grade D/HH children's production of classifiers in narrative retells. The authors concluded that repeated viewings of strong ASL models paired with teacher mediation has the potential to improve classifier use in narrative retell, but there were also effects of a child's ASL experience. There were also variable effects of mediation across students; some required more scaffolding.

Kelley and McCann (2021) reported sign language outcomes with a deaf child with DSILD following a seven-week intervention. The child had native access to ASL through his deaf family and attended an ASL/English bilingual school for the deaf. Assessments revealed language difficulties in the absence of cognitive, motor, or neurological impairments. Weaknesses were noted in the use of subject-predicate sentences, third person pronouns, lexical diversity, using noun phrases with descriptors, and responding to wh-questions. Focused stimulation was used with treatment stimuli selected and implemented following the three principles of statistical learning: high-density input, consistency, and variability (Plante & Gomez, 2018). Following intervention, increased lexical diversity as measured by the number of different verbs used in structured activities was observed. While the child did not increase frequency of SV/SVO structures during probe tasks, a review of his productions during intervention interactions revealed qualitative differences across sessions. He increased his frequency of third person subjects (as opposed to primarily first-person "I" during baseline and early sessions) and incorporated referents for classifier complements.

Suggestions for clinicians working with children with DSILD

For bilingual children acquiring their home language and spoken English, there are questions about when and how the home language should be integrated into therapy. For D/HH children whose primary language is ASL, intervention in their accessible visual language is warranted. Given the need for intervention in ASL and the differences that exist between signed and spoken languages, clinicians should consider the linguistic structure of ASL and developmental considerations when identifying intervention targets. Collaboration with fluent users of the signed language is critical and may be supported by the following considerations.

The purpose of this section is not to discuss assessment for eligibility for services. Language intervention eligibility varies across jurisdictions and may include specific or unique requirements. There are issues related to the availability of diagnostic assessments that differentiate between typical and atypical development which is beyond the scope of this chapter (see Henner et al., 2018, for more information). We focus on how to identify potential treatment targets and strategies to support children with DSILD based on the linguistic features of ASL. We provide a checklist of ASL structures that serves as a guide for the clinician to identify potential areas for intervention (see Appendix 5.1). This checklist highlights structures that are motivated by the visual–spatial nature of signed languages.

Checklist to guide target selection

A checklist to guide the clinician in identifying target structures of ASL is provided in Appendix 5.1 (see descriptions of other sign languages for comparable structures). The first step in identifying potential targets for intervention is to gather a language sample with stimuli that provide opportunities for the child to demonstrate the range of skills included on the checklist. Using a wordless video or picture book with multiple characters provides contexts for the child to demonstrate language skills in the visual modality that may not be necessary in conversational contexts (see also Quinto-Pozos, 2022 for other suggestions about signed language assessment). For older clients, an explanation of how to play a game or sport elicits higher level language skill that will support identification of areas of need.

We suggest evaluating verb types for agreement early in the analysis. As mentioned earlier, there are three classes of verbs: plain, agreeing, and locative. A plain verb generally does not inflect (i.e., there is no change to aspects of handshape or location) based on agent-theme roles or how an action takes place in space. While plain verbs may be inflected for aspect, this modulates the movement without reference to agent-theme considerations and can be considered separately. An agreeing verb is inflected for agent-theme roles by changing the movement path between entities that have been established/

referenced in the signer's space (either present/real or absent/imagined). For example, a signer could sign TEACHER and reference the left side of their signing space followed by CHILD and a subsequent reference the right side of their signing space. The movement of the verb from one of those locations to the other indicates the agent (beginning location) and theme (ending location) roles. A locative verb is inflected to indicate how an object or entity moves in space between locations (real or imagined). For example, a signer may establish two locations, for example, HOME (on the right) and SCHOOL (on the left), and then signs the target verb, DRIVE-TO indicating the origin and destination. Examples of different types of ASL verbs are provided in Table 5.1. If a client uses agreeing or locative verbs in their citation form (i.e., uninflected) but the context specifies agreement, the use of space/agreement is warranted for intervention. For a subset of these verbs, it is important to identify movement in space and selection of handshape to match the entity that is being acted on. For example, when a large book is the entity being moved, the signer would use a C handshape, whereas an apple may be represented by the "claw" handshape.

The clinician should also consider evaluating the use of different sentence types. Children with typically developing language skills will demonstrate flexibility in sentence type with increasing complexity expected with age. Considering the "hands before faces" pattern of acquisition suggested by Reilly (2006), SLPs should examine what sentence types are used and how they are encoded (i.e., through lexical signs in certain orders, non-manual signals, or both). Different possibilities for target selection exist. If the child demonstrates difficulty with non-manual signal production, the SLP could prioritize a communicative intent/context for which the child does not have a lexical option. As previously discussed, the preverbal object use (OSV sentence structure) may be motivated by the use of topicalization. If the non-manual marker is not present, the sentence might not be understood as intended. Targeting non-manual features of topic OSV structure could be expected to have positive outcomes on reducing ambiguity of agent and theme roles. The use of non-manuals as an obligatory marker may then generalize to other structures. If a child has a strategy for a communicative intent, but is not integrating non-manual

Table 5.1 Sample verbs for each of the three categories.

Plain	Agreeing	Locative
LIKE	HELP	PUT
WANT	SHOW	MOVE
HAVE	GIVE-TO	THROW
COOK	FORCE	DRIVE-TO
PLAN	SUMMON	FLY-TO
READ	INFORM	HURT

Note: Some verbs (GIVE-TO, PUT, and MOVE) may also incorporate size/shape characteristics.

markers (e.g., they use wh-questions words without the associated non-manual features), a target of intervention could be the integration of the manual and non-manual components. Given the lack of research on the topic, it is difficult to know which target priority would result in the most effective and efficient change to the child's language system. Iconicity has been presented as a potential scaffold for the use of space and classifiers. For non-manuals, it does not appear that communicative non-manuals facilitate the acquisition of grammatical forms (Chen-Pichler, 2012) so focusing on communicative/affective use is not advised as a strategy for determining targets or during intervention.

Similar to spoken languages, signed languages may expand on utterance complexity by combining propositions. ASL not only shares some conjunctions with English (e.g., BUT), but also has signs that are unique to ASL in joining utterances (e.g., UNDERSTAND, FRUSTRATE, HIT, WRONG). ASL commonly uses the pronoun SELF and space and/or non-manual markers to encode relative clauses (in addition to the lexical signals WHO and THAT) or for copula use (Sampson & Mayberry, 2022). If the child demonstrates a limited frequency or repertoire of expanded utterances, intervention for this area is warranted.

When children have difficulty with classifiers, the clinician should evaluate what elements are missing, have errors, or are poorly coordinated. The checklist in Appendix 5.1 identifies classifiers of three types: semantic, size and shape, and handling, and provides example skills to look for when observing classifier use. As indicated earlier, classifier acquisition begins as early as 2–3 years old, but continues to develop throughout early-school years (and into adolescence, in some cases). If the child struggles to use classifiers within the language sampling context, additional tasks may be warranted such as picture description or narrative retelling (e.g., with soundless video prompts). The documentation of production ability includes phonological features of the signs (e.g., handshape, palm orientation, location, and movement) how referents are established by the child (e.g., with full nouns, pronominal points, role/referential shift), and the appropriate use of space. Observations of how figure/ground relationships are integrated and use of space and perspective should also be documented.

Intervention considerations

Several factors will determine the therapy approach including the child's age and metalinguistic skill (the ability to think and talk about language). The choice of stimuli for intervention depends on knowledge of ASL linguistics, however. For example, not all verbs incorporate subject–theme roles or locative information. The goal of implicit approaches, such as focused stimulation and recasting, is to provide high-density modeling of a target language form and provide a context that encourages the child to use the target construction. To achieve the frequency and diversity in modeling, the clinician should consider candidate verbs in planning and set up the environment so that multiple opportunities are available for those agreeing or locative verbs. Explicit approaches use direct instruction of target language structures. Direct instruction may include explanations of subject and object roles with inclusion of verbs that change in phonological form (e.g., from subject–object agreement or information about the location of the goal) and those that do not.

The clinician is encouraged to leverage the visual nature of ASL. If a child has difficulty with both present and absent referents, they may start by setting up contexts where referents are visually available through manipulatives, drawings, or people in the environment. Once a child is successful with present referents, they may begin to remove those referents as a scaffold for agreement for absent referents. This same strategy may support pronoun use when the child exhibits difficulty with stacking errors (i.e., locating multiple referents in the same area of the signing space) or maintaining referent locations during discourse. Initially visual anchors (concrete objects in the environment) may be employed and then removed as the child experiences success. While this suggestion is not based on previous intervention research, it could build upon linguistic strengths/abilities that the child may have, and then presents a new, potentially more challenging, discourse context for the child. There are both linguistic and gestural ways to communicate in ASL. The SLP may design interventions that take advantage of iconicity as a scaffold for acquiring a new skill but consider the transition to more abstract contexts.

While "breaking-down and building-up" utterances is a familiar practice to most SLPs, clinicians may not be aware that this approach may be applied to classifier constructions or constructed action. The SLP may model a classifier construction, break it down into isolated propositions, and then build it back up to the complex construction. They may also use vertical structuring by taking a child's production, eliciting additional information, and then model a classifier construction combining those ideas. The propositions could include the representation of the focus object or person, the movement involved (e.g., for depicting path and manner), and ground referents. While constructed action is a common structure in ASL and other signed languages, children who lack sign or classifier use may depend primarily on affective gesture or facial expression.

Conclusion

Recent research has shed some light on language characteristics of DSILD, although there are comparatively few publications in this area of child development. Additionally, minimal research and few resources exist on how to guide clinicians' identification of targets and intervention. To assist clinicians, we have provided a checklist of signed language structures including sentence and verb types, pronouns and their use, classifiers, and role shift, that could serve as potential targets for language intervention. We suggest that assessment and intervention require collaboration with fluent users of the language, and we encourage SLPs to work closely with Deaf professionals, when possible. As can be expected, a basic understanding of the linguistic structure of ASL (or the ambient sign language) is a must. Moreover, knowledge of phonological, morphological, and syntactic differences between signed and spoken languages could be a valuable tool to support the SLP's decision-making as part of the interprofessional team.

References

Beal-Alvarez, J., & Easterbrooks, S. R. (2013). Increasing children's ASL classifier production: A multi-component intervention. *American Annals of the Deaf, 158*(3), 311–333. https://doi.org/10.1353/aad.2013.0028

Boyes-Braem, P. (1990). Acquisition of the handshape in American sign language: A preliminary analysis. In V. Volterra & C. J. Erting (Eds.), *From gesture to language in hearing and deaf children* (pp. 107–127). Springer. https://doi.org/10.1007/978-3-642-74859-2_10

Cheek, A., Cormier, K., Repp, A., & Meier, R. (2001). Prelinguistic gesture predicts mastery and error in the production of early signs. *Language, 77*(2), 292–323. httsp://doi.org/10.1353%2Flan.2001.0071

Chen-Pichler, D. (2012). Acquisition. In R. Pfau, M. Steinbach, & B. Woll (Eds.), *Sign language: An international handbook* (pp. 647–686). De Gruyter Mouton. https://doi.org/10.1515/9783110261325

Cripps, J. H., Cooper, S. B., Supalla, S. J., & Evitts, P. M. (2016). Meeting the needs of signers in the field of speech and language pathology: Some considerations for action. *Communication Disorders Quarterly, 37*(2), 108–116. https://doi.org/10.1177%2F1525740115576955

Dostal, H. M., & Wolbers, K. A. (2014). Developing language and writing skills of deaf and hard of hearing students: A simultaneous approach. *Literacy Research and Instruction, 53*(3), 245–268. https://doi.org/10.1080%2F19388071.2014.907382

Emmorey, K., & Reilly, J. (1998). The development of quotation and reported action: Conveying perspective in ASL. In E. Clark (Ed.), *The proceedings of the twenty-ninth annual child language research forum* (pp. 81–90). CLSI Publications.

Hall, W. C., Levin, L. L., & Anderson, M. L. (2017). Language deprivation syndrome: A possible neurodevelopmental disorder with sociocultural origins. *Social Psychiatry and Psychiatric Epidemiology, 52*(6), 761–776. https://doi.org/10.1007%2Fs00127-017-1351-7

Henner, J., Novogrodsky, R., Reis, J., & Hoffmeister, R. (2018). Recent issues in the use of signed language assessments for diagnosis of language disorders in signing deaf and hard of hearing children. *Journal of Deaf Studies and Deaf Education, 23*(4), 307–316. https://doi.org/10.1093%2Fdeafed%2Feny014

Kelley, L. E., & McCann, J. P. (2021). Language intervention isn't just spoken: Assessment and treatment of a deaf signing child with SLI. *Language, Speech, and Hearing Services in Schools, 52*(4), 978–992. https://doi.org/10.1044/2021_LSHSS-21-00038

Klima, E. S., & Bellugi, U. (1979). *The signs of language*. Harvard University Press. https://doi.org/10.2307/413507

Lillo-Martin, D., & Henner, J. (2021). Acquisition of sign languages. *Annual Review of Linguistics, 7*, 395–419. https://doi.org/10.1146/annurev-linguistics-043020-92357

Lillo-Martin, D., & Quadros, R. M. de. (2011). Acquisition of the syntax—discourse interface: The expression of point of view. *Lingua, 121*(4), 623–636. https://doi:10.1016/j.lingua.2010.07.001

Loew, R. (1984). *Roles and reference in American sign language: A developmental perspective* (Publication No. 8418508) [Doctoral dissertation, University of Minnesota]. ProQuest Dissertations Publishing.

Mason, K., Rowley, K., Marshall, C. R., Atkinson, J. R., Herman, R., Woll, B., & Morgan, G. (2010). Identifying specific language impairment in deaf children acquiring British sign language: Implications for theories and practice. *British Journal of Developmental Psychology, 28*(1), 33–49. https://doi.org/10.1348%2F026151009x484190

Meier, R. P. (1982). *Icons, analogues, and morphemes: The acquisition of verb agreement in American Sign Language* (Publication No. 8224525) [Doctoral dissertation, University of California]. ProQuest Dissertations Publishing.

Morgan, G., Herman, R., & Woll, B. (2007). Language impairments in sign language: Breakthroughs and puzzles. *International Journal of Language and Communication Disorders, 42,* 97–105. https://doi.org/10.1080/13682820600783178

Padden, C. (1983). *Interaction of morphology and syntax in American sign language* [Unpublished doctoral dissertation, University of California].

Plante, E., & Gomez, R. L. (2018). Learning without trying: The clinical relevance of statistical learning. *Language, Speech, and Hearing Services in Schools, 49*(3S), 710–722. https://doi.org/10.1044%2F2018_lshss-stlt1-17-0131

Quadros, R. M. de, & Lillo-Martin, D. (2007). Gesture and the acquisition of verb agreement in sign languages. In H. Caunt-Nulton, S. Kulatilake, & I. Woo (Eds.), *Proceedings of the 31st annual Boston University conference on language development* (Vol. 1, pp. 520–531). Boston University Press.

Quinto-Pozos, D. G. (2002). *Contact between Mexican sign language and American sign language in two Texas border areas* (Publication No. 3082889) [Doctoral dissertation, University of Texas]. ProQuest Dissertations Publishing.

Quinto-Pozos, D. G. (2014). Considering communication disorders and differences in the signed language modality. In D. Quinto-Pozos (Ed.), *Multilingual aspects of signed language communication and disorder* (pp. 1–42). Multilingual Matters, Ltd. https://doi.org/10.21832/9781783091317-004

Quinto-Pozos, D. G. (2022). Developmental language disorder and the assessment of signed language. In T. Haug, W. Mann, & U. Knoch (Eds.), *The handbook of language assessment across modalities.* Oxford University Press. https://doi.org/10.1093/oso/9780190885052.003.0015

Quinto-Pozos, D. G., & Cooley, F. (2020). A developmental disorder of signed language production in a native deaf signer of ASL. *Languages, 5*(4), 40. https://doi.org/10.3390%2Flanguages5040040

Quinto-Pozos, D. G., Forber-Pratt, A. J., & Singleton, J. L. (2011). Do developmental communication disorders exist in the signed modality? Perspectives from professionals. *Language, Speech, and Hearing Services in Schools, 42*(4), 423–443. https://doi.org/10.1044%2F0161-1461%282011%2F10-0071%29

Quinto-Pozos, D. G., Singleton, J. L., & Hauser, P. C. (2017). A case of specific language impairment in a deaf signer of American sign language. *Journal of Deaf Studies and Deaf Education, 30*(5), 332–359. https://doi.org/10.1093%2Fdeafed%2Fenw074

Quinto-Pozos, D. G., Singleton, J. L., Hauser, P. C., Levine, S., Garberoglio, C. L., & Hou, L. (2013). Atypical signed language development: A case study of challenges with visual-spatial processing. *Cognitive Neuropsychology, 30,* 332–359. https://doi.org/10.1080/02643294.2013.863756

Reilly, J. (2006). How faces come to serve grammar: The development of nonmanual morphology in American sign language. In B. Schick, M. Marschark, & P. E. Spencer (Eds.), *Advances in the sign language development of deaf children* (pp. 262–290). Oxford University Press. https://doi.org/10.1093/acprof:oso/9780195180947.003.0011

Sampson, T., & Mayberry, R. I. (2022). An emerging SELF: The copula cycle in American Sign Language. *Language, 98*(2), 327–358. doi:10.1353/lan.2022.0005

Schembri, A. (2003). Rethinking "classifiers" in signed languages. In K. Emmorey (Ed.), *Perspectives on classifier constructions in sign languages* (pp. 3–34). Lawrence Erlbaum Associates, Inc.

Scott, J. A., & Dostal, H. M. (2019). Language development and deaf/hard of hearing children. *Education Sciences, 9*(2), 135. https://doi.org/10.3390/educsci9020135

Siedlecki, T., & Bonvillian, J. D. (1993). Location, handshape & movement: Young children's acquisition of the formational aspects of American sign language. *Sign Language Studies, 78*, 31–52. https://doi.org/10.1353/sls.1993.0016

Simms, L., Baker, S., & Clark, M. D. (2013). The standardized visual communication and sign language checklist for signing children. *Sign Language Studies, 14*(1), 101–124. https://doi.org/10.1353/sls.2013.0029

Slobin, D. I., Hoiting, N., Kuntze, M., Lindert, R., Weinberg, A., Pyers, J., Anthony, M., Biederman, Y., & Thumann, H. (2003). A cognitive/functional perspective on the acquisition of "classifiers." In K. Emmorey (Ed.), *Perspectives on classifier constructions in sign languages* (pp. 271–296). Lawrence Erlbaum Associates, Inc.

Steinbach, M. (2021). Role shift. In J. Quer, R. Pfau, & A. Hermann (Eds.), *The Routledge handbook of theoretical and experimental sign language research* (pp. 351–377). Routledge. https://doi.org/10.4324/9781315754499-16

Woll, B., & Morgan, G. (2012). Language impairments in the development of sign: Do they reside in a specific modality or are they modality-independent deficits? *Bilingualism, Language and Cognition, 15*(1), 75–87. https://doi:10.1017/S1366728911000459

Wolsey, J. A., Clark, M. D., & Andrews, J. F. (2018). ASL and English bilingual shared book reading: An exploratory intervention for signing deaf children. *Bilingual Research Journal, 41*(3), 221–237. https://doi.org/10.1080%2F15235882.2018.1481893

Appendix 5.1

Checklist for identification of language targets for children with DSILD

The following aspects of ASL linguistic structure may be observed within language samples collected using a variety of strategies including wordless picture books, wordless videos, or prompts to explain the rules of a game. A verbatim transcription of the entire language sample is not needed to complete the checklist.

Background information

Appendix Table 5.2

Child's Name:	Child's Age:
Age of Exposure to Signed Language:	Language(s) Used:
Prior Signed Language Interventions:	
Language Sample Context:	

Appendix Table 5.3

Area	Look-for		Example of appropriate use	Example of error
Phonology				
Handshape	C, A, S, 1, 5, L			
	B, F, O			
	W, D, P, 3, V, H, I, Y			
	X, R, M, N, T, 7, 8			
Movement	Sign Path			
	Sign Internal			
Orientation				
Location				

Area	Look-for		Example of appropriate use	Example of error
Sentence Types				
SVO	SVO			
Topic Structure	Non-manual marker (raised eyebrow)			
Yes/No Question	Non-Manual Marker (raised eyebrow)			
	Lexical Marker (QM-"question mark")			
Wh-Question	Non-Manual Marker (furroughed eyebrows)			
	Lexical Marker (Wh-question signs)			
Rhetorical Question	Non-Manual Marker (raised eyebrow)			
	Lexical Marker (Wh-question signs)			
Negation	Non-Manual Marker (headshake)			
	Lexical Marker (e.g., NOT, NONE, DON'T-WANT)			
Verb Type Use				
Plain Verbs	Uninflected			
Agreement Verbs (e.g., HELP, INFORM)	Use of space			
	Present Referents			
	Absent Referents			
	Handshape modification			
Spatial Verbs (e.g., MOVE, PUT, DRIVE-TO)	Location Agreement			
	Handshape modification			
Aspect Markers Distribution • To each • To all Temporal • Continuous • Repeated	Movement marker			
	Use of Space			
	Lexical Markers (e.g., ALL-DAY, EVERYDAY)			
Expanding sentences				
Conjunctions (e.g., FINISH, UNDERSTAND, #OR)	Lexical Markers			

(*Continued*)

Appendix Table 5.3 (Continued)

Area	Look-for		Example of appropriate use	Example of error
Relative Clauses (e.g., SELF, WHO, THAT)	Lexical Markers			
	Non-manual markers (eye-brow, space)			
Conditionals (e.g., #IF, SUPPOSE)				
Pronoun Use				
Present Referents	Eye-gaze Indexing Use of space			
Absent Referents	Eye-gaze Indexing Use of Space			
Numerical Incorporation	(e.g., TWO-OF-US)			
Classifiers				
Semantic	Established referent			
	Use of handshape for object, entity			
	Movement of entity Path Manner			
Size and Shape	Established referent			
	Handshape selection			
	Size shape movement			
	Use of space			
Handling	Established referent			
	Handshape selection			
	Movement			
	Use of space			
Discourse Functions	Primary object, entity			
	Background objects, entities			
	Movement			
	Constructed Action			
	Maintenance of space reference			
Role-shift/constructed action				
Identification of Referents	Referents			
Shifting	Eye Gaze			
	Head/Shoulder Shift			
	Body Shifting (e.g., to show size/height)			
	Facial Expression			
Discourse maintenance	Referent location/Pronouns			

Part II

Applications to adult speech and language differences and disorders

6 Phonetics and Phonology

The phonetics and phonology of intelligibility: The functional importance to intelligibility of speech sounds

Naomi Gurevich and Heejin Kim

Abstract

Most undergraduate curricula in Communication Disorders require the foundational course of Phonetics, where future clinicians are taught to classify sounds by place and manner of articulation, and to transcribe speech using the international phonetic alphabet. Phonology is not typically required as part of communication disorders curricula. As such, clinicians are missing an important piece of the puzzle with respect to speech intelligibility. In this chapter, we support a conceptual hierarchy of functional importance to intelligibility based on four phonological properties of sounds (contrast, context, frequency, and functional load). We then explain the use of this concept in clinical practice to both diagnose and treat intelligibility disorders in adults.

Statement to the reader

As a clinician, you already know that articulatory accuracy is relevant to intelligibility: you know that misarticulated phonemes can make it hard to understand one's speech. But if you have a list of consonants a speaker has problems producing, do you know which ones are most important to intelligibility? This decision is rooted in the phonological properties of speech sounds. In this chapter we provide a basic overview of these properties without assuming any formal education in this area of linguistics. We explain how these properties influence speech intelligibility and provide the clinician with a resource to help prioritize treatment targets to improve intelligibility of adults with dysarthria.

Introduction

A listener's ability to understand speech depends on the ability to perceive and decode acoustic signals. Acoustic clarity of speech sounds (phones) within

DOI: 10.4324/9781003045519-8

words plays an important part in the decoding process, but this importance varies depending on linguistic properties. That is, the level of acoustic clarity required for a phone to be correctly perceived may vary depending on the following phonological factors: (1) contrast, (2) context, (3) frequency, and (4) functional load. Given that communication is the primary function of language, and verbal communication depends on spoken words being correctly perceived, or intelligible, these factors can be thought of as having a *functional importance to intelligibility* (FITI). These linguistic properties with FITI are not independent from each other but rather are interrelated. Considering these factors is central to investigating consonant production and perception because consonants are particularly critical to word-level intelligibility in speech perception (Fogerty et al., 2012; Toro et al., 2008) as well as in language acquisition (Hochmann et al., 2011).

An adult with acquired dysarthria may have difficulty with certain consonants in some (or all) positional contexts. It should be noted that adult speakers have mastered the full phonemic inventory and have internalized the phonological rules and patterns of their language. Thus, the goal of treatment is not analogous to speech therapy with pediatric speech-sound clients for whom a key goal might be to target filling in the full inventory of phonemes to match same-age peers in developing speech (please see Chapter 1 by Velleman and Abbiati in this volume for a discussion of the full complexities of child speech sound therapy). For adults with acquired disorders, we must go beyond thinking only about *which* sounds are difficult for a given speaker and consider also *where* those sounds are difficult, as well as how disruptive the difficulty is to verbal communication.

All sounds in a given language are not equally important to intelligibility. As we examine the four phonological properties of sounds (contrast, context, frequency, and functional load), patterns emerge that shape the phonemic inventory of a language into a hierarchy of FITI to help identify key articulation targets and prioritize them for treatment to improve intelligibility. We conclude the chapter with a section on Clinical Use where we offer the FITI Table as a resource for clinicians to help them recognize *which* sounds and *where* are most important to a client's intelligibility.

Phonological contrast

The perception of phones fluctuates depending on phonological contrast (Boomershine et al., 2008; Noguchi & Kam, 2018; Trubetzkoy, 1939). The distinction across phones that are contrastive (*phonemes*) has been shown to be perceived better than across phones that are not contrastive (phonetic variants of phonemes, or *allophones*) (Boomershine et al., 2008; Harnsberger, 2001; Noguchi & Kam, 2018). We know that exposure to the system of contrasts of one's native language affects perception across phones, reducing the ability to perceive the difference between non-contrastive phones as early as six months old (Kuhl et al., 1992). Additional evidence that contrast affects perception and that listeners are more sensitive to acoustic differences between sounds that are contrastive in their own language is provided from studies involving Malayalam, English, Spanish, and Korean:

Malayalam. Dental and alveolar nasals (n̪, n) are in complementary distribution (i.e., in mutually exclusive contexts, which for phonetically related sounds usually implies they are allophones of the same phoneme), and are perceived as less distinct than bilabial and velar nasals (m, ŋ) which are contrastive in this language (Harnsberger, 2001).

English and Spanish. English /ð/ is distinct from /d/, of which [ɾ] is a positional allophone: that is, the /d/ is produced as the voiced tap [ɾ] in post-stressed, intervocalic positions (e.g., "Adam" [ˈærəm], and "kiddo" [ˈkɪɾo]). On the other hand, in Spanish [ð] is an allophone of /d/, and /ɾ/ is distinct. Speakers are more sensitive to the differences between the sounds that are distinct in their own language than to differences between the sounds that are in complementary distribution (Boomershine et al., 2008).

Korean and English. Unlike English, Korean does not have voicing contrasts for stop consonants. Instead, voiced stops occur as allophones between voiced segments such as vowels (Cho & Park, 2006; Lee, 1999). Korean learners of English are not used to phonological-level voicing contrasts and therefore have difficulties producing and perceiving voiced stops in English (Kim & Duanmu, 2004).

Role in FITI. There is a hierarchy of phonological contrasts in which phonemic distinctions are more important than allophonic ones for the purposes of comprehension. For example, the acoustic clarity of nasality is necessary to distinguish /b/ from /m/ (e.g., "bat" versus "mat") but is not as crucial for the various allophonic variations of /t/ (e.g., aspirated [tʰ] or tapped [ɾ]) to identify the word "atom." A motor speech disorder that affects a speaker's ability to produce sufficient acoustic cues for phonemic distinctions is expected to have a significant effect on intelligibility. On the basis of this, materials used to elicit speech for clinical purposes must include all phonemes in a language.

Phonological context

The perception of phones fluctuates based on phonological context (Trubetzkoy, 1939), such as the positions of consonants in a syllable or in a word, the type of surrounding sounds, and whether a consonant is in a stressed or unstressed syllable. For example, there is cross-linguistic evidence that distinctions between phonemes are generally more perceptible in pre-vocalic contexts than in pre-consonantal ones (Jun, 2011; Silverman, 1995; Steriade, 1999). Phonetic processes such as lenition[1] are less likely to neutralize phonetic

---

1. *Lenition* is usually defined as a weakened articulation of a sound and is a category of phonetically conditioned changes that are quite common in human languages and are similar to each other across languages. For more information, see Gurevich (2004, 2011).

distinctions[2] in onset (consonants that occur before the nucleus of a syllable) positions than in coda (consonants after the nucleus of a syllable) (Gurevich, 2004, 2011). Additionally, second language acquisition studies report better performance in both perception and production of non-native consonants in onset position than in codas (Cheng & Zhang, 2015).

The importance of acoustic clarity of a phone to speech perception is also dependent on word position. Phonetic neutralization resulting from word-final devoicing is a common phenomenon in languages (Guitart, 1976) and in general phonemes are more likely to be deleted word-finally (Harris, 2011). In foreign-accented speech, word-initial phonemic errors have been found to interfere with intelligibility to a higher degree than word-final errors (Bent et al., 2007; Bent et al., 2001; Scharenborg et al., 2016). Also, most word-initial consonants are acquired first during language development (Bleile, 2015; Jusczyk, 1999; Kessler & Treiman, 1997; Stokes & Surendran, 2005; To et al., 2013), and children perform better at discriminating word-initial contrasts (Cilibrasi et al., 2015). Certain consonants, however, are acquired in word-final position earlier than in initial positions. For example, in American English, children acquire fricatives, velars, and the /r/[3] in syllable- and word-final positions before word-initial ones (Dyson, 1986; Kent, 1982; McGowan et al., 2004; Rockman & Elbert, 1984). In addition, consonant production errors in dysarthric speech are shown to be influenced by word positions (Antolík & Fougeron, 2013; Kim & Gurevich, 2021). For example, in CP-associated dysarthric speech produced by native speakers of American English, fewer production errors were found in word-initial positions compared to medial and final positions for stop, liquid, and nasal consonants, while fricatives did not exhibit such positional effects (Kim & Gurevich, 2021).

Positional contexts related to prosody can also affect the production and perception of consonants. For example, lexical stress in English plays an important communicative function, by disambiguating word meaning, and stressed positions are indisputably more prominent than unstressed ones (Jun, 2011). Specifically, sounds in stressed syllables are more strongly articulated (referred to as prosodic strengthening), as evidenced by faster, longer, or bigger speech gestures (Beckman & Edwards, 1994; Cho, 2001; de Jong, 1995). In developmental linguistics, children (both typical and atypical) are found to repeat stressed syllables more accurately than unstressed ones, and stressed environments also improved discrimination of this contrast (Cilibrasi et al., 2015; Marshall & van der Lely, 2009).

Role in FITI. The acoustic clarity of sounds is more important for comprehension in some positions than in others. For example, the intelligibility of an

---

2. *Phonetic neutralization* indicates the distinction between two sounds has been obliterated. For example, if a tʰ and a t are both produced as a [t], the aspirated/unaspirated distinction between them is lost.

3. For the sake of convenience, as there is no trill in English, the English ɹ is written as r throughout our chapter. We also acknowledge that some researchers and clinicians treat syllable or word-final ɹ and rhotic diphthongs as vowels.

individual with dysarthria who has problems maintaining voicing distinctions at word-final positions (e.g., due to breath support for phonation) may not be as affected as that of an individual who has difficulty maintaining voicing distinctions in word-initial positions (e.g., due to weakness or incomplete vocal fold adduction). In other words, it is important to discover in which context contrasts are compromised. Therefore, materials used to elicit speech for clinical purposes must include phonemes in all allowable positional contexts in that language: that is, word-initial (#_), word-final (_#), and combinations of pre-vocalic (_V), pre-consonantal (_C), post-vocalic (V_), and post-consonantal (_C), in both stressed and unstressed syllables. Once speech data is collected for all positions, it can help prioritize treatment of positions that are most important for comprehension.

Frequency

Trubetzkoy (1939) distinguishes token frequency (how often a phoneme occurs in speech) from type frequency (the number of words that depend on a phoneme to be distinguished from each other; this is *functional load* discussed next). These two properties of speech have a complex relationship and can sometimes have opposing effects on speech. With respect to token frequency, phonemes that are more frequent in a language are less dependent on acoustic clarity to be decoded by listeners (Gurevich, 2004; Moates et al., 2006). Frequency at the word level is also relevant, as words that are more frequent or common in a language can be more easily recognized from lesser signals (Kingston, 2008) and are regularly perceived as less accented in foreign-accented speech (Levi et al., 2007). In general, words that are more frequent are more familiar, and hence can be more intelligible (Owens, 1961). However, a misarticulated frequent phoneme also has the potential to affect a greater number of words that depend on it for distinction (related to functional load, discussed next) and therefore may have a greater impact on intelligibility.

The potential effect of frequency on intelligibility is disrupted in the case of the most frequent common words in a language: function words. These are words that serve a grammatical purpose, such as auxiliary verbs, prepositions, articles, and conjunctions. These words sidestep dependence on acoustic clarity to be decoded or intelligible because they can largely be predicted from context (Bell et al., 2003; Gregory, 2001; Gurevich, 2004; Jurafsky et al., 2001; Lieberman, 1963).

Role in FITI. The most frequent words in English (and really, in any language) are function words and compared to content words, these do not depend as much on acoustic clarity to be decoded because they are predictable from grammar. An articulation disorder that affects the /ð/ phoneme, extremely common in function words but one of the least common phonemes in content words, is unlikely to affect one's overall intelligibility. Given a client who fatigues easily, phonemes that are more frequent in content words should be prioritized for treatment.[4] On the basis of this, materials used to elicit speech for clinical purposes should have a hierarchy of phonemes by frequency in content words only, excluding function words.

Functional load

The functional load of a phoneme, referred to as type frequency in Trubetzkoy (1939), is defined as the number of words that depend on this phoneme to be distinguished from each other. The acoustic clarity of a phoneme with a higher functional load may be more important for decoding speech than the acoustic clarity of a phoneme with a lower functional load (Bent et al., 2007; Bybee, 1994; Gurevich, 2004). As noted earlier, this effect can be mitigated by high frequency of the phoneme in the language or increased by high frequency of the phoneme in content words. That is, a frequent token in general may have reduced reliance on acoustic clarity to be perceived, but when misarticulated, it also has the potential to affect a greater number of words that rely on it for distinction, and therefore may have a greater impact on intelligibility.

To be truly dependent on an opposition between phonemes for lexical distinction, the lexical items must be minimal pairs. For an example of a phoneme with a high functional load, consider the importance of perceiving the /t/ in a word like "tap" to distinguish it from "cap," "sap," "rap," "gap," "nap," "pap," and other similar words in English. Compare with the importance of perceiving the contrast between /ʃ/ and /ʒ/ in English, a contrast that distinguishes very few words from each other (Hockett, 1967). Another example of low functional load involves glides in Blackfoot (or *Siksiká*, a North American Plains Algonquian language) that can only occur in two suffixes that relate to obligatorily possessed nouns: -*wa* and -*ji* (Frantz, 1971); perceiving the acoustic signal of either glide is not crucial for decoding meaning, and in fact, both phonemes are lost in post-consonantal context with little consequence for meaning (Gurevich, 2004).

Clearly, functional load is intimately related to phonological contrast, but its effect on communication (its FITI) is also influenced by phonological context and token frequency. To illustrate, consider the consequence of phonetic neutralization: The risk of this obliteration of acoustic and perceptual distinction resulting in the obliteration of meaning distinction (phonological neutralization) is nonexistent for non-contrastive phones (e.g., between the allophones [p] and [pʰ] in stressed-syllable initial position in English). In the case of contrastive phones, the risk of obliterating meaning distinction is lower for (a) oppositions with low functional loads (e.g., the Blackfoot glides example); (b) in contexts where the opposition is harder to perceive (e.g., in coda over onset positions); and (c) oppositions involving very frequent phonemes (e.g., the t/d

---

4. Note that we are discussing intelligibility goals. A misarticulated /ð/ in English would be very noticeable given its frequency in definite articles ('the') but its effect on intelligibility is predicted to be minimal. However, if a client wishes to focus on the naturalness of their speech, /ð/ becomes a high priority target.

opposition in American English carries a substantial functional load and yet was neutralized intervocalically between a stressed vowel and an unstressed one (Hockett, 1967)). With respect to the t/d opposition in American English, presumably, the load of the opposition was mitigated by its frequency, reducing the need for a clear acoustic distinction to decode lexical items.[5]

Role in FITI. An opposition that is highly used in a language is more important to distinguishing words because it is the main distinction between more words. However, this importance can be mitigated by frequency. The importance of functional load to intelligibility is well supported but also complex, and it is not always possible to predict which oppositions are more important (not to mention, this importance can change over time). We can predict, mostly, that phonemes that are rare in certain positions in a language, hence having low functional load in those positions, are not likely to depend on the clearest acoustic signals for comprehension. Hence, a misarticulation of these sounds is not likely to cause misunderstanding. On the basis of this, materials used to elicit speech for clinical purposes should include and prioritize high functional load elements and downgrade, or omit, low functional load ones.

Incorporating FITI properties into speech materials

In order to incorporate the four phonological properties of sounds (contrast, context, frequency, and functional load) into materials to elicit speech for clinical purposes, we compiled a word list of 308 unique words, constructed from a corpus of the 5,000 most frequent words in American English (but only content words were used, leaving a corpus of 4,706 words once function words were omitted). The corpus we used is based on data from ten large corpora of English (*Word frequency data*, 2019) and its printed version, the Frequency Dictionary of Contemporary American English (Davies & Gardner, 2010). We organized our word list into all allowable contexts for each English phoneme, by employing the following principles.

The word list includes every phoneme in English in order to incorporate **phonological contrast**. Additionally, every allowable **phonological context** in English is included achieving significant coverage of allophonic variation. All contrastive features, including voicing and stress, are well-represented. **Frequency** and **functional load** of oppositions in English are represented in our list in several ways. First, since function words are to a large degree predictable from context, they rarely truly depend on any opposition to be recognized. As such they have very low functional load and therefore omitting them from the list improves its overall representation of this linguistic factor. Second, inasmuch as type frequency is related to token frequency (which it is inherently, since type frequency is defined as the number of words that depend on the distinction),

---

5. This is a prime example of the opposing forces of functional load and frequency: While a higher functional load suggests that an opposition is more integral to comprehension, the frequency of the phonemes involved may make them less dependent on acoustic signals.

functional load is represented in the distribution of phonemes across included words. Third, for some allowable contexts, no example word token exists in the corpus of 4,706 words. These allowable but rare contexts indicate a lower functional load of a phoneme (another example of the opposing forces of frequency and functional load discussed in footnote 5) and demonstrate positional dependence of the functional load of certain oppositions (i.e., the direct interaction between context and functional load).

The FITI table, a clinical tool

In the previous section, we proposed a conceptual hierarchy of FITI based on the four phonological properties of sounds (contrast, context, frequency, and functional load) and explained the construction of a word list with all four phonological properties. In this section, we offer the FITI Table that presents the importance to intelligibility hierarchy of these properties with respect to each other. The FITI Table is a clinical tool to be used during assessment and treatment. We provide instructions on how to use this tool in treatment and discuss how to create a similar resource in other languages. The table is provided in Appendix 6.1.

Organization of the FITI table

This table allows the clinician to identify treatment targets that are most likely to affect intelligibility and to help create a prioritized list for intervention. It is not meant as a treatment activity: The words in the table are provided for assessing phonemes in specific positional contexts. Once a treatment target is identified, for example the word-initial pre-vocalic /r/ ('really'), the clinician should find additional tokens to work on this target (any words that start with /r/ followed by a vowel, which in English means any words that start with /r/ because, as can be seen in the table, /r/ is not allowed in English in word-initial pre-consonantal position). The table is organized as follows:

Rows. The rows of the table are all the phonemes of the language (in this case English) in order of frequency of their use in common content words, ordered from most frequent to least. The phoneme /r/ is the most frequent phoneme in English content words. The phoneme /ʒ/ is the least frequent phoneme in English content words. The phoneme /ð/ is extremely frequent in English function words, but scarce (second to last in frequency) in content words. A speaker who has difficulty with this sound may seem to have a severe articulation deficit, but its effect on the speaker's intelligibility will in fact be minor given that most function words are predictable from grammar, so a clear acoustic signal is not essential for communication to be understood.

Columns. The columns are ranked in three tiers. Tier 1 includes the most prominent positional contexts: pre-vocalic. This is where the distinctions between phonemes are most perceptible from the acoustic signal. It is also where consonants are less likely to be weakened. Pre-vocalic positions are most consequential for production and perception performance. Within this tier, word-initial (#_V) is most prominent, followed by post-vocalic, which is in turn followed by post-consonantal. Tier 2 includes the word-initial pre-consonantal context (#_C). And Tier 3 has the least prominent contexts including the pre-consonantal context and the word-final context: for both, post-vocalic contexts (V_C, V_#) take precedence over post-consonantal ones (C_C, C_#).

Gray Cells. Empty gray cells are disallowed contexts in English. Starred gray cells are allowed, but rare (in fact, rare enough that no representative words among frequent content words could be found). As such, phonemes in these locations have very low FITI, and should only be targeted for intervention if the client requests them or if no higher FITI targets are identified.

The full list of positional contexts in our work also includes stress and syllable boundaries. However, these contexts were not incorporated within the current resource in order to prioritize efficiency and convenience for clinical use.

How to use the table (the hierarchies)

The ranking is related to the relative FITI (functional importance for intelligibility): The higher the row, the higher the FITI, and tiers 1, 2, and 3 are provided in order of importance (left-to-right). Within tiers, the columns are also organized in order of importance, but here the clinicians are encouraged to use their own judgment to prioritize intervention targets based on individual needs. There may be individual differences; a person may have frequent need of a phoneme or context that does not match the rest of the language, for example, for an uncommon name or if their vocation involves specialized jargon including a lot of foreign borrowings. It is also possible that the inter-consonantal (C_C) context is selected over other columns in tier 3 because it is more difficult to produce and as such may be especially useful to work on practicing intelligibility strategies such as hyper-articulating or slowing down the rate of speech. In general, the information ranked in rows is considered more consequential to intelligibility than the information ranked in columns (the tiers) because it is inherently tied to frequency of occurrence in the language. As such, a Tier 3 context for /t/ (row 2) may be expected to have higher FITI than a Tier 1 /g/ (row 14).

Example of Using Hierarchy to Prioritize Initial Treatment Goals. Imagine a client who has difficulty with /dʒ/, /θ/, and /ʃ/, and can only handle short sessions due to fatigue or impaired focus. According to their ranking in the FITI Table, the order of treatment should be /ʃ/ first, then /dʒ/, followed by /θ/. A client who has difficulties with /n/ in prevocalic position, as well as in word-final position, should work on prevocalic first (Tier 1).

Creating the FITI table in other languages

In order to create a similar table in a different language or dialect, a list of phonemes ranked by order of frequency in common content words is needed. It is imperative that only content words (and not function words) are used. The tiers and columns within tiers are based on universal properties and therefore should apply across languages. The gray cells will be different for each language and as such, disallowed contexts in the target language will need to be identified. For example, the velar nasal does not appear in word- or syllable-initial positions in English, but it can in other languages, and similarly, the /h/ does not occur in word-final or pre-consonantal positions in English but can in other languages. Word tokens with the target phonemes in the specific contexts should be added to the table. The starred gray cells (i.e., allowable but infrequent contexts) may be different in other languages. Similar to our method, these can be determined by the absence of an example word token in the common content word corpus in the target language.

Future directions

The conceptual hierarchy of FITI is well motivated by theory and is supported in clinical data. The next step is to investigate the intelligibility outcomes of intervention that selects treatment targets using the FITI Table.

Summary

In this chapter, we presented a novel approach to assessing and treating intelligibility disorders in adults: one that recognizes the fact that there is a hierarchy of functional importance to intelligibility (FITI) of consonants in a language. This hierarchy depends on four phonological properties of sounds (contrast, context, frequency, and functional load) that are explained in the chapter along with their importance to intelligibility. We also offer a novel clinical resource to help prioritize treatment targets that will have the most important consequence for a client's speech.

Acknowledgments

This work was supported by grants funded by Purdue Research Foundation and Purdue University Fort Wayne Research and Innovation.

References

Antolík, T. K., & Fougeron, C. (2013, August). Consonant distortions in dysarthria due to Parkinson's disease, amyotrophic lateral sclerosis and cerebellar ataxia. *Interspeech*. www. halshs.archives-ouvertes.fr/halshs-01401418

Beckman, M. E., & Edwards, J. (1994). Articulatory evidence for differentiating stress categories. In P. A. Keating (Ed.), *Papers in laboratory phonology III: Phonological structure and phonetic form* (pp. 7–33). Cambridge University Press.

Bell, A., Jurafsky, D., Fosler-Lussier, E., Girand, C., Gregory, M., & Gildea, D. (2003). Effects of disfluencies, predictability, and utterance position on word form variation in English conversation. *The Journal of the Acoustical Society of America, 113*(2), 1001–1024. https://doi.org/10.1121/1.1534836

Bent, T., Bradlow, A. R., & Smith, B. L. (2007). Phonemic errors in different word positions and their effects on intelligibility of non-native speech. In O. S. Bohn & M. J. Munro (Eds.), *Language experience in second language speech learning: In honor of James Emil Flege* (pp. 331–347). John Benjamins Publishing Company. https://doi.org/10.1075/lllt.17.28ben

Bent, T., Smith, B. L., Lodewyck, D., & Bradlow, A. R. (2001). Non-native speech production (II): Phonemic errors by position-in-word and intelligibility. *The Journal of the Acoustical Society of America, 110*(5), 2684. https://doi.org/10.1121/1.4777206

Bleile, K. M. (2015). *The manual of speech sound disorders: A book for students & clinicians* (3rd ed.). Cengage Learning.

Boomershine, A., Currie Hall, K., Hume, E., & Johnson, K. (2008). The impact of allophony versus contrast on speech perception. In P. Avery, B. E. Dresher, & K. Rice (Eds.), *Contrast in phonology: Theory, perception, acquisition* (pp. 145–171). Mouton de Gruyter.

Bybee, J. L. (1994). A view of phonology from a cognitive and functional perspective. *Cognitive Linguistics, 5*(4), 285–305.

Cheng, B., & Zhang, Y. (2015). Syllable structure universals and native language interference in second language perception and production: Positional asymmetry and perceptual links to accentedness [Original Research]. *Frontiers in Psychology, 6*(1801). https://doi.org/10.3389/fpsyg.2015.01801

Cho, J., & Park, H. K. P. (2006). A comparative analysis of Korean-English phonological structures and processes for pronunciation pedagogy in interpretation training. *Meta: Translators' Journal, 51*, 229–246. https://doi.org/10.7202/013253ar

Cho, T. (2001). *Effects of prosody on articulation in English.* University of California.

Cilibrasi, L., Stojanovik, V., & Riddell, P. (2015). Word position and stress effects in consonant cluster perception and production. *Dyslexia, 21*(1), 50–59. https://doi.org/10.1002/dys.1488

Davies, M., & Gardner, D. (2010). *A frequency dictionary of contemporary American English: Word sketches, collocates, and thematic lists.* Routledge.

de Jong, K. J. (1995). The supraglottal articulation of prominence in English: Linguistic stress as localized hyperarticulation. *The Journal of the Acoustical Society of America, 97*(1), 491–504. https://doi.org/10.1121/1.412275

Dyson, A. T. (1986). Development of velar consonants among normal two-year-olds. *Journal of Speech, Language, and Hearing Research, 29*(4), 493–498. https://doi.org/10.1044/jshr.2904.493

Fogerty, D., Kewley-Port, D., & Humes, L. E. (2012). The relative importance of consonant and vowel segments to the recognition of words and sentences: Effects of age and hearing loss. *The Journal of the Acoustical Society of America, 132*(3), 1667–1678. https://doi.org/10.1121/1.4739463

Frantz, D. G. (1971). *Toward a generative grammar of blackfoot (with particular attention to selected stem formation processes).* Summer Institute of Linguistics of the University of Oklahoma.

Gregory, M. L. (2001). *Linguistic informativeness and speech production: An investigation of contextual and discourse-pragmatic effects on phonological variation.* University of Colorado.

Guitart, J. M. (1976). *Markedness and a Cuban dialect of Spanish.* Georgetown University Press.

Gurevich, N. (2004). *Lenition and contrast: Functional consequences of certain phonetically conditioned sound changes.* Routledge.

Gurevich, N. (2011). Lenition. In M. Oostendorp, C. J. Ewen, E. Hume, & K. Rice (Eds.), *The Blackwell companion to phonology* (Vol. 3). Wiley-Blackwell.

Harnsberger, J. D. (2001). The perception of Malayalam nasal consonants by Marathi, Punjabi, Tamil, Oriya, Bengali, and American English listeners: A multidimensional scaling analysis. *Journal of Phonetics, 29*(3), 303–327. https://doi.org/10.1006/jpho.2001.0140

Harris, J. (2011). Deletion. In M. Oostendorp, C. J. Ewen, E. Hume, & K. Rice (Eds.), *The Blackwell companion to phonology* (Vol. 3). Wiley-Blackwell. https://doi.org/10.1002/9781444335262.wbctp0068

Hochmann, J. R., Benavides-Varela, S., Nespor, M., & Mehler, J. (2011). Consonants and vowels: Different roles in early language acquisition. *Developmental Science, 14*(6), 1445–1458. https://doi.org/10.1111/j.1467-7687.2011.01089.x

Hockett, C. F. (1967). The quantification of functional load. *Word, 23*(1–3), 300–320. https://doi.org/10.1080/00437956.1967.11435484

Jun, J. (2011). Positional effects in consonant clusters. In M. Oostendorp, C. J. Ewen, E. Hume, & K. Rice (Eds.), *The Blackwell companion to phonology* (Vol. 2). Wiley-Blackwell. https://doi.org/10.1002/9781444335262.wbctp0046

Jurafsky, D., Bell, A., Gregory, M. L., & Raymond, W. D. (2001). Probabilistic relations between words: Evidence from reduction in lexical production. In J. Bybee & P. Hopper (Eds.), *Frequency and the emergence of linguistic structure* (pp. 229–254). John Benjamins.

Jusczyk, P. W. (1999). How infants begin to extract words from speech. *Trends in Cognitive Sciences, 3*(9), 323–328. https://doi.org/10.1016/S1364-6613(99)01363-7

Kent, R. D. (1982). Contextual facilitation of correct sound production. *Language, Speech, and Hearing Services in Schools, 13*(2), 66–76. https://doi.org/10.1044/0161-1461.1302.66

Kessler, B., & Treiman, R. (1997). Syllable structure and the distribution of phonemes in English syllables. *Journal of Memory and Language, 37*(3), 295–311. https://doi.org/10.1006/jmla.1997.2522

Kim, H., & Gurevich, N. (2021). Positional asymmetries in consonant production and intelligibility in dysarthric speech. *Clinical Linguistics & Phonetics*, 1–18. https://doi.org/10.1080/02699206.2021.2019312

Kim, M. R., & Duanmu, S. (2004). "Tense" and "lax" stops in Korean. *Journal of East Asian Linguistics, 13*(1), 59–104. https://doi.org/10.1023/B:JEAL.0000007344.43938.4e

Kingston, J. (2008). Lenition. In L. Colantoni & J. Steele (Eds.), *Proceedings of the third conference on laboratory approaches to Spanish phonology* (pp. 1–31). Cascadilla Press.

Kuhl, P. K., Williams, K. A., Lacerda, F., Stevens, K. N., & Lindblom, B. (1992). Linguistic experience alters phonetic perception in infants by 6 months of age. *Science, 255*(5044), 606–608. www.jstor.org/stable/2876832

Lee, H. B. (1999). Korean. In The International Phonetic Association (Ed.), *Handbook of the international phonetic association* (pp. 120–123). Cambridge University Press.

Levi, S. V., Winters, S. J., & Pisoni, D. B. (2007). Speaker-independent factors affecting the perception of foreign accent in a second language. *Journal of the Acoustical Society of America, 121*(4), 2327–2338. https://doi.org/10.1121/1.2537345

Lieberman, P. (1963). Some effects of semantic and grammatical context on the production and perception of speech [Article]. *Language and Speech, 6*(3), 172–187. https://doi.org/10.1177/002383096300600306

Marshall, C. R., & van der Lely, H. K. J. (2009). Effects of word position and stress on onset cluster production: Evidence from typical development, specific language impairment, and dyslexia. *Language, 85*(1), 39–57. www.jstor.org/stable/40492845

McGowan, R. S., Nittrouer, S., & Manning, C. J. (2004). Development of [r] in young, midwestern, American children. *The Journal of the Acoustical Society of America, 115*(2), 871–884. https://doi.org/10.1121/1.1642624

Moates, D. R., Watkins, N. E., Bond, Z. S., & Stockmal, V. (2006). Frequency effects in phoneme processing. *The Journal of the Acoustical Society of America, 120*(5), 3252. https://doi.org/10.1121/1.4788313

Noguchi, M., & Kam, C. L. H. (2018). The emergence of the allophonic perception of unfamiliar speech sounds: The effects of contextual distribution and phonetic naturalness. *Language Learning, 68*(1), 147–176. https://doi.org/10.1111/lang.12267

Owens, E. (1961). Intelligibility of words varying in familiarity. *Journal of Speech and Hearing Research, 4*(2), 113–129. https://doi.org/10.1044/jshr.0402.113

Rockman, B. K., & Elbert, M. (1984). Untrained acquisition of /S/ in a phonologically disordered child. *Journal of Speech and Hearing Disorders, 49*(3), 246–253. https://doi.org/10.1044/jshd.4903.246

Scharenborg, O. E., Coumans, J. M. J., Kakouros, S., & Hout, R. W. N. M. V. (2016). Does the importance of word-initial and word-final information differ in native versus non-native spoken-word recognition? *Proceedings of Interspeech 2016*, 858–862.

Silverman, D. (1995). *Phasing and recoverability* University of California Press.

Steriade, D. (1999). Alternatives to the syllabic Interpretation of consonantal phonotactics. In O. Fujimura, B. Joseph, & B. Palek (Eds.), *Proceedings of the 1998 linguistics and phonetics conference* (pp. 205–242). The Karolinum Press.

Stokes, S. F., & Surendran, D. (2005). Articulatory complexity, ambient frequency, and functional load as predictors of consonant development in children. *Journal of Speech, Language and Hearing Research, 48*(3), 577–591. https://doi.org/10.1044/1092-4388(2005/040)

To, C. K. S., Cheung, P. S. P., & McLeod, S. (2013). A population study of children's acquisition of Hong Kong Cantonese consonants, vowels, and tones. *Journal of Speech, Language and Hearing Research (Online), 56*(1), 103–122. https://doi.org/10.1044/1092-4388(2012/11-0080)

Toro, J. M., Nespor, M., Mehler, J., & Bonatti, L. L. (2008). Finding words and rules in a speech stream: Functional differences between vowels and consonants. *Psychological Science, 19*(2), 137–144. https://doi.org/10.1111/j.1467-9280.2008.02059.x

Trubetzkoy, N. S. (1939). *Principles of phonology* (C. A. M. Baltaxe, Trans.). University of California Press.

Word frequency data. (2019, May). www.wordfrequency.info

Appendix 6.1
The FITI Table

Prioritize articulatory targets

Rows: ranked by frequency of phonemes in corpus of most frequent content words

Columns: ranked by tiers related to relative functional importance for intelligibility (FITI); within tiers—use your clinical judgment to prioritize based on individual strengths/needs. For example, C_C is more difficult but useful to work on to practice intelligibility strategies such as hyperarticulation and slow rate.

Other notes:

Gray cells—not allowed in English; starred gray cells allowed but very rare
Within tiers—post-vocalic is more salient for listener; post consonantal is least salient

Appendix 6.1

	Tier 1			Tier 2	Tier 3			
	#_V	V_V	C_V	#_C	V_C	V_#	C_C	C_#
/r/	really	around	problem		service	appear		
/t/	teacher	return	student	treatment	treatment	about	control	result
/n/	never	enough	technology	*	only	begin	concerned	return
/s/	system	decide	consider	student	suggest	produce (v)	understand	perhaps
/l/	little	believe	include		also	control	girlfriend	girl
/k/	country	become	discuss	question	actually	attack	include	think
/p/	people	appear	important	problem	perhaps	escape	explain	help
/d/	different	today	condition	driver	address	provide	hardly	understand
/m/	mister	remain	information	music	company	become	firmly	perform
/f/	family	effect	performance	future	reflect	enough	confront	golf
/b/	business	about	baseball	brother	subject (n)	describe	embrace	absorb
/ʃ/	shoulder	machine	insurance	shrimp	freshman	push	*	harsh
/v/	very	development	involve	viewer	movement	receive	involved	involve
/g/	government	begin	forget	global	agree	fatigue	congressional	*
/w/	woman	away	question					
/z/	zodiac	result	exactly	*	business	disease	transmit	sometimes
/dʒ/	general	majority	enjoy	*	judgment	engage	largely	change
/ŋ/		singer			single	along		
/j/	usually	crayola	community					
/tʃ/	challenge	achieve	exchange		approached	approach	researched	lunch
/h/	happen	behavior	perhaps	*				
/θ/	theory	authority	enthusiasm	threaten	athletic	both	birthday	month
/ð/	therefore	within	northern	*	breathes	breathe	*	*
/ʒ/		decision	version	*		garage	*	*

7 Morphosyntax

Verb and sentence impairments in aphasia: theory, assessment, and treatment

Roelien Bastiaanse

Abstract

For a long time, treatment of word retrieval impairments has focused on nouns as single words. However, we speak in sentences and sentences are built around the verb. The verb describes the event and defines the structure of the sentence, so word retrieval and sentence construction are integrated to make a sentence. This makes verbs particularly vulnerable: the use of verbs is affected in aphasic individuals with word retrieval deficits as well as in those with grammatical deficits.

This role of the verb in the sentence also shows that it is important to find the underlying deficit when an aphasic speaker demonstrates problems with sentence production: is it word retrieval, the inability to use the verb to build a sentence frame, or problems with inflecting the verb for tense and agreement? This implies the need for sensitive assessment tools as well as treatment programs that address the locus of impairment. This chapter will discuss the representation of verbs and how they are used to construct a sentence and will then show how the stages of verb and sentence production can be addressed for successful remediation.

Statement to the reader

As a clinician, you are aware of the different aphasia types and disorders at the phoneme, word, and sentence levels. Much research, as well as assessment and treatment of aphasias, focuses on the retrieval of nouns and sentence production. Verbs as a word class are often ignored. In this chapter, the pivotal role of the verb in sentence production is emphasized and the implications for assessment and treatment of verb and sentence production are extensively described. Fortunately, several specific tests and treatment programs are available nowadays, to train verbs and sentence production.

DOI: 10.4324/9781003045519-9

Introduction

Aphasia may manifest itself at different levels and in different modalities of language processing, dependent on the size and the site of the brain lesion. This chapter addresses impairments at the grammatical level and how they can be diagnosed, and provides a description of treatment methods to address these impairments. For that, a theoretical background is required, sketched by a model that describes the processes needed for sentence production. This model will serve as a framework to discuss assessment tools and treatment methods (including their efficacy). However, let us start with a short introduction to explain some grammatical terminology.

Grammatical background

Verbs are the core of a sentence; sentences without a verb are, at least in English, ungrammatical (unless in an ellipse). Verbs are a very complex word class, much more complex than, for example, nouns. Verbs have *argument structure*, that is, their meaning includes the number of other entities that are needed for the action expressed by that verb. For example, a verb like "swimming" implies that someone, a human being or an animal, is performing this action. We call this a "one argument" or "intransitive" verb. Other verbs need more word groups, for example "reading." There must be a person doing the action, but there should also be an entity that is read. We call this a "two argument" or transitive verb. There are also "three argument" verbs, like "giving," "sending," and "donating" (*Zack gives flowers to Sophie*), also known as "ditransitive verbs." Notice that these arguments are not always obligatory realized: one can say "I have been reading all night," without mentioning what has been read. This is perfectly grammatical, but still something has been read, even though it is not explicitly mentioned.

These arguments fulfill so-called thematic roles, which are also defined by the verb. "Swimming," "reading," "giving," and so on all require someone who is performing the action. This is the "agent." The person, animal, or thing undergoing the action is called the "theme." Again, argument structure and thematic roles are inherent to the meaning of the verb. This makes verbs not only a complex but also a very interesting word class.

When humans use language, they speak in sentences, that is, a string of words—nouns, verb, pronouns, adjectives—tied together in a language-specific way. For example, in a simple English sentence like "the cat is chasing the dogs," the grammatical subject is the animal that is doing the chasing. We call this the "agent." The dogs are the grammatical object, the ones being chased and we call that the "theme." Such a sentence can be linguistically described as in (1).

(1) cat$_{subj,agent,sg}$ chase$_{pres.progr.,3rd\ sg}$ dog$_{obj,theme,pl}$
(subj=subject; sg=singular; pres.prog.=present progressive; obj=object; pl.=plural)

A more or less similar meaning can be expressed by the sentence "the dogs are chased by the cat." The dogs are now the grammatical subject of the sentence and the cat is in the *by*-phrase. Notice that the dogs are still the theme and the cat is still the agent. Here, some grammatical operations have taken place, to form a similar sentence in a different form. English uses a specific verb form (*is* V-*ed*) combined with the preposition "by" to form this sentence structure; other languages, like Finnish, use case and still others, like German use both. The point is that similar meanings can be expressed by different grammatical structures that are language dependent.

A model of verb and sentence production

The knowledge of words and grammar allows human beings to speak in meaning full sentences. But how do they do this? How do they make sentences? This can be sketched by a model for sentence production, given in Figure 7.1. This model is based on earlier ones from Ellis and Young (1996) and Levelt (1989).

When a *concept* is triggered, it activates a *lemma*. A lemma is a unit that contains not only information about the meaning of a word, but also information about word class and, in the case of verbs, information about argument structure; thematic roles, and subcategorization (what sentence structure is needed

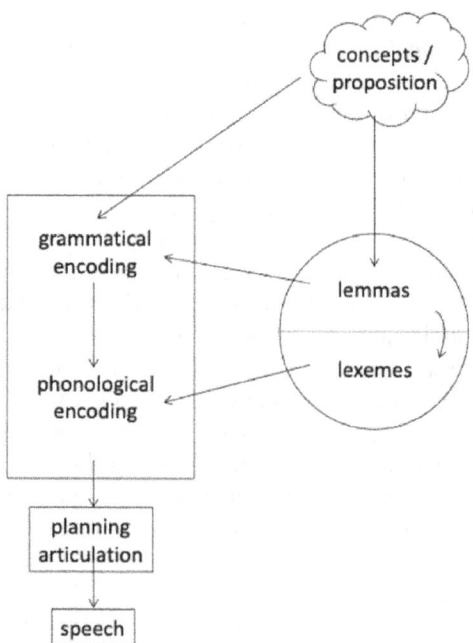

Figure 7.1 A model for sentence production (Bastiaanse et al., 2016b; based on Levelt, 1989).

for the thematic roles?). For example, for an intransitive verb, a verb with only one argument like "to smile," the lemma contains the information that it is a verb with one argument, an agent, that is subcategorized for a simple subject—verb sentence. Transitive verbs, verbs with two arguments like "to read" have two arguments, an agent (the person who is writing) and a theme (that which is being written), as in *the girl is reading a letter*. Verbs that have three arguments are called "ditransitives," such as *giving* and *sending*. There is one verb with four arguments, *exchanging*: *the woman exchanges her boat with her neighbor for his car*.

During *grammatical encoding*, input comes from two sources, and this information is used to form a sentence frame: the event to be expressed (which can be not only an action, but can also be a complete proposition) and the lemma. The grammatical encoder uses the verb-argument structure that is represented in the lemma to generate a sentence frame that suits the intention of the speaker (the concept/proposition). Notice that grammatical encoding is always needed, even when a single word is produced. A single word is seen as a minimal sentence. Let us use an example of a transitive verb, "to write." This verb requires two arguments: an agent and a theme. When the preverbal message is that a specific girl is writing letters, then the lemma "to write" is retrieved by the grammatical encoder, together with the lemmas of "girl" and "letter," and it will encode the following structure (2):

(2) $girl_{subj,agent,sg}$ $write_{pres.progr.,3rd sg}$ $letter_{obj,theme,pl}$

In this case, the subject is the agent and is singular, the verb is the third person singular of the progressive and the direct object is the theme and plural.

However, a similar message, but with a slightly different emphasis, may be expressed by a passive structure (2):

(3) $letter_{subj,theme,pl}$ $write_{pass.pres.pl}$ $girl_{by\ -phrase,agent,sg}$

In this case, the subject is the theme and is plural, the verb should be inflected with the passive form in the third person plural and the agent is singular and is expressed with a *by*-phrase.

Once the lemma has been retrieved, it activates the *lexeme*, that is, the underlying spoken word form. The lexeme is inserted in the sentence frame that has been constructed by the grammatical encoder. This is the process of *phonological encoding*. In case of example (2), this will result in (4):

(4) The girl is writing the letters

whereas the phonological encoding of (3) will result in (5):

(5) The letters are written by the girl

These examples show that, at least in English, the order of the arguments may vary on the basis of the perspective of the sentence. They also show that both lemmas and grammatical encoding can be not only fairly simple, as with an intransitive verb and an active sentence, but also quite complex, as is the case with ditransitive verbs and passive sentences. We know that in aphasia this variation in complexity may be reflected in the performance of the aphasic speaker, not only in those with a grammatical impairment, but also when word retrieval is compromised.

Impairments in verb retrieval and sentence construction

In the case of an impairment in word retrieval in general, a speaker will also encounter problems with sentence production. This holds for nouns as well as verbs, but the effect on sentence production may vary. For some aphasic speakers, construction of a sentence requires extra effort resulting in diminished word retrieval, that is, retrieving the lexeme from the lexicon. For others, a sentence frame may help to find the intended lexemes. This illustrates the interaction between lexeme retrieval and grammatical encoding. In the case of a pure grammatical impairment (as is often the case in agrammatic speakers), this is already visible in the retrieval of verbs, like in the answer to the question "what will you do tomorrow?" "biking." As mentioned earlier, the verb "biking" needs to be grammatically encoded, even though it is only a single word and grammatical encoding is the problem for agrammatic speakers. The more information is included in the lemma of a verb, the harder it is for agrammatic speakers to produce this verb (Kim & Thompson, 2004; Thompson et al., 1997).

An impairment in grammatical encoding can manifest itself in different ways. It may be the case that the aphasic speaker cannot construct complex sentences and will, hence, speak in short, simple sentences with verbs not inflected for tense and agreement. Sometimes, sentence production is restricted to one- and two-word utterances, and sometimes longer sentences will be used, but these may be incorrect. This is known as "agrammatic speech" and is characteristic of agrammatic aphasia. Other aphasic speakers may produce longer and more complex sentences, but will make errors, for example, in word order and/or use incorrect inflections. This not only occurs in Broca's aphasia, but is also common in Wernicke's aphasia (paragrammatic speech).

Considering the wide spectrum of impairments in aphasia, be it a grammatical impairment, poor word finding, problems with phonological encoding or a combination of the two, sentence production in aphasia is always compromised. In order to treat these impairments at the sentence level, it is important to understand which process is affected. This can be assessed by several instruments, which will be discussed in the next section.

Diagnosis of sentence production impairments

In order to identify the level(s) of impairment, thorough diagnosis is needed. It is rather surprising that there is little material available for this purpose. The two most extensive test batteries are the Northwestern Assessment of Verbs and

Sentences (NAVS; Thompson, 2012) and the Verb And Sentence Test (VAST; Bastiaanse et al., 2002). Both batteries assess production and comprehension at the word (verb) and the sentence level. For the NAVS and the VAST, the emphasis is on the lexical characteristics of verbs (age of acquisition, instrumentality, transitivity, etc.), as well as on verb inflection and the position of the verb in the sentence (in languages where this is relevant, like Dutch and Norwegian). The NAVS focuses on verb–argument structure. Furthermore, both tests assess comprehension and production of sentences with specific attention to word order. First, the assessment of verb production will be presented, followed by the production of sentences.

Verb production

As shown earlier, the verb plays a pivotal role in the sentence; the characteristics of the verb determine the grammatical roles and, hence, the structure of the sentence. This is illustrated by an example. Depending on the perspective of the speaker, to express that flowers went from Zack to Sophie, two different verbs can be used:

(6) $\text{Zack}_{\text{subj,agent}}$ gave $\text{flowers}_{\text{obj,theme}}$ to $\text{Sophie}_{\text{indirect obj, recipient}}$
(7) $\text{Sophie}_{\text{subj,recipient}}$ got $\text{flowers}_{\text{obj,theme}}$ from $\text{Zack}_{\text{adverbial phrase,source}}$

It is clear that the choice of the verb is decisive for the grammatical and thematic structure of the sentence. This implies that grammatical encoding of the sentence structure is dependent on the verb lemma that the speaker selects. Thus, in order to test all aspects of sentence production, verb retrieval needs to be assessed. Although verb retrieval in isolation may not be the best way to do that—verbs are rarely used in isolation—this stage is included in the NAVS and VAST, but only as an intermediary step.

The VAST includes tasks for producing infinitives and finite verbs in a sentence context. This implies that the arguments are provided and the aphasic speaker has to fill in the verb. An example is given in Figure 7.2.

With a set of tasks like these, clinicians can analyze what the cause of the verb problems of an aphasic speaker is: is it accessing the lemmas or lexemes of the verbs in the lexicon (performance on all three tasks will be impaired)?, is it integrating the verb in a sentence (retrieving verbs in isolation will be relatively spared, but producing verbs in a sentence context will impaired)? or is it retrieving a verb and inflecting it for tense and agreement (both producing verbs in isolation and in infinitival form in a sentence context will be relatively good, but retrieving a finite verb in a sentence context will be poor)? Experience tells us that all kinds of patterns of impairment are possible, but that for most aphasic speakers, regardless of aphasia type, retrieving a verb and inflecting it, that is, integrating verb retrieval and grammatical encoding, is most difficult. This is exactly what we need to do when we speak in daily life: all sentences contain a finite verb.

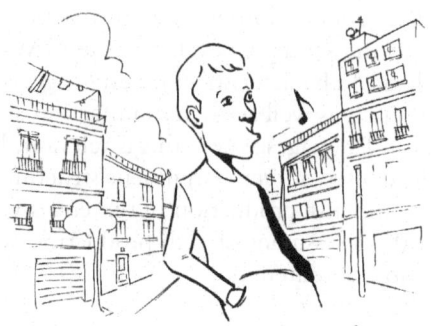

The boy likes to ... in the street

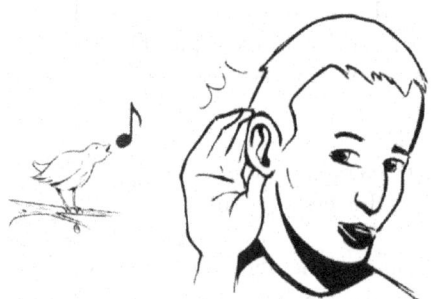

Every morning the boy ... to the bird

Figure 7.2 Example of the tasks *filling in infinitives* (top) and *filling in finite verbs* (bottom) of the VAST (App version; Bastiaanse et al., 2016a). Art work by Victor Xandri Antolin. © Roelien Bastiaanse, University of Groningen.

The items of the VAST are all action verbs and have been matched and controlled for on several linguistic factors: transitivity, name relation to a noun, instrumentality, word frequency, age of acquisition, and imageability, because it is known that these factors may influence word retrieval (be it verbs or nouns). However, in a study on a large group of aphasic speakers, not selected for aphasia type, only age of acquisition was shown to play an important role; later acquired verbs are harder to retrieve for aphasic speakers (Bastiaanse et al., 2016b).

The NAVS is designed to evaluate the influence of argument structure, because it contains not only transitive and intransitive action verbs, but also ditransitive verbs. Earlier studies showed that these factors influenced verb retrieval in agrammatic aphasia (e.g., Kim & Thompson, 2004; Thompson et al., 1997) and fluent aphasic (Whitworth, 1995) speakers. In the NAVS, verb retrieval is only tested in isolation, but recently the Northwestern Assessment of Verb Inflection (NAVI; see Lee et al., 2015) was published that allows for systematic testing of verb inflection. Apart from all these tasks for verbs, both the NAVS and the VAST allow for testing at the sentence level as well, as will be discussed in the next section.

Production of sentences

As previously mentioned, we speak in sentences and in order to do so, grammatical encoding is needed. During this process, the constituents are ordered around the verb, following the grammatical rules of a language. For languages like Dutch and English (and many other Germanic and Romance languages), the information provided by the order of the constituents is decisive for assigning thematic and grammatical rules. In a sentence like (8), the first constituent (*Sophie*) is supposed to be the subject and the agent of the sentence, and the final constituent (*book*) is the direct object and the theme. The reverse order of the grammatical and thematic roles would render the sentence ungrammatical, as shown in (9).

(8) Sophie$_{subj,agent}$ is reading a book$_{obj,theme}$
(9) *A book$_{obj,theme}$ is reading Sophie$_{subj,agent}$

However, in many languages (e.g., German, all Slavic languages), there is much more variation in word order, because the grammatical roles are expressed by case rather than by sentence position. This is important because the way in which grammatical encoding should be tested and treated is, thus, dependent on the linguistic characteristics of a particular language. In this chapter, word order is discussed as the critical factor. Unfortunately, little has been written about assessing grammatical encoding in languages with relatively free word order.

Classically, word order has been assessed mainly for comprehension and for semantically reversible sentences. Although this taught us the fundamentals of grammatical impairments (even though the theories about why semantically reversible sentences are difficult to comprehend are almost as numerous as the studies done; Drai & Grodzinsky, 2006; Grodzinsky, 2000, and responses on those papers), semantically reversible sentences are hardly used in daily life. Still, they should be tested in order to understand the underlying sentence production disorder. Therefore, word order is the key variable for the sentence production tasks both in the VAST and in the NAVS.

It would be easy if we could just ask the aphasic speaker to produce a sentence corresponding to a presented picture. However, in this way, we run into the key characteristic of language: the number of options to describe a picture of, for example, a man digging a hole, is endless, so it is hard to elicit exactly the sentence the test developer had in mind. For that reason, the NAVS uses

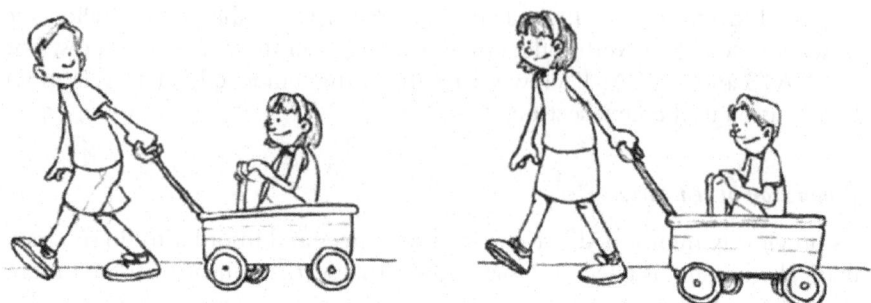

Figure 7.3 Example of an item for sentence production of the NAVS. Here [pointing to the picture on the left] you can ask: "who is pulling the girl?" and here [pointing to the picture on the right] you can ask: Who is the girl pulling? [picture used with permission].

a "sentence prompting" paradigm. Two pictures are presented to the aphasic speaker, and the experimenter produces a sentence with the first picture. For the second picture, in which the thematic roles have been reversed, the aphasic speaker needs to use the same sentence structure. See Figure 7.3 for an example. In this way, a number of sentence structures are tested.

The sentence production task of the VAST gives the aphasic speaker more freedom; a picture is shown and s/he is invited to produce one sentence that covers what is in the picture. This task includes structures with intransitive and transitive verbs, the latter including semantically reversible and irreversible sentences. Of course, the problem here is how to score the responses. Is the use of pronouns instead of nouns correct? What if past tense is used? Non-brain-damaged speakers don't use these kinds of sentences on this test, but that does not mean that they are incorrect. The directions for the VAST sentence construction task are to count a sentence as correct when the response is a grammatically correct sentence that expresses what is in the picture. For both the NAVS and the VAST, a thorough error analysis is essential. This will reveal more about the underlying disorder than a simple correct/incorrect score. The score forms of both tests are designed in a way that the most common error types can be identified. The VAST includes three anagram tasks for sentence construction that elicit alternative sentence structures: one without pictures for irreversible active and passive sentences and two with pictures, one with pictures for semantically irreversible and reversible sentences and one for wh-questions (*who-, what, where-* and *when-*questions). In this way, awareness of word order in relation to meaning can be assessed. In 2012, the NAVS was extended with the Northwestern Anagram Test (NAT; Thompson et al., 2012) that also assesses the ability to construct sentences with different structures.

In Table 7.1 the NAVS and VAST are compared.

Table 7.1. A comparison of the VAST and NAVS.

	VAST	*NAVS*
Target group	All aphasia types	Agrammatic aphasia
Focus on **verb** production	Verb position verb inflection	Argument structure
Focus on **sentence** production	Word order in relation to verb position Verb inflection	Word order

It may be clear that testing sentence structures, and even more, interpreting the aphasic individuals' ability to produce a wide array of sentence structures is hard, and thorough knowledge of grammar is needed to interpret the results, which should be done in relation to the performance on the verb production tasks. Still, such a test is the most important part of assessing sentence production in aphasia; as previously mentioned, we speak in sentences and the final aim of aphasia treatment is to do this as well as possible.

How to interpret the results of the assessment?

The hardest part of the assessment is to interpret the test data, but this is, of course, the most important part. When the underlying disorder is understood, treatment can be fine-tuned and will be more effective. This will be illustrated by an example.

AK was a 46-year-old, right-handed male when he suffered a stroke in the left temporo-parietal region. He suffered from fluent aphasia. His spontaneous speech was characterized by word finding problems and included several semantic and phonological paraphasias, but usually he succeeded in expressing what he wished to say. Executive and motor skills were intact. Initial treatment focused on word finding problems. When no further improvement occurred, he was tested with the VAST and a spontaneous speech sample of 300 words was linguistically analyzed according to the method of Bastiaanse and Jonkers (1998). The spontaneous speech analysis revealed that the mean length of utterances was low, but the number of nouns and verbs was within normal limits. The diversity of the nouns was normal as well, but the diversity of verbs was extremely low. The latter implies that, in combination with the normal overall number of verbs, he used the same verbs over and over again, thus providing little information. This is illustrated in the excerpt in (10) which is his answer to a question about how his speech was just after his stroke. The lexical verbs are underlined (. . . indicates pauses).

(10) only sentences . . . only sentences . . . yes beginning that was nothing, basically . . .. yes, not even not even not even my name not even, no numbers nothing and then I <u>thought</u>, well, yes . . . then I <u>thought</u> . . . a day I <u>thought</u> then I <u>thought</u> two days well and not even newspapers then I

thought okay you can with your legs and arms that is okay but only those sentences and a newspaper, that doesn't work.

The results of the relevant variables are given in Table 7.2. Action naming and his ability to use infinitives in sentences were quite well preserved relative to the average of aphasic individuals. Filling in finite verbs was severely impaired and the task elicited semantic and phonological paraphasias, but the verb was always correctly inflected for tense and agreement. Sentence construction was severely affected and most of the errors concerned the verbs. He produced semantic paraphasias, incorrect verb argument structures, and inflectional errors and turned nouns into verbs (*the man goalied* for a goalie catching a ball).

The finding of the assessment was that, although AK's access to lexical verbs was relatively well-preserved both at the word level and in sentence context, integrating verb retrieval and inflecting the verb for tense and agreement was too hard for him. In spontaneous speech, this impairment was reflected by a very limited number of verbs (that, in fact, were all inflected correctly), resulting in classical "empty speech". The speech rate was normal, but little information was provided. This, quite rare, phenomenon was only detected by careful screening for verb retrieval and grammatical processing.

Treatment of verb and sentence deficits

As previously stated, verbs are the core of the sentence and, therefore, we do not think it is useful to train verb retrieval in isolation. Studies that have focused on training verbs at the word level do show some improvement on trained items, but hardly any generalization to untrained verbs, nor to spontaneous speech or language use in daily life; those studies that focused on verbs in a sentence context do show improvement (see three systematic reviews: De Aguiar et al., 2016; Hickin et al., 2020; Webster & Whitworth, 2012).

ACTION! (Bastiaanse et al., 2006; Links et al., 2010) is meant to train verb production in a sentence context, with emphasis on the integration of (uninflected and inflected) verbs and grammatical structure. Another treatment program focusing on the production of verbs in a sentence context is *Verb Network*

Table 7.2 Performance of AK on the relevant variables of the spontaneous speech analysis and the VAST.

Spontaneous speech	AK	Healthy speakers (range)
Diversity of nouns	0.61	0.54–0.88
Diversity of verbs	0.23	0.63–0.86
VAST		*Maximum*
Action naming	31	40
Filling in infinitives	8	10
Filling in finite verbs	5	10
Sentence construction	7	20

Strengthening Treatment (VNeST; e.g., Edmonds et al., 2014). Both ACTION! and VNeST are meant for treating fluent as well as non-fluent aphasic speakers. Two treatment methodologies that have word order in relation to verb argument structure as a central element are *Mapping Therapy* (Byng et al., 1994; Jones, 1986; Rochon, 2005, among others) and *Treatment of Underlying Forms* (TUF; Thompson & Shapiro, 2005). These two methods are meant for treatment of agrammatic aphasia. These four treatment methods have been selected because efficacy data on connected speech and/or communication in daily life are available.

ACTION!

ACTION! (Bastiaanse et al., 1997, 2016a) is a treatment program developed to train verb production step by step. It was originally developed for Dutch, a language where the position of the verb varies per structure. Nevertheless, it has successfully been used in other languages as well (De Aguiar et al., 2015). Action! consists of four steps:

(i) lexical retrieval: verb selection
(ii) using a verb (infinitive) in a sentence context
(iii) inflecting the verb for tense and agreement
(iv) constructing a sentence

The materials are the same for all four steps: action pictures (with a sentence underneath in steps 2 and 3). Apart from simple sentences with a subject and an object/adjunct, several other more complex sentence structures can be elicited (for an extended description, see Bastiaanse et al., 2006).

The idea behind the program is that aphasic speakers are not trained to produce sentences that are too complex for them. However, they are supported to make sentences that they can handle. This may be sentences with finite verbs, but in case this is too difficult, the focus can be on step 3: they are encouraged to use light verbs (like *do* or *is*) and modals (verbs like *can, may* etc.) and carrying structures to avoid verb inflection (or at least, in English, finite lexical verbs). For example, instead of training sentences like "the man reads a book," the structure "the man is reading a book" or "the man can read a book" is trained. The speaker with fluent aphasia, introduced earlier, was trained on step 3 (followed by step 4). We taught him that sentences without finite lexical verbs were much easier for him. After treatment, his verb production was much better, both on the tests and in spontaneous speech (see Table 7.3).

Links et al. (2010) performed a group study, including 11 agrammatic speakers. Both at the group level and at the individual level, several relevant variables of spontaneous speech (utterance length, verb diversity, percentage of finite verbs) and verbal communication in daily life improved significantly, which is exactly what aphasia therapy should do. In 2016, an App version of ACTIION! was released, with which aphasic speakers can do exercises independently, with

Table 7.3 Performance of AK before and after treatment with ACTION! (*significant improvement).

Spontaneous speech	Before treatment	After treatment	Healthy speakers (range)
Diversity nouns	0.61	0.63	0.54–0.88
Diversity verbs	0.23	0.57	0.63–0.86
VAST			Maximum
Action naming	31	31	40
Filling in infinitives	8	10	10
Filling in finite verbs	5	10*	10
Sentence construction	7	15*	20

the support of their therapist. An extra step was added to train verb inflection for different time frames (past, present, and future). So far, this version is only available in Dutch (Bastiaanse et al., 2016a).

Verb network strengthening treatment (VNeST)

VNeST has been developed by Edmonds (Edmonds et al., 2009; Edmonds, 2014). The idea is that emphasizing the meaning as well as the role of the verb and its arguments may facilitate verb retrieval. The therapist selects a number of verbs that the aphasic individual will work with; nouns that can be used in relation to these verbs are presented as well. For example, the therapist selects the verb *to measure* and presents it with agents that can measure (*chef, carpenter, surveyor*) and things that can be measured (*sugar, lumber, land*; example from Edmonds et al., 2009). In this way, "networks" are built for each of the verbs and the meaning of the verb is deepened. Notice that one of the gains of VNeSt is that nouns are trained at the same time as the arguments of the verb. Slowly, sentence becomes longer, although not necessarily more complex. The focus is on teaching the aphasic speaker to produce verbs with their arguments in relatively simple sentences. This is very different from, for example, TUF (see later), that focuses more on sentence structure than on verb retrieval.

In 2014 Edmonds and colleagues studied VNeST in four individuals to show that in connected speech, more complete sentences were produced after treatment, but lexical retrieval did not improve. Most importantly, the Communicative Effectiveness Index (CETI; Lomas et al., 1989) showed improvement.

Mapping therapy

Mapping Therapy was developed by Eirian Jones (1986), who described its methodology in a case study. Jones (1986) only trained sentence comprehension, but others have trained production as well (Byng, 1988; Nickels et al., 1991). The term "mapping" refers to the fact that thematic roles (e.g., agent, theme) should be mapped onto grammatical roles (subject, direct object) and that this process is impaired in agrammatic aphasia. Mapping therapy has been used for training both sentence comprehension and production. The central idea is to make the aphasic individual aware of the verb argument structure and then teach the patients how to relate ("map") thematic roles onto grammatical roles and vice versa. Rochon et al. (2005) applied it successfully to train sentence production of a number of agrammatic speakers. Some of them improved in connected speech (which was the Cinderella story). No information is available on generalization to narrative/spontaneous speech or verbal communication in daily life. Since word order is the crucial variable here, mapping therapy is less useful in languages other than English and its effects have mainly been described for English speakers with agrammatic aphasia.

Treatment of underlying of forms (TUF)

This training program is based on the idea that sentences have a base word order and that other word orders are derived by grammatical operations. For example, a *wh*-object-question is derived from an active sentence by putting the questioned object in sentence initial position, as shown in (11).

(11) the girl is reading ___$_i$ → what$_i$ is the girl reading?

Treatment starts with training the simple underlying form and then the therapist shows how other sentence structures, like *wh*-question as in (10), are derived from this structure. This way of treatment has been shown to be quite successful for sentence production. However, the most remarkable aspect of TUF is that very interesting generalization patterns appear. For example, when production of *who*-questions is trained, production of *what*-questions improves as well, but not of *when*-questions. The reason is that *when*-questions, like *where*-questions are derived in a different way; they do not question the direct object in the sentence, which is an argument of the verb, but an adjunct, that does not belong to the argument structure of the verb. Hence, in *when*- and *where*-questions, a different operation is involved. This operation is the same in *when*- and *where*-questions and generalization between these two adjunct questions does occur.

Another interesting generalization pattern observed in TUF is generalization among structures with the same underlying form, but different complexity. For example, a *wh*-object-question has the same underlying structure as an object cleft sentence, as shown in (12) and (13).

(12) who is reading the book ___?
(13) it is the girl [who is reading the book ___].

Thompson et al. (1998, 2010) showed that training production of complex structures generalizes to production of simpler structures if the derivation is similar. This finding is counter-intuitive in aphasia treatment; therapists have the tendency to start easy and then to slowly build up to more complex structures. TUF suggests that when treatment starts at a higher level, the lower level comes for free, but only if it concerns the same kind of derivation. If the structures are not similar, no generalization appears; training tense inflection results in better production of agreement inflection and vice versa, but it does not result in better production of complementizers (words introducing an embedded sentence, such as *because, while*) or the other way around (Thompson et al., 2006). This is explained by the fact that Tense and Agreement inflection both take place in the Inflectional position, and complementizers are in the complementizer position. Interestingly, in the ACTION! study on Dutch by Links et al. (2010), training production of finite verbs in the inflectional position did not generalize to better production of infinitives, that are in a different position, or the other way around, even though both are verbs. This is in line with the findings of Thompson et al. (2006).

The TUF methodology has been shown to be quite effective for English agrammatic speakers; improvement on tests like the NAVS as well as in connected speech (storytelling) has been reported (Thompson & Shapiro, 2005; Thompson et al., 2010). No information is available for improvement of daily communication.

In Table 7.4, the four treatment methods are compared.

Table 7.4 A comparison of four treatment methods.

	VNeST	ACTION!	Mapping therapy	TUF
Target group	All aphasia types	All aphasia types	Agrammatic aphasia	Agrammatic aphasia
Focus	Sentence structure around verbs	Verb and verb inflection in sentences	Word order in relation to thematic roles	Word order in relation to underlying structure

Conclusions

Studies on the treatment of verb and sentence production mainly focus on agrammatic aphasia. Although this taught us a lot about the effects of these kinds of treatment for this type of aphasia, the incidence of agrammatic aphasia is rather low. Studies on sentence production in fluent aphasia are rare, even though these aphasic speakers often produce ungrammatical sentences as well. In general, studies of verb and sentence remediation do result in improvement of trained and untrained materials, but there is only limited evidence that this improvement generalizes to spontaneous speech, let alone to communication in daily life. One of the reasons for this lack of evidence is that this kind of improvement is hardly ever measured. Studies on Mapping Therapy and TUF have used storytelling as a source for narrative speech analysis, which is a useful method for analysis at the discourse level, but not representative for language use in daily life. The studies of ACTION! (Links et al., 2010) and VNeST (Edmonds et al., 2014) used narrative speech. Both studies show generalization to narrative speech, although for VNeST, it is limited to the number of complete sentences. For both studies, improvement of communicative abilities was found after therapy.

All four treatment methods described here have now been transformed to electronic versions:

ACTION! so far, only available for Dutch (Bastiaanse et al., 2016a)
VNeST-C (Furnas & Edmonds, 2014)
Mapping Therapy (Beveridge & Crerar, 2002)
TUF → *Sentactics*® (Thompson et al., 2010)

References

Bastiaanse, R., De Aquiar, V., & Satoer, D. D. (2016a). *ACTIE! Een therapie App voor de training van werkwoordproductie.* App Store.

Bastiaanse, R., Edwards, S., & Rispens, J. (2002) *The verb and sentence test (VAST).* Thames Valley Test Company.

Bastiaanse, R., Hurkmans, J., & Links, P. (2006) The training of verb production in Broca's aphasia: A multiple-baseline across-behaviours study. *Aphasiology, 20,* 298–311. https://doi.org/10.1080/02687030500474922

Bastiaanse, R., & Jonkers, R. (1998). Verb retrieval in action naming and spontaneous speech in agrammatic and anomic aphasia. *Aphasiology, 12,* 951–969. https://doi.org/10.1080/02687039808249463

Bastiaanse, R., Jonkers, R., Quak, C., & Varela Put, M. (1997). *Werkwoordproduktie op Woord- en Zinsniveau: Een Linguïstische Oefenprogramma voor Afasiepatiënten.* Lisse, Swets Test Publishers.

Bastiaanse, R., Wieling, M., & Wolthuis, N. (2016b). The role of frequency in the retrieval of nouns and verbs. *Aphasiology, 30,* 1221–1239. https://doi.org/10.1080/02687038.2015.1100709

Beveridge, M. A., & Crerar, M. A. (2002). Remediation of asyntactic sentence comprehension using a multimedia microworld. *Brain and Language, 82,* 243–295. https://doi.org/10.1016/s0093-934x(02)00015-9

Byng, S. (1988). Sentence processing deficits: Theory and therapy. *Cognitive Neuropsychology, 5,* 629–676. https://doi.org/10.1080/02643298808253277

Byng, S., Nickels, L., & Black, M. (1994). Replicating therapy for mapping deficits in agrammatism: Remapping the deficit? *Aphasiology, 8,* 315–341. https://doi.org/10.1080/02687039408248663

De Aguiar, V., Bastiaanse, R., Capasso, R., Gandolfi, M., Smania, N., Rossi, G., & Miceli, G. (2015). Can tDCS enhance item-specific effects and generalization after linguistically motivated aphasia therapy for verbs? *Frontiers Behavioral Neuroscience.* https://doi.org/10.3389/fnbeh.2015.00190

De Aguiar, V., Bastiaanse, R., & Miceli, G. (2016). Improving production of treated and untreated verbs: A meta-analysis. *Frontiers in Human Neuroscience, 10,* 1–17. https://doi.org/10.3389/fnhum.2016.00468

Drai, D., & Grodzinsky, Y. (2006). A new empirical angle on the variability debate: Quantitative neurosyntactic analyses of a large data set from Broca's aphasia. *Brain and Language, 96,* 157–170. https://doi.org/10.1016/j.bandl.2004.10.016

Edmonds, L. A., Mammino, K., & Ojeda, J. (2014). Effect of verb network strengthening treatment (VNeST) in persons with aphasia: Extension and replication of previous findings. *American Journal of Speech-Language Pathology*, *23*, S312–S329. https://doi. org/10.1044/2014_AJSLP-13-0098

Edmonds, L. A., Nadeau, S. E., & Kiran, S. (2009). Effect of verb network strengthening treatment (VNeST) on lexical retrieval of content words in sentences in persons with aphasia. *Aphasiology*, *23*, 402–424. https://doi.org/10.1080/02687030802291339

Ellis, A. W., & Young, A. W. (1996). *Human cognitive neuropsychology*. Taylor and Francis. https://doi.org/10.4324/9780203727041

Furnas, D. W., & Edmonds, L. A. (2014). The effect of computerized verb network strengthening treatment on lexical retrieval in aphasia. *Aphasiology*, *28*, 401–420. https://doi.org /10.1080/02687038.2013.869304

Grodzinsky, Y. (2000). The neurology of syntax: Language use without Broca's area. *Behavioral and Brain Sciences*, *13*, 388–393. https://doi.org/10.1017/s0140525x00002399

Hickin, J., Cruice, M., & Dipper, L. (2020). A systematically conducted scoping review of the evidence and fidelity of treatments for verb deficits in aphasia: Verb-in-isolation treatments. *American Journal of Speech and Language Pathology*, *29*, 530–559. https://doi. org/10.1044/2019_AJSLP-CAC48-18-0234

Jones, E. V. (1986). Building the foundations for sentence production in a nonfluent aphasic. *British Journal of Disorders of Communication*, *21*, 63–82. https://doi. org/10.3109/13682828609018544

Kim, M., & Thompson, C. K. (2004). Verb deficits in Alzheimer's disease and agrammatism: Implications for lexical organization. *Brain and Language*, *88*, 1–20. https://doi. org/10.1016/s0093-934x(03)00147-0

Lee, J., Yoshida, M., & Thompson, C. K. (2015). Grammatical planning units during real-time sentence production in agrammatic aphasia and healthy speakers. *Journal of Speech, Language, and Hearing Sciences*, *58*, 1182–1194. https://doi.org/10.1044/2015_JSLHR-L-14-0250

Levelt, W. J. M. (1989). *Speaking: From intention to articulation*. MIT Press.

Links, P., Hurkmans, J., & Bastiaanse, R. (2010). Training verb and sentence production in agrammatic Broca's aphasia. *Aphasiology*, *24*, 1303–1325. https://doi. org/10.1080/02687030903437666

Lomas, J., Pickard, L., Bester, S., Elbard, H., Finlayson, A., & Zoghaib, C. (1989). The communicative effectiveness index: Development and psychometric evaluation of a functional communication measure for adult aphasia. *Journal of Speech and Hearing Disorders*, *54*, 113–124. https://doi.org/10.1044/jshd.5401.113

Nickels, L., Byng, S., & Black, M. (1991). Sentence processing deficits: A replication of therapy. *British Journal of Disorders of Communication*, *26*, 175–199. https://doi. org/10.3109/13682829109012002

Rochon, E., Laird, L., Bose, A., & Scofield, J. (2005). Mapping therapy for sentence production impairments in nonfluent aphasia. *Neuropsychological Rehabilitation*, *15*, 1–36. https://doi.org/10.1080/09602010343000327

Thompson, C. K. (2012). *Northwestern assessment of verbs and sentences (NAVS)*. Northwestern University. http://northwestern.flintbox.com/public/project/9299/

Thompson, C. K., Ballard, K. J., & Shapiro, L. P. (1998). The role of syntactic complexity in training wh-movement structures in agrammatic aphasia: Optimal order for promoting generalization. *Journal of the International Neuropsychological Society*, *4*, 661–674. https:// doi.org/10.1017/S1355617798466141

Thompson, C. K., Choy, J. J., Holland, A., & Cole, R. (2010). Sentactics®: Computer-automated treatment of underlying forms. *Aphasiology*, *24*, 1242–1266. https://doi. org/10.1080/02687030903474255

Thompson, C. K., Lange, K. L., Schneider, S. L., & Shapiro, L. P. (1997). Agrammatic and non-brain-damaged subjects' verb and verb argument structure production. *Aphasiology*, *11*, 473–490. https://doi.org/10.1080/02687039708248485

Thompson, C. K., Milman, L. H., Dickey, M. W., O'Connor, J. E., Bonakdarpour, B., Fix, S., Arcuri, D. F., & Choy, J. J. (2006). Functional category production in agrammatism: Treatment and generalization effects. *Brain and Language*, *99*, 79–81. https://doi.org/10.1016/j.bandl.2005.07.066

Thompson, C. K., & Shapiro, L. P. (2005). Treating agrammatic aphasia within a linguistic framework: Treatment of underlying forms. *Aphasiology*, *19*, 1021–1036. https://doi.org/10.1080/02687030544000227

Thompson, C. K., Weintraub, S., & Mesulam, M. M. (2012). *Northwestern anagram test (NAT)*. http://northwestern.flintbox.com/public/project/19927/

Webster, J., & Whitworth, A. (2012). Treating verbs in aphasia: Exploring the impact of therapy at the single word and sentence levels. *International Journal of Language and Communication Disorders*, *47*, 619–636. https://doi.org/10.1111/j.1460-6984.2012.00174.x

Whitworth, A. (1995). Characterising thematic role assignments in aphasic sentence production: Procedures for elicited and spontaneous output. *International Journal for Language and Communication Disorders*, *30*, 384–399. https://doi.org/10.3109/13682829509021450

8 Semantics

Contextual variability of word meaning: implications for the treatment of acquired language disorders

Christopher M. Grindrod

Abstract

Lexical semantics is concerned with the nature of word meaning, the semantic relations between words, as well as the ways in which word meanings vary with the context in which they occur. This chapter highlights these different aspects of semantics by focusing on lexical ambiguity. Major concepts such as homonymy and polysemy, the organization of multiple word meanings in our mental lexicon, and contextual variability of word meaning are first reviewed. The impact of acquired language disorders, such as aphasia and right hemisphere brain injury, on understanding words with contextually variable interpretations is examined next. Finally, current treatment approaches are reviewed along with recommendations for best practices in treating context-based semantic impairments. Given that most, if not all, meaning is context-dependent, contextual variability should be considered whenever possible in the treatment of acquired lexical–semantic disorders.

Statement to the reader

As a clinician, you are well aware of the different meaning relations between words, such as synonymy and antonymy. However, you may not have realized that a large number of common English words have multiple meanings, which often leads to lexical ambiguity. In this chapter, an overview of different types of ambiguity is provided along with a discussion of how word meaning can vary depending on the surrounding linguistic context. The impact of acquired brain injury on lexical ambiguity processing is also discussed as well as suggestions for incorporating context into treatment approaches. As a resource for the clinician, two lists of homonyms and brief sentence contexts to reinforce different interpretations of the ambiguous words are provided. These lists can be used

DOI: 10.4324/9781003045519-10

to either assess understanding of a specific meaning, or train identification of alternative interpretations of ambiguous words.

Introduction

Semantics is the study of how meaning is conveyed through language. Despite many years of investigation, we still know very little about the nature of meaning or how it is represented in the human mind. In fact, a major focus of semantics to this day is to determine what meaning is and how best to specify it. Another key question is to understand how meanings vary with the context in which they occur, which is the focus of this chapter. Within the field of semantics, there are several theoretical approaches, including *formal semantics*, which studies meaning in natural languages using techniques from symbolic logic, mathematics, and mathematical logic, *grammatical semantics*, which studies aspects of meaning relevant to syntax, and *pragmatics*, which studies the interpretation of meaning in situational context. As these approaches to the study of meaning require considerable knowledge of other disciplines (particularly logic, mathematics, and philosophy), the focus of this chapter will be on an area of semantics that is most relevant to communication disorders: *lexical semantics*, the study of how meaning is encoded in words, and how word meaning relates to sentence meaning.

In the first part of this chapter, key concepts of lexical semantics are reviewed, including lexical ambiguity, such as homonymy and polysemy, the organization of multiple word meanings in our mental lexicon, and the related phenomenon of contextual variability of word meaning (i.e., how the interpretation of words with multiple meanings or senses can vary based on the surrounding linguistic and/or situational context). In the second section, the impact of acquired language disorders, such as aphasia and right hemisphere brain injury, on understanding words with contextually variable interpretations is discussed. In the last section, current treatment approaches are described along with recommendations for best practices in treating context-based semantic impairments. Given that most, if not all, meaning is context-dependent, contextual variability should be considered whenever possible in designing treatment approaches for individuals with acquired lexical–semantic disorders.

Lexical ambiguity

In trying to determine a word's meaning, one problem we often encounter is that the interpretation of a word can vary greatly from one context to another. These variations in meaning can be quite obvious or very subtle in nature. In some cases, there is little or no connection between the interpretations, as with *bank* in *He got a loan from the **bank**.* compared to *The boat was sitting at the **bank**.* In other cases, there is a clear relationship between the interpretations, as with *school* in *The town decided to build a new **school**.*, which refers to the physical building, compared to *John's* **school** *won the football game.*, which refers to a subset of the individual students. Finally, yet other cases demonstrate relatively subtle variations in interpretations, as with *path* in *She came down the* **path** *to meet me at the front gate.* compared to *They followed a winding* **path** *through the woods.*, where the mental image of a path is slightly different in the two sentences.

The aforementioned examples illustrate what is known as lexical or semantic ambiguity. Many words are ambiguous, in that the same written or spoken form can have multiple senses, and often completely unrelated meanings. In fact, it has been estimated that at least 80% of common English words have more than one meaning or dictionary definition (Parks et al., 1998; Rodd et al., 2002). For the most part, ambiguity goes unnoticed and does not disrupt language comprehension because we use contextual cues and our own linguistic experience to quickly resolve any ambiguity that arises. Before describing the most common types of lexical ambiguity, it is important to consider two points. First, not all ambiguity is lexical in nature. Another well-known type is syntactic ambiguity, as in the example *wealthy men and women*, where only the men are wealthy or both the men and women are, depending on how the sentence structure is interpreted. Non-lexical ambiguity can also arise from alternative interpretations of a simile or metaphor, as in *Steve works like lightning.* (i.e., very fast) compared to *Steve works like lightning, in brief flashes with lots of noise.* Second, ambiguity does not account for all possibilities of contextual variation. For example, *doctor* is interpreted differently in *Leah's doctor is on maternity leave.* compared to *Leah's doctor is on paternity leave.* The gender of *doctor* is clearly influenced by the presence of *maternity* and *paternity*, respectively, in the context. This word, however, is not considered to be ambiguous because there is no clear sense boundary between the interpretations.

The presence of a sense boundary is a key feature of true lexical ambiguity. Sense boundaries are identified using specific criteria. Each of these criteria can be considered as different ways in which an interpretation may be autonomous, that is ways in which it plays an individual semantic role in a language (Cruse, 2011). Two interpretations demonstrate attentional autonomy if they are mutually incompatible, that is they are in competition for attention and cannot both be held simultaneously at the center of attention. For example, if a speaker produces the sentence, *Laura is wearing a light jacket.*, only one interpretation (i.e., a light-weight jacket or a light-colored jacket) is intended, and the listener must determine that interpretation based on contextual cues. If they are unable to do so, they must ask for further clarification. Crucially, only one interpretation is possible and has to share attentional focus by the speaker and listener. Two interpretations demonstrate relational autonomy if they have independent sets of sense relations. For example, the two interpretations of *light* have distinct opposites, namely *dark* and *heavy*. The fact that these sense relations are completely unrelated indicates the presence of a sense boundary. The two interpretations of *bank* also have independent sense relations. The *river bank* interpretation refers to the land next to the water and is related to *mouth, source,* and *bed.* In contrast, the *money bank* interpretation refers to a type of financial institution, and is related to *manager, building,* and *ATM.* Lastly, two interpretations demonstrate compositional autonomy if they can be obtained independently through the process of composition. For example, modification of a noun by an adjective, a compositional process, leads to independent interpretations of *bank,* as in *a steep bank* or *a commercial bank.* Compositional autonomy in addition to attentional and relational autonomy can therefore be used as evidence of a sense boundary between the various possible meanings of a word.

Homonymy

Homonyms are words with multiple *unrelated meanings* which share the same phonology (homophones), orthography (homographs), or both. Homophones share the same pronunciation, but a different spelling, as in *right* versus *write,* and *piece* versus *peace.* Homographs share the same spelling, but can have a similar or different pronunciation. For example, *bank* is pronounced the same regardless of whether it refers to the financial institution or the side of a river. In contrast, *bow* has a different pronunciation depending on whether it refers to a weapon for shooting arrows or the act of bending at the waist. While most homographs have unrelated meanings from the same grammatical class (e.g., noun–noun homographs; *palm-hand, palm-tree*), some have unrelated meanings from different grammatical classes (e.g., noun–verb homographs; *swallow-bird, swallow-digest*). In most standard dictionaries, homographs are listed as distinct lexical entries, such as *bank¹* and *bank²*, to reflect the fact that the meanings are unrelated. It is also possible that the frequency of use of each of the meanings varies to an extent, with some words having a highly dominant or frequent meaning (i.e., unbalanced homonyms) and other words having more equally frequent meanings (i.e., balanced homonyms). Fortunately, we do not have to determine the frequency of use of these meanings, as this information has already been documented for hundreds of homonyms in different languages (e.g., Armstrong et al., 2012, 2016; Haro et al., 2017; Twilley et al., 1994).

Polysemy

Polysemy occurs when a word has two or more *related senses.* Notice here that we refer to senses rather than meanings to capture the relatedness of the interpretations. Polysemy has received significant attention in research on lexical semantics due to the inherent difficulty in distinguishing between these alternations in meaning and describing how related senses are represented and generated in the lexicon (for further details, see Apresjan, 1974; Cruse, 1986, 1995; Nunberg, 1979). A good example of polysemy is the word *mark,* as it has several related senses, including:

- a visible spot or line on a surface (e.g., *His boots left black marks on the floor.*)
- a written symbol (e.g., *You need to add a punctuation mark.*)

- a grade in an academic course or on an exam (e.g., *He got a good mark on the test.*)
- a goal or target (e.g., *She hit the mark every time.*)
- an indication of some quality or property (e.g., *The mark of a good leader is humility.*)
- the intended victim or target of a scam (e.g., *He was gullible and an easy mark.*)

Like homonyms, some polysemous words share the same grammatical class (e.g., noun–noun polysemy; *belt-clothing, belt-mechanical*), while others can function as either denominal verbs or their root nouns (e.g., noun–verb polysemy; *hammer-tool, hammer-hit*). In most standard dictionaries, polysemous words are listed under one entry to reflect the fact that the senses are related. The frequency of use of the related senses may vary although to a lesser extent than with homonyms. It is also more difficult to determine the frequency of use of each sense as this information is not as widely available for polysemous words (e.g., Durkin & Manning, 1989).

Polysemous words can be further divided based on whether there is a linear or nonlinear relationship between their senses (Cruse, 2011). Linear polysemy describes words where one sense covers a more specific area within the area covered by the other, as is the case when one sense denotes a subtype or part of the other. Autohyponymy and automeronymy are two types of linear polysemy. Autohyponymy occurs when a sense denotes a subtype of another sense. For example, *drink* has two senses, a general sense "to consume a liquid" as in *You shouldn't drink anything before surgery.*, and a more specific sense "to consume alcohol" as in *You shouldn't drink while driving*. Automeronymy occurs when a sense denotes a subpart of another sense. For example, *arm* has two senses, one that refers to the whole arm as in *She lost an arm in the accident.*, and another that refers to a part of the arm as in *The cat scratched her arm.*, which typically means the non-hand part of the arm. Nonlinear polysemy describes words where there is no relationship of inclusion between the senses, as is the case with metaphor and metonymy. In metaphor, the senses are related based on analogy (see Kovecses, 2010, for further discussion). For example, *position* clearly has a number of senses which indicate whether someone is literally or figuratively in a certain location or situation, as illustrated by its various uses in *I slept in an uncomfortable position.*, *The principal is in a position of authority.* and *You put me in an awkward position.* In metonymy, the name of an object or concept is replaced by a word closely related to it. For example, *mouth* is interpreted nonliterally in *There are too many mouths to feed.*, where *mouths* is substituted for *children*, and literally in *You shouldn't talk with your mouth full.*

Dynamic construal approach to contextual variability of word meaning

The discussion so far may lead one to think that words are associated with a fixed number of meanings and/or senses with varying degrees of overlap.

Recent approaches, however, argue that our mental lexicon does not store words with a fixed number of senses, but instead it acts as an active generator of new senses. For the most part, such generative lexicon approaches assume that a core set of senses is used to generate a larger set of senses when individual words are combined together (Copestake & Briscoe, 1995; Cruse, 1986, 1995; Pustejovsky, 1995). One proposal, the dynamic construal approach (Croft & Cruse, 2004), assumes that words do not have a fixed set of meanings permanently assigned to them, but that word meanings emerge in actual use through various mental processes of meaning construal or construction. What a word does map onto is a body of conceptual content (i.e., memories of previous experiences of the contextualized use of a word), but the exact meanings themselves are underspecified or underdetermined. Meaning construction takes place in context, but is also subject to a number of contextual constraints, which make some interpretations of a word more likely than others. Many aspects of context can constrain meaning construal or construction, including:

- *Linguistic Context*: The linguistic expressions surrounding the word, including both the immediately adjacent words (local context) and more distant sentences in the same utterance (global context).
- *Physical Context*: The physical environment in which the participants share a communicative exchange.
- *Cognitive Context*: The individual knowledge and experiences of the participants which may or may not be shared with each other.
- *Sociolinguistic Context*: The social function of the communicative exchange, including its level of formality (e.g., formal or informal) and purpose (e.g., clinical, educational, legal, medical, or political).
- *Personal Context*: The personal dynamics of the participants, including perceived power or status roles, prior relationships, and gender differences.

The dynamic construal approach does not exclude the possibility that some interpretations have a default status, that is, a specific interpretation will emerge if there is not enough context to guide the process of construal. This does not mean, however, that default interpretations are the real, inherent, meanings of words; they still have to be construed based on the available context.

Understanding context-dependent word meanings after acquired brain injury

The ability to understand lexical ambiguity in context has been well-studied in individuals with acquired brain injury. There is substantial evidence that individuals with aphasia or right brain injury have difficulty determining which interpretation of an ambiguous word is contextually appropriate. In people with aphasia (PWA), this finding may be surprising given that these individuals typically benefit from context. For example, PWA better understand syntactically complex sentences when these sentences are embedded in semantically supportive contexts (Cannito et al., 1986; Hough et al., 1989; Pierce, 1988).

They can also use context to build expectations about upcoming words in a sentence (Friederici, 1983, 1985; Wayland et al., 1996). In people with right brain injury, this finding is less surprising given the well-known issues these individuals have in interpreting alternative meanings and understanding higher level discourse. Importantly, both groups do not have difficulty understanding ambiguous words more so than other types of words when no context is provided. For example, when these words are presented in word pairs such as *bank-river* and *bank-money*, individuals with aphasia or right brain injury show evidence of understanding each of the alternative meanings (Katz, 1988; Klepousniotou & Baum, 2005a). It is only when the interpretation of these words becomes context-dependent, and the meaning must be derived based on contextual cues that difficulties can emerge.

Aphasia

A number of studies have examined how PWA interpret ambiguous words in a linguistic context (Grindrod, 2012; Grindrod & Baum, 2003, 2005; Henderson & Wright, 2016; Klepousniotou & Baum, 2005b; Laurinavichyute et al., 2014; Prather et al., 1994; Swaab et al., 1998; Swinney et al., 1989, 2000). Three main findings are most relevant to the current discussion. First, PWA take longer to determine the contextually appropriate meaning. At early stages, these individuals are still considering both meanings regardless of the context (Grindrod & Baum, 2003; Klepousniotou & Baum, 2005b; Swaab et al., 1998). Given more time, they are eventually able to determine which meaning is most appropriate. Thus, it appears that their ability to use context is intact, but somewhat delayed. Second, PWA only benefit from specific types of contexts while other contexts can actually have a detrimental effect on their understanding. For example, understanding of ambiguity in PWA is better with short, highly constrained contexts where a noun or a verb biases a specific interpretation (e.g., *His nose bled after the powerful **punch**.* versus *For the party, she prepared a **punch**.*; Klepousniotou & Baum, 2005b). Highly constrained discourse contexts, where biasing information is repeated across several sentences to reinforce a specific interpretation, also seem to be beneficial (e.g., *Dan went to the **dentist**. He had to get a **cavity** filled. The **dentist** examined his **teeth**. Then, he pulled out a **drill**.* versus *Kristin wants to be the best **player** on the **team**. She goes to the **gym** every day. There, she shoots **baskets**. Every day, she practices this **drill**.*; Henderson & Wright, 2016). In contrast, less-constrained contexts, or those where the biasing information is separated from the ambiguous word by some distance, are less effective (Grindrod, 2012; Grindrod & Baum, 2005). PWA therefore seem to benefit most from strongly constrained contexts that contain multiple sources of biasing information. Lastly, PWA may experience persistent difficulty understanding less frequent interpretations of ambiguous words. These individuals often only demonstrate understanding of the dominant, more frequent meaning even in cases where the context supports an interpretation consistent with the less frequent meaning (e.g., *Due to supply shortages, General*

*Motors decided to shut down production at every **plant**.*; Grindrod & Baum, 2005; Prather et al., 1994; Swinney et al., 1989). It is unclear whether these interpretations are in general more difficult to retrieve, if they require a stronger context to be reinforced, or the more frequent interpretation of many of these words is simply too difficult to override. On the whole, it does seem that even with adequate linguistic context, less frequent meanings are more difficult for PWA to understand.

The difficulties described previously can lead to misinterpretations during communication and a potential inability for PWA to recover from these misinterpretations. In a typical conversation, only minimal context is needed to understand a homonym. Context, however, is also building up over time such that the interpretation of a word early on impacts how subsequent words are interpreted. If a PWA is slower to determine the contextually appropriate meaning, they may still be considering alternative meanings at a point when they encounter another word or phrase whose meaning is dependent on the interpretation of the previous word. If they fail to derive the appropriate interpretation of the initial word in time, any attempt at understanding later information could be severely disrupted. Slowed context processing also leaves very little time for PWA to revise their initial interpretation, which may be necessary when a homonym has a highly frequent meaning, but is ultimately resolved toward the less frequent meaning (e.g., *The **ball** was crowded*). Finally, delayed interpretation of word meanings in context could also have a detrimental effect on higher level language comprehension processes such as syntactic and discourse comprehension in PWA.

Right hemisphere brain injury

Individuals with right hemisphere disorder (RHD) have also been studied with respect to their ability to understand alternative meanings of ambiguous words in context (Fassbinder & Tompkins, 2001; Grindrod, 2012; Grindrod & Baum, 2003, 2005; Klepousniotou & Baum, 2005b; Tompkins et al., 1997, 2000, 2002). Their deficits have been characterized in one of two ways. Some research has argued that these individuals generate multiple meanings but cannot suppress contextually inappropriate interpretations over time. Similar to people with aphasia, RHD individuals consider both meanings regardless of context early on. Over time, they are, however, unable to determine the correct interpretation and continue to entertain the contextually inappropriate meaning (Klepousniotou & Baum, 2005b; Tompkins et al., 1997, 2000, 2002). Some models of language comprehension assume that healthy adults generate multiple interpretations initially and that any meanings which over time become incompatible with the context or final interpretation are eventually eliminated or suppressed (Gernsbacher, 1990; Gernsbacher & Faust, 1991). As RHD individuals are unable to eliminate these meanings, they are considered to have a suppression deficit. In contrast to the above findings, other research has argued that RHD individuals are insensitive to context and must rely on other cues to determine the interpretation of an ambiguous word. These studies have shown that RHD individuals generate only the more frequent meaning of homonyms regardless of context (Grindrod, 2012; Grindrod & Baum, 2003). This pattern of performance is observed across short, single-sentence contexts to larger, discourse contexts. To account for these results, it has been argued that RHD individuals have inefficient context use and when unable to fully rely on context, they determine the final interpretation based on their linguistic experience with the expression by choosing the more familiar or frequent meaning. Although current research suggests two competing accounts for RHD individuals' difficulty in understanding ambiguous words in context, it is clear that generating the more frequent meaning interferes with their ability to understand alternative, less frequent meanings.

Both of the impairments described previously could negatively impact language comprehension processes in RHD individuals. For example, a suppression deficit may lead to poor narrative comprehension. Rapid, efficient suppression of contextually inappropriate interpretations generally leads to better understanding of a text as a whole. The generation and maintenance of inappropriate meanings could slow down the overall comprehension process. This may be particularly problematic for auditory comprehension as opposed to reading comprehension when the individual cannot stop the incoming speech stream in order to fully process the intended meaning. If RHD individuals generate only more frequent, familiar interpretations due to inefficient context use, they may have a too narrow or literal interpretation of what the speaker intended. It is also possible that what is a more familiar interpretation for the RHD individual may not necessarily be the same as that of their conversational partner which could lead to misunderstandings. For example, if an RHD individual were to use *quarters* with the intended meaning of living quarters, as opposed to the more frequent meaning of coins, a communication breakdown would result which could only be repaired by recognizing that the word has alternative meanings and by using it in context. Finally, inefficient context use could exacerbate other well-known deficits associated with right brain injury, such as inferencing, and the appreciation of humor or sarcasm, in which ambiguity often plays a prominent role.

Current treatment approaches

Despite the aforementioned difficulties in people with aphasia, no treatments have been targeted specifically at improving understanding of contextually appropriate meanings. Context has been incorporated into some treatments for word retrieval deficits such as anomia (Edmonds & Babb, 2011; Edmonds et al., 2014; Raymer & Kohen, 2006). In RHD individuals, a recent treatment approach has been developed by Tompkins and colleagues (Blake et al., 2015; Tompkins et al., 2011, 2012). This approach, known as contextual constraint treatment, is described in more detail next.

Contextual constraint treatment was originally designed to improve suppression of inappropriate meanings in RHD individuals. Unlike other treatments, which tend to be more metalinguistic in nature, this restorative therapy is implicit and indirect. As such, individuals perform a speeded judgment task during treatment, which promotes more automatic language processing and does not require an explicit response about the meaning of the words. Treatment stimuli are simple sentences that end in a homonym and contain a verb that biases the interpretation toward the less frequent meaning. The treatment hierarchy consists of three different contexts which vary in their level of constraint:

- Strong constraint context: She put on the beautiful gown. She was excited about the dance. She went to a BALL.
- Moderate constraint context: She was excited about the dance. She went to a BALL.
- Minimal constraint context: She went to a BALL.

Target words, presented one second after sentence offset, are related to the unbiased, more frequent meaning of the homonym (e.g., kick). Individuals must respond as quickly as possible via button press on a response box whether the target word is related to the sentence. The goal is to boost the contextually appropriate meaning while helping the individual to suppress the contextually inappropriate meaning. In measuring response times, it is assumed that faster responses indicate an increased ability to rule out inappropriate interpretations while slower responses indicate a decreased ability and more interference from the inappropriate meaning.

The treatment begins with auditory presentation of the strong constraint context followed by the target word. The individual's RT to the target word is compared to a preset RT criterion, defined as one standard deviation below the mean RT achieved by healthy older adults based on previous research (Tompkins et al., 2000). If the RT criterion is met, then the individual is presented with the moderate constraint context. If the RT criterion for this context is met, then the individual is presented with the minimal constraint context. If the individual meets the final RT criterion (i.e., they have moved through all three levels of constraint), then they move back up the hierarchy to the moderate and strong constraint contexts. After one full cycle of the hierarchy has been completed, they then move on to the next treatment stimulus. If at any point in the hierarchy, the individual does not meet the RT criterion, they move back to the previous level of constraint or in the case of the strong constraint context, it is repeated. If the RT criterion is not met after two repetitions, treatment for that stimulus is discontinued and the individual moves on to the next stimulus.

Results of this treatment are limited as it has only been tested on a few RHD individuals who were in early stages of their recovery (5–6 months post-stroke). In a single-subject design, Tompkins et al. (2011) found that one client improved their ability to achieve the RT criterion from 40–50% at baseline to 80–90% after ten treatment sessions, arguing that they were better able to suppress inappropriate meanings after a relatively short treatment period. The other client, who exhibited more severe difficulties interpreting ambiguity in context, improved from 20–30% accuracy in reaching the RT criterion at baseline to 50–60% after 9 treatment sessions, showing some degree of improvement although with more variability. This treatment shows some promise, but it remains to be seen if treatment gains are maintained long-term and whether other types of constraining contexts may be more beneficial.

Recommendations for treatment

Currently, there is little evidence to guide treatment of context-based meaning impairments in people with aphasia or right brain injury. The next section provides recommendations for each of these clinical populations. These recommendations mainly focus on the design of treatment stimuli, specifically strategies to develop supportive contexts. Many of these stimuli could be adapted for activity-based treatments by including more personally meaningful information or material that is relevant for completing activities of daily living or more functional tasks. As a resource for the clinician, two lists of homonyms and brief sentence contexts to reinforce different interpretations of the ambiguous words are provided in Appendices 8.1 and 8.2. These lists can be used to either assess understanding of a specific meaning or train identification of alternative interpretations of ambiguous words.

Aphasia

For people with aphasia, treatment should focus on providing enough contextual support and time to facilitate understanding of contextually appropriate interpretations. There are a number of ways to create highly constrained linguistic contexts for use in therapy although they may need to be adapted depending on the severity and type of aphasia. In individuals with agrammatic aphasia, it is recommended that short, active sentences be used, where both a noun and a verb bias a particular interpretation (e.g., *The player swung the bat.* or *The biologist caught the bat.*). These contexts could be adjusted for individuals with grammatical category deficits such that only a constraining noun or verb is used depending on the client's strengths and weaknesses (e.g., *He swung the bat.* or *The player saw the bat.*; see the appendices for more examples). One advantage is that these types of materials provide a simple, effective way to constrain the context instead of adding more sentences, which could increase working memory and sentence comprehension demands. The main goal should be to improve the client's accurate interpretation of ambiguity with the least amount of context over time, starting with the most constrained contexts first and then moving to those that are less constrained. An alternative approach for people with aphasia, especially those with syntactic impairments, is to use a visual context instead. Many ambiguous word meanings can be easily captured by a concrete object or image, so visual cues could be incorporated into therapy as a way to reinforce a specific interpretation. As with a linguistic context, several pictures could be used initially to strengthen a specific interpretation and faded over time such that only minimal visual cues are used in later stages if improvement in the clients' understanding is demonstrated.

Right hemisphere brain injury

For individuals with right hemisphere brain injury, treatment should focus on manipulating different aspects of the linguistic context to promote understanding of alternative, less frequent meanings. One strategy to increase the strength of the context is to increase the number of sentence cues (see the treatment approach by Tompkins et al. (2011) discussed earlier). An alternative method, which could be equally effective, is to increase the number of related words or contextual cues in a shorter, single-sentence context. To promote the ability to switch from one interpretation to another, contexts could also be constructed such that they are initially neutral with respect to a particular interpretation, but then resolved toward the less frequent meaning (e.g., *He was finally able to locate the bat. He found it difficult to see in the cave.*). Treatment with a linguistic context is highly recommended for RHD individuals given their relative strengths in general lexical and syntactic processing. In contrast, a visual context may not be appropriate for this population because of possible visual or attentional deficits, such as neglect. More metalinguistic tasks, where clients are asked to make explicit judgments or decisions about contextually variable interpretations, could also be used to increase awareness of alternative meanings. For example, after presenting an ambiguous word in context, the clinician could ask the individual to give their initial interpretation. The clinician would then provide an explicit context which reinforces the alternative interpretation and ask the client to explain why or why not the initial interpretation is still appropriate, and what contextual cues influenced their decision. Individuals who have difficulty explaining their interpretations may need to work on associating, organizing, and identifying relationships between treatment stimuli and contextual information. Alternatively, at a more elementary level, they may need to work on identifying, recognizing, or discriminating parts of the stimuli and contexts or even deciding what is most relevant or crucial to determining the appropriate interpretation.

Conclusion

The interpretation of most words is highly context dependent. Lexical ambiguity provides a clear case of how context is needed to quickly determine an appropriate interpretation with no disruption to the comprehension process. Individuals with acquired brain injury exhibit specific difficulties in understanding ambiguous words only when these words occur in a linguistic context.

Despite these well-documented impairments, few treatment approaches have been targeted at promoting context-based understanding in individuals with aphasia or right brain injury. This chapter argues that contextual variability should be considered whenever possible in the treatment of acquired lexical–semantic disorders. Future treatment approaches should consider employing different types of contexts to support language comprehension as well as examining more carefully which aspects of the context provide the most benefit to individuals with acquired brain injury.

References

Apresjan, J. D. (1974). Regular polysemy. *Linguistics, 14*, 5–32.

Armstrong, B. C., Tokowicz, N., & Plaut, D. C. (2012). eDom: Norming software and relative meaning frequencies for 544 English homonyms. *Behavior Research Methods, 44*, 1015–1027.

Armstrong, B. C., Zugarramurdi, C., Cabana, Á., Valle Lisboa, J., & Plaut, D. C. (2016). Relative meaning frequencies for 578 homonyms in two Spanish dialects: A cross-linguistic extension of the English eDom norms. *Behavior Research Methods, 48*, 950–962.

Blake, M. L., Tompkins, C. A., Scharp, V. L., Meigh, K. M., & Wambaugh, J. (2015). Contextual constraint treatment for coarse coding deficit in adults with right hemisphere brain damage: Generalization to narrative discourse comprehension. *Neuropsychological Rehabilitation, 25*, 15–52.

Cannito, M. P., Jarecki, J. M., & Pierce, R. S. (1986). Effects of thematic structure on syntactic comprehension in aphasia. *Brain and Language, 27*, 38–49.

Croft, W., & Cruse, D. A. (2004). *Cognitive linguistics*. Cambridge University Press.

Copestake, A., & Briscoe, T. (1995). Semi-productive polysemy and sense extension. *Journal of Semantics, 12*, 15–67.

Cruse, D. A. (1986). *Lexical semantics*. Cambridge University Press.

Cruse, D. A. (1995). Polysemy and related phenomena from a cognitive linguistic viewpoint. In P. Saint-Dizier & E. Viegas (Eds.), *Computational lexical semantics* (pp. 33–49). Cambridge University Press.

Cruse, D. A. (2011). *Meaning in language: An introduction to semantics and pragmatics*. Oxford University Press.

Durkin, K., & Manning, J. (1989). Polysemy and the subjective lexicon: Semantic relatedness and the salience of intraword senses. *Journal of Psycholinguistic Research, 18*, 577–612.

Edmonds, L. A., & Babb, M. (2011). Effect of verb network strengthening treatment in moderate-to-severe aphasia. *American Journal of Speech-Language Pathology, 20*, 131–145.

Edmonds, L. A., Mammino, K., & Ojeda, J. (2014). Effect of verb network strengthening treatment (VNeST) in persons with aphasia: Extension and replication of previous findings. *American Journal of Speech-Language Pathology, 23*, S312–S329.

Fassbinder, W., & Tompkins, C. A. (2001). Slowed lexical-semantic activation in individuals with right hemisphere brain damage? *Aphasiology, 15*, 1079–1090.

Friederici, A. D. (1983). Aphasics' perception of words in sentential context: Some real-time processing evidence. *Neuropsychologia, 21*, 351–358.

Friederici, A. D. (1985). Levels of processing and vocabulary types: Evidence from on-line comprehension in normals and agrammatics. *Cognition, 19*, 133–166.

Gernsbacher, M. A. (1990). *Language comprehension as structure building*. Lawrence Erlbaum Associates.

Gernsbacher, M. A., & Faust, M. E. (1991). The mechanism of suppression: A component of general comprehension skill. *Journal of Experimental Psychology: Learning, Memory, and Cognition, 17,* 245–262.

Grindrod, C. M. (2012). Effects of left and right hemisphere damage on sensitivity to global context during lexical ambiguity resolution. *Aphasiology, 26,* 933–952.

Grindrod, C. M., & Baum, S. R. (2003). Sensitivity to local sentence context information in lexical ambiguity resolution: Evidence from left- and right-hemisphere-damaged individuals. *Brain and Language, 85,* 503–523.

Grindrod, C. M., & Baum, S. R. (2005). Hemispheric contributions to lexical ambiguity resolution in a discourse context: Evidence from individuals with unilateral left and right hemisphere lesions. *Brain and Cognition, 57,* 70–83.

Haro, J., Ferre, P., Boada, R., & Demestre, J. (2017). Semantic ambiguity norms for 530 Spanish words. *Applied Psycholinguistics, 38,* 457–475.

Henderson, A., & Wright, H. H. (2016). Lexical ambiguity resolution using discourse contexts in persons with and without aphasia. *American Journal of Speech-Language Pathology, 25,* S839–S853.

Hough, M. S., Pierce, R. S., & Cannito, M. P. (1989). Contextual influences in aphasia: Effects of predictive versus nonpredictive narratives. *Brain and Language, 36,* 325–334.

Katz, W. F. (1988). An investigation of lexical ambiguity in Broca's aphasics using an auditory lexical priming technique. *Neuropsychologia, 26,* 747–752.

Klepousniotou, E., & Baum, S. R. (2005a). Unilateral brain damage effects on processing homonymous and polysemous words. *Brain and Language, 93,* 308–326.

Klepousniotou, E., & Baum, S. R. (2005b). Processing homonymy and polysemy: Effects of sentential context and time-course following unilateral brain damage. *Brain and Language, 95,* 365–382.

Kovecses, Z. (2010). *Metaphor: A practical introduction.* Oxford University Press.

Laurinavichyute, A. K., Ulicheva, A., Ivanova, M. V., Kuptsova, S. V., & Dragoy, O. (2014). Processing lexical ambiguity in sentential context: Eye-tracking data from brain-damaged and non-brain-damaged individuals. *Neuropsychologia, 64,* 360–373.

Nunberg, G. (1979). The non-uniqueness of semantic solutions: Polysemy. *Linguistics and Philosophy, 3,* 143–184.

Parks, R., Ray, J., & Bland, S. (1998). *Wordsmyth English dictionary-thesaurus* [online]. www.wordsmyth.net

Pierce, R. S. (1988). Influence of prior and subsequent context on comprehension in aphasia. *Aphasiology, 2,* 577–582.

Prather, P. A., Love, T., Finkel, L., & Zurif, E. (1994). Effects of slowed processing on lexical activation: Automaticity without encapsulation. *Brain and Language, 47,* 326–329.

Pustejovsky, J. (1995). *The generative lexicon.* MIT Press.

Raymer, A., & Kohen, F. (2006). Word-retrieval treatment in aphasia: Effects of sentence context. *Journal of Rehabilitation Research and Development, 43,* 367–378.

Rodd, J. M., Gaskell, G., & Marslen-Wilson, W. (2002). Making sense of semantic ambiguity: Semantic competition in lexical access. *Journal of Memory and Language, 46,* 245–256.

Swaab, T. Y., Brown, C. M., & Hagoort, P. (1998). Understanding ambiguous words in sentence contexts: Electrophysiological evidence for delayed contextual selection in Broca's aphasia. *Neuropsychologia, 36,* 737–761.

Swinney, D. A., Prather, P. A., & Love, T. (2000). The time-course of lexical access and the role of context: Converging evidence from normal and aphasic processing. In Y. Grodzinsky, L. Shapiro, & D. A. Swinney (Eds.), *Language and the brain: Representation and processing* (pp. 273–292). Academic Press.

Swinney, D. A., Zurif, E., & Nicol, J. L. (1989). The effects of focal brain damage on sentence processing: An examination of the neurological organization of a mental module. *Journal of Cognitive Neuroscience, 1,* 25–37.

Tompkins, C. A., Baumgaertner, A., Lehman, M. T., & Fossett, T. R. D. (1997). Suppression and discourse comprehension in right brain-damaged adults: A preliminary report. *Aphasiology, 11,* 505–519.

Tompkins, C. A., Baumgaertner, A., Lehman, M. T., & Fassbinder, W. (2000). Mechanisms of discourse comprehension impairment after right hemisphere brain damage: Suppression in lexical ambiguity resolution. *Journal of Speech, Language and Hearing Research, 43,* 62–78.

Tompkins, C. A., Lehman-Blake, M. T., Baumgaertner, A., & Fassbinder, W. (2002). Characterizing comprehension difficulties after right brain damage: Attentional demands of suppression function. *Aphasiology, 16,* 559–572.

Tompkins, C. A., Lehman-Blake, M. T., Wambaugh, J., & Meigh, K. (2011). A novel, implicit treatment for language comprehension processes in right hemisphere brain damage: Phase I data. *Aphasiology, 25,* 789–799.

Tompkins, C. A., Scharp, V. L., Meigh, K., Blake, M. L., & Wambaugh, J. (2012). Generalization of a novel, implicit treatment for coarse coding deficit in right hemisphere brain damage: A single subject experiment. *Aphasiology, 26,* 689–708.

Twilley, L. C., Dixon, P., Taylor, D., & Clark, K. (1994). University of Alberta norms of relative meaning frequency for 566 homographs. *Memory and Cognition, 22,* 111–126.

Wayland, S. C., Berndt, R. S., & Sandson, J. R. (1996). Aphasic patients' sensitivity to structural and meaning violations when monitoring for nouns and verbs in sentences. *Neuropsychology, 10,* 504–516.

Appendix 8.1

Appendix Table 8.1 Balanced homonyms (i.e., ambiguous words with two relatively equally frequent meanings).

Homonym	M1 Associate	M1 Frequency	M1 Context	M2 Associate	M2 Frequency	M2 Context
advance	attack	0.65	He led the advance.	payment	0.35	He received the advance.
bat	ball	0.61	He swung the bat.	animal	0.39	He killed the bat.
bolt	screw	0.66	He tightened the bolt.	thunder	0.34	He heard the bolt.
cape	coat	0.56	He wore the cape.	island	0.44	He visited the cape.
case	court	0.55	She defended the case.	luggage	0.45	She emptied the case.
cast	arm	0.56	She autographed the cast.	actors	0.44	She interviewed the cast.
cell	jail	0.55	He entered the cell.	nucleus	0.45	He magnified the cell.
change	new	0.54	He implemented the change.	coins	0.46	He counted the change.
charm	bracelet	0.54	She engraved her charm.	wit	0.46	She exploited her charm.
chest	body	0.65	He bared his chest.	treasure	0.35	He unlocked the chest.
court	judge	0.60	She presided over the court.	basketball	0.40	She walked onto the court.
crane	machine	0.57	He operated the crane.	bird	0.43	He fed the crane.
fall	down	0.60	She broke the fall.	autumn	0.40	She preferred the fall.
gag	choke	0.64	He removed the gag.	joke	0.36	He told the gag.
iron	metal	0.59	He melted the iron.	clothes	0.49	He unplugged the iron.
major	minor	0.67	He declared his major.	army	0.33	He saluted his major.
marble	tile	0.59	He repaired the marble.	ball	0.41	He rolled the marble.
mass	weight	0.60	He calculated the mass.	church	0.40	He attended the mass.
match	flame	0.64	She lit the match.	game	0.36	She won the match.
model	pretty	0.59	He dated a model.	toy	0.41	He built a model.

(Continued)

Appendix Table 8.1 (Continued)

Homonym	M1 Associate	M1 Frequency	M1 Context	M2 Associate	M2 Frequency	M2 Context
mole	animal	0.64	She caught the mole.	face	0.36	She covered the mole.
nail	hammer	0.62	He dropped a nail.	finger	0.38	He broke a nail.
nut	shell	0.62	She ate a nut.	crazy	0.38	She was a nut.
organ	kidney	0.52	He transplanted the organ.	piano	0.48	He tuned the organ.
panel	wood	0.59	He installed the panel.	judges	0.41	He interrogated the panel.
pass	catch	0.61	He intercepted the pass.	ticket	0.39	He bought the pass.
pipe	smoke	0.61	He lit the pipe.	water	0.39	He installed the pipe.
pitcher	water	0.51	He spilled the pitcher.	baseball	0.49	He coached the pitcher.
pupil	student	0.67	He quizzed his pupil.	eye	0.33	He dilated his pupil.
ring	diamond	0.68	He bought a ring.	phone	0.32	He heard a ring.
screen	computer	0.67	He brightened the screen.	door	0.33	He closed the screen.
seal	animal	0.56	He trained the seal.	envelope	0.44	He licked the seal.
sling	shot	0.59	He loaded the sling.	arm	0.41	He wore the sling.
speaker	speech	0.65	He greeted the speaker.	stereo	0.35	He rewired the speaker.
straw	hay	0.66	He gathered the straw.	drink	0.34	He bent the straw.
temple	church	0.67	He entered the temple.	head	0.33	He rubbed his temple.
tick	flea	0.55	She killed the tick.	tock	0.45	She heard the tick.
tip	top	0.61	She broke the tip.	money	0.39	She left the tip.
trip	vacation	0.68	He was delighted by the trip.	fall	0.32	He was injured by the trip.
yard	house	0.68	He cleaned his yard.	meter	0.32	He bought one yard.

Note: M1 = primary meaning. M2 = secondary meaning. Meaning frequency is based on Twilley et al. (1994).

Appendix 8.2

Appendix Table 8.2 Unbalanced homonyms (i.e., ambiguous words with a highly frequent meaning).

Homonym	M1 Associate	M1 Frequency	M1 Context	M2 Associate	M2 Frequency	M2 Context
arm(s)	legs	0.95	He bent his arms.	weapons	0.05	He fired his arms.
ball	bounce	0.98	She grabbed the ball.	dance	0.02	She catered the ball.
bar	drink	0.92	He frequented the bar.	metal	0.08	He grabbed the bar.
battery	power	0.93	He purchased the battery.	assault	0.07	He committed battery.
belt	pants	0.92	He loosened the belt.	hit	0.08	He avoided the belt.
bill	check	0.93	He paid the bill.	law	0.07	He supported the bill.
bluff	lie	0.92	She called his bluff.	cliff	0.08	She climbed the bluff.
boil	water	0.95	She adjusted the boil.	blister	0.05	She bandaged the boil.
break	crack	0.90	He patched the break.	rest	0.10	He needed a break.
cap	hat	0.93	He wore the cap.	bottle	0.07	He unscrewed the cap.
coat	jacket	0.95	He lost the coat.	paint	0.05	He applied a new coat.
corn	cob	0.99	She ate the corn.	foot	0.01	She bandaged the corn.
dive	pool	0.99	He performed the dive.	dump	0.01	He renovated the dive.
finish	line	0.97	He approached the finish.	stain	0.03	He scratched the finish.
flight(s)	airport	0.98	She booked two flights.	stairs	0.02	She climbed two flights.
flush	toilet	0.94	She heard a flush.	poker	0.06	She was dealt a flush.
game	play	0.97	He explained the game.	hunt	0.03	He hunted the game.
ham	meat	0.97	He sliced the ham.	comic	0.03	He was a ham.
jam	jelly	0.96	She spread the jam.	traffic	0.04	She caused the jam.
key	door	0.96	She turned the key.	code	0.04	She wrote the key.

(Continued)

Appendix Table 8.2 (Continued)

Homonym	M1 Associate	M1 Frequency	M1 Context	M2 Associate	M2 Frequency	M2 Context
letter(s)	mail	0.91	He received the letters.	alphabet	0.09	He capitalized the letters.
log	wood	0.95	He chopped the log.	math	0.05	He computed the log.
passage	tunnel	0.92	She exited the passage.	text	0.08	She read the passage.
pen	ink	0.96	She lost the pen.	pig	0.04	She locked the pen.
pitch	baseball	0.93	He threw the pitch.	sound	0.07	He raised his pitch.
plane	fly	0.93	He flew the plane.	geometry	0.07	He calculated the plane.
record	album	0.94	She played the record.	diary	0.06	She updated the record.
scoop	ice-cream	0.96	He washed the scoop.	news	0.04	He reported the scoop.
shot	gun	0.94	He fired the shot.	alcohol	0.06	He drank the shot.
shower	bath	0.98	He took a shower.	rain	0.02	He forecasted a shower.
spare	tire	0.98	He found a spare.	bowling	0.02	He threw a spare.
square	circle	0.91	He drew a square.	root	0.09	He calculated the square.
state	country	0.91	She governed her state.	mind	0.09	She altered her state.
sting	bee	0.96	He felt the sting.	police	0.04	He organized the sting.
stories	books	0.98	He read five stories.	floors	0.02	He climbed five stories.
suit	tie	0.98	He bought a suit.	law	0.02	He filed a suit.
switch	light	0.97	He flipped the switch.	change	0.03	He encouraged the switch.
tie	suit	0.96	He loosened the tie.	score	0.04	He broke the tie.
toast	bread	0.91	He ate the toast.	speech	0.09	He rehearsed the toast.
top	bottom	0.96	She reached the top.	spin	0.04	She wound the top.

Note: M1 = primary meaning. M2 = secondary meaning. Meaning frequency is based on Twilley et al. (1994).

9 Pragmatics

Discourse assessment and treatment in traumatic brain injury

Shaun R. Stephens, Carl Coelho, and Michael S. Cannizzaro

Abstract

Discourse is commonly occurring and encompasses many forms of everyday communication. Within the context of traumatic brain injury (TBI) and associated cognitive-communication disorders (CCD), it is critical that clinicians include analysis of discourse production, in genres relevant to the client, when forming their assessment protocol. For clinicians unfamiliar with assessing discourse this can be a daunting task due to the time involved and the myriad of analysis techniques that are possible. In an effort to facilitate the use of discourse analysis for the management of CCD after TBI, this chapter provides an overview of elicitation techniques and several types of analyses. Treatment directed toward improving functional communication is dependent on client-focused discourse assessment using ecologically valid forms of communication.

Statement to reader

This chapter is intended to encourage and facilitate the use of discourse analysis by clinicians when assessing cognitive-communication disorders after TBI. The authors provide a synopsis of the literature on discourse deficits following TBI, as well as elicitation and analysis techniques. The chapter ends with suggestions for assessment and treatment techniques.

Background: discourse is important

Discourse is the central form of human communication. It is functional language, used to persuade, to inspire, to tell stories, to procure something, to explain, to share ideas. We make sense of the world and our place in it through the stories we tell. Discourse is defined as the sequential organization of language beyond the sentence level (Galski et al., 1998; Müller et al., 2009). This chapter summarizes recent research on discourse from a "functionalist"

DOI: 10.4324/9781003045519-11

perspective. Discourse is considered primarily as a semantic unit rather than a grammatical one (Armstrong, 2000), organized around units of meaning, rather than grammatical structures. Discourse is embedded within a particular communicative context that varies from genre to genre.

There are a variety of discourse genres used for social or "pragmatic" purposes: conversation, expository (explaining or stating an opinion), procedural, persuasive, personal narrative, and fictional narratives (Aboud et al., 2019; Hill et al., 2020; Nippold et al., 2014; Scott & Windsor, 2000). Despite the variety of genres used in daily life, most research on discourse has focused on fictional narratives (Hill et al., 2021; Sherratt, 2007). Due to the diversity of discourse genres used in daily and professional life, clinicians need to assess an individual's performance across genres, rather than in a single genre (Hill et al., 2020). This chapter provides guidance on efficient and valid methods for assessing and treating discourse across genres.

The theoretical framework proposed by Dipper and colleagues (2021) for characterizing how individuals formulate and process oral discourse (*Linguistic Underpinnings of Narrative in Aphasia; LUNA*) proposes four processing components: Pragmatic, which includes contextual and interpersonal variables; Macrostructural planning, which involves an organizational frame for the discourse; Propositional, which transforms macro-level structure into micro-level action plans for individual utterances; and the Linguistic component, which translates propositional action plans into utterances.

These components of discourse are dependent on the cognitive domains of executive functioning, memory, social cognition, and theory of mind (ToM; Jacoby & Fedorenko, 2020; Mar, 2011). There is overlap among all these skills; however, discourse must be addressed as its own entity. In other words, improvements in executive functioning, memory, or ToM will not necessarily translate into improvements in discourse. Because discourse overlaps with cognitive domains, it is characterized as cognitive communication (ASHA, 2003).

Discourse and brain injury

Traumatic brain injury (TBI) is the most common cause of disability and death in young adults under 45 years (Marcotte et al., 2020).[1] In the United States, TBI accounts for approximately 2.4 million emergency department visits and hospitalizations per year, and 61,000 deaths per year (Centers for Disease Control and Prevention, 2015). The long-term effects of TBI include both physical symptoms (headache, vision impairments, fatigue), emotional and personality changes, and cognitive-communication symptoms. TBI often results in poor psychosocial outcomes: social isolation, difficulty reintegrating into paid work, and lack of independence. Elbourn and colleagues (2019) found significant correlations between psychosocial outcomes and discourse performance across

---

1. Throughout this chapter we will refer to TBI, but most of the applied clinical information will be equally relevant for non-traumatic acquired brain injuries (ABI).

the first-year post-injury; and discourse performance at 6 months significantly predicted 12-month psychosocial outcomes. Brain injury, even moderate or mild, can affect formulation and comprehension of discourse in individuals without aphasia, and normal performance on aphasia assessments does not rule out discourse impairment (Brown & Knollman-Porter, 2019; Crewe-Brown et al., 2011; Dikmen et al., 2017; Kintz et al., 2018; Marini et al., 2017; Stout et al., 2000). Nor is injury severity on its own an accurate predictor of functional recovery (physical or communicative); among individuals with moderate to severe TBI, initial severity did not correlate with functional independence measures at discharge (Al-Hassani et al., 2018).

Discourse impairments are common after TBI. Conversation skills are impaired in 60% of individuals with moderate to severe TBI (Marcotte et al., 2020), and impairments in productivity (fewer utterances and shorter length utterances) and fluency (more pauses, more unfilled pauses) have also been reported in the oral discourse of adolescents with moderate to severe TBI (Lundine & Barron, 2019). Impaired discourse is a more common cognitive-communication impairment after TBI than aphasia, a fact which has been recognized for over 40 years (Holland, 1982). Discourse impairment after TBI results in poor functional outcomes, even in the absence of aphasia including social isolation, difficulty with reintegration into work, problems with relationships (Ponsford et al., 2014), lower independence, and lower quality of life (QoL) (Douglas et al., 2016; Elbourn et al., 2019). Impairments in discourse are associated with higher incarceration rates among teenagers and young adults. In studies from the United States, the United Kingdom, Australia, and New Zealand, rates of language disorder among youth offenders ranged from 25% to 67%, compared to 3% to 4% in the general age-matched cohort (Anderson et al., 2016; Snow, 2019). Discourse-level skills have been shown to discriminate between adults with stable employment compared to those with unstable employment after moderate to severe TBI (Meulenbroek & Turkstra, 2016). Further, among school-age children, discourse formulation (particularly measures of productivity and fluency) distinguishes children with developmental language disorder from typically developing children (Scott & Windsor, 2000). Among adults, long-term difficulties with social communication after brain injury occur primarily at the level of interactional discourse (Elbourn et al., 2019; Worrall et al., 2011). In short, cognitive-communication disorders after TBI are commonly observable as discourse-level impairments, which are associated with poor psychosocial, vocational, and avocational outcomes.

Discourse is neurologically diffuse and highly susceptible to disruption following brain injury (Coelho, 2007; Tremblay & Dick, 2016; Ylvisaker, et al., 2008). The cognitive-communicative impairments associated with disordered discourse are a result of widely distributed disruptions of neural networks that support the content organization necessary for clear and efficient communication (Wood & Grafman, 2003; Ylvisaker, et al., 2008). Following brain injury, there is a decreased ability to plan, organize, control, and execute the cognitive processes and linguistic components that contribute to a coherent message, on both micro- and macro-structural discourse levels (Coelho et al., 2005;

Coelho, 2002; Ylvisaker et al., 2008). It is not the purpose of this chapter to delve into the minute details of the neuroanatomy underlying discourse; however, a brief summary is provided to illustrate the complexity of the neural architecture underlying these abilities. Discourse processing activates a large network of brain regions bilaterally, which are influenced by a multitude of factors including the temporal characteristics of the discourse message, the genre, the inferencing required, perspective taking, and coherence requirements (Cannizzaro et al., 2012; Cannizzaro & Stephens, 2019; Cannizzaro et al., 2016; Crozier et al., 1999; Ferstl et al., 2008; Ferstl & von Cramon, 2001; Jacoby & Fedorenko, 2020; Tremblay & Dick, 2016). This widespread activity has been described as an extended language network (ELN) that includes and extends far beyond the left peri-sylvian language zone (Ferstl et al., 2008). It entails contributions from the anterior temporal lobes, the dorsomedial prefrontal cortex, parahippocampal gyrus, precuneus, cuneus, lingual gyrus, and portions of the right hemisphere (Ferstl et al., 2008; Tremblay & Dick, 2016). Investigations using functional near-infrared spectroscopy (fNIRS) have revealed activation patterns during discourse production that are greater than those observed during sentence-level language production, and these activation patterns change according to the elicitation task or genre (Cannizzaro et al., 2016). Cortical activation also reflects the complexity, efficiency, and informativeness of the message (Cannizzaro & Stephens, 2019).

After TBI or acquired brain injury (ABI), impairments in executive functions are thought to affect the allocation and control of cognitive resources, resulting in deficits in discourse formulation on multiple levels. Peach and Hanna (2021) found support for this "resource model" of discourse processing in the discourse of adults with moderate to severe TBI, but without aphasia. All discourse samples contained microlinguistic deficits in their narratives regardless of story completeness, and participants whose narratives were mostly complete or mixed complete/incomplete also had deficits in inter-sentential cohesion and intra-sentential pausing. These findings fit with the expected pattern, that "speakers with TBI may focus more on the overall coherence of their narratives (i.e., producing complete stories) and, as a result, are unable to devote sufficient attention to inter-sentential cohesion and sentence production" (Peach & Hanna, 2021, p. 10). Reduced resource allocation and subsequent communication disruptions clearly impact the complex processes of discourse generation, and these challenges are appreciable on both the structural levels (e.g., story completeness) and the sentence-level and inter-sentential-level processing.

Discourse can be complex and time-consuming to measure

Orthographic transcription-based language sample analysis (LSA) has been the "gold standard" of discourse analysis for many years (Bloom & Lahey, 1978; Brown, 1973; Piaget, 1926). This approach to examining language formulation has numerous advantages in that, once it's transcribed, it can be analyzed in many ways. For example, if the clinician is interested in studying grammatical complexity or simply sentence length, there are numerous micro-linguistic measures for that purpose. If the focus is broader, such as how meaning is linked across sentences, macro-linguistic measures such as cohesive adequacy are used. When larger segments of discourse, such as the organization of narratives are the target, macro-structural measures such as story grammar and global coherence may be measured (Cannizzaro & Coelho, 2002; Liles, 1985; Merritt & Liles, 1987). A recent review of the literature on discourse analysis and aphasia reported as many as 536 potential measures (Bryant et al., 2016). In addition, LSA is ecologically valid as it can examine language that occurs in functional, real-world contexts (Heilmann et al., 2010; Miller et al., 2016). Language samples can be elicited from individuals of any age, are sensitive to change over time, can minimize cultural bias, and may be repeated frequently. Discourse from any genre of interest can be studied, making this an ultimately flexible tool to meet the communication needs of almost any individual client.

Despite the usefulness of discourse analysis in the diagnostic process for individuals with TBI, the time-consuming nature of these procedures has proven to be a barrier to widespread clinical adoption. Software advances have streamlined the process somewhat (Miller & Iglesias, 2020) and there are several speech-to-text programs available for transcription. However, Miller et al. report that the *Systematic Analysis of Language Transcripts (SALT)* software staff have examined several of these programs, and concluded that, in some cases, correcting the resulting transcripts can take more time than an experienced transcriber to complete a language sample (i.e., 7–8 minutes to transcribe each minute of an audio recording of a language sample; Miller et al., 2016). Reportedly, only 6.2% of speech-language pathologists across clinical settings use specific tools for examining discourse and 4% report using discourse for measuring treatment outcomes. The primary reasons are the lack of normative data and time required for transcription and analysis (Bryant et al., 2017; Dalton et al., 2020; Frith et al., 2014). Although there have been efforts to find methods that do not rely on transcription analysis (Dalton et al., 2020), most discourse analyses do require transcription and specialized software (Fromm et al., 2020). Other attempts at decreasing the amount of time necessary for discourse analyses have involved comparing the validity of shorter versus longer language samples. For example, samples containing 100, 50, 25, and 12 utterances were found to be highly correlated for mean length of utterance for morphemes and words (MLUu & MLUw; Thordardottir, 2015). Fortunately, 1- and 3-minute samples were found to be as reliable as 7-minute samples for certain discourse measures (Heilmann et al., 2010).

Although there are discourse assessment tools normed for use with children (Gillam & Pearson, 2017; Gillam et al., 2017) and for adults with aphasia (Doyle et al., 2000; McNeil et al., 2001), none are currently available for adults with TBI. Therefore, it may be more accurate and valid to create empirically derived combinations of tools, as this has been effectively implemented in child language assessment (see Chapter 4 as well as Oetting et al., 2008; Spaudling et al., 2006). Such a battery would be most particularly useful to assess discourse across genres, as some individuals may have difficulty with some genres (e.g., social transactional genres such as a conversation or persuasion) and not with others (i.e., monologic genres such as procedural, expository, or narrative stories). In addition, much of the research on discourse formulation has used stimuli that are arguably too simple and potentially overly familiar, including picture description tasks, retelling fictional narratives (e.g., Cinderella), procedural narrative tasks (e.g., how to make a peanut butter and jelly sandwich) yielding an impression that discourse abilities are intact. Discourse has a variety of genres (conversation, expository, procedural, persuasive, personal narrative, and fictional narrative) that arguably have a broad utility, but research has primarily focused on story narratives with much less ecological validity. For example, expository narratives were found to be equally or more neurologically demanding than story narratives (Jacoby & Fedorenko, 2020) and have much higher legitimacy as part of everyday communication. Outside the world of professional writers, it is a much less frequent occurrence that an adult is tasked with the communication demands of generating a fictional narrative.

Regarding the measurement of discourse performance, there is a great deal of variation in the analyses used. Pritchard and colleagues reported on the psychometric properties of acceptability, reliability, and validity of discourse measures of information content. The authors described 58 measures and found no reports on acceptability, little information on reliability (i.e., test-retest, intra- and inter-rater), but overall high content validity (Pritchard et al., 2017). This same group also examined properties of a non-fiction discourse measure derived from the "Autobiographical incident memories" section of the *Autobiographical Memory Interview* (AMI; Kopelman et al., 1990). The measure includes three genres: descriptive (two picture descriptions), procedural (two procedural discourses), and personal (nine personal discourses). They used this measure to examine microstructural and macrostructural characteristics among 17 adults with mild to moderate aphasia, and found high levels of acceptability, reliability, and validity (Pritchard et al., 2018). Along similar lines, Boyle (2020) introduced a seven-question procedure to help clinicians determine which outcome measure would be best suited for different clients. The questions focus on linguistic variables (e.g., micro- versus macrostructure), discourse genre, and psychometric properties (e.g., reliability, sensitivity) of the specific measures, all of critical importance to help direct clinical decision-making. Discourse analysis has recently been applied for the detection of subtle differences between mild cognitive impairment and healthy aging (Kim, B. S. et al., 2019). This same research team also identified a short list (25 words) of core function words and noted that persons with aphasia produced fewer of the core function words than the control group, and that core function word use was strongly correlated with aphasia severity. While not directly focused on CCD, there is clear applicability to discourse impairments occurring in the absence of aphasia. Clearly more attention needs to be focused on developing a core set of psychometrically sound discourse measures that are widely used by researchers so findings across studies can be readily compared.

Elicitation techniques

Research remains sparse on discourse genres other than fictional narrative, but it is critical for clinicians to assess more than a single discourse type (Sherratt, 2007), and several discourse genres can provide clinicians with more ecologically valid language samples (e.g., personal narratives, event recasts, complex procedural discourse, conversation). These genres appear frequently in everyday communication (Cannizzaro & Stephens, 2019; McCabe et al., 2008). Genres are defined as "different ways of using language to achieve different culturally established tasks" (Eggins & Martin, 1997, p. 234). Therefore, different genres of discourse will have different social purposes and pressures, communicative contexts, as well as different word use, syntax demands, organizational patterns, and pragmatic intentions.

Sampling a variety of discourse genres comes with challenges related to multiple elicitation methods and assessment techniques necessary to collect and analyze communication samples for clinical and research purposes. This is further exacerbated by the fact that non-standardized assessment measures may better capture the subtle nature of the cognitive-communication impairments for many of the discourse deficits experienced after TBI (Coelho et al., 2005; Lundine & Hall, 2020). This may be challenging for the clinician who wants to characterize the communication impairment for assessment and treatment purposes, but is not familiar with the great variety of standardized and non-standardized tools often used for these purposes (Coelho et al., 2005). It can be problematic to compare different genres unless content and structural differences are accounted for. Fortunately, tools such as the *Curtin University Discourse Protocol* (CUDP) have been developed to elicit multiple genres, in a standard, replicable manner (Whitworth et al., 2015). These genres have organizational structures that introduce and conclude the discourse, with elements in the body of the discourse that provide steps, facts, events, or opinion statements. The CUDP includes a multi-genre design that can be easily applied to healthy adults, to provide a common framework to characterize the organization and structure of communication across genres. Assessing communication across genre provides a wealth of information, and evidence suggests that genre exerts significant influence on discourse production (Cannizzaro & Stephens, 2019; Hill et al., 2021). Self- and other report measures also provide a method for the analysis of discourse that is not necessarily dependent on genre.

Analysis methods

Analysis of discourse samples is organized into three levels summarized later, with examples of measures:

1. Microlinguistic (or microstructural) measures: word- or sentence-level processes, such as word choice, syntactic complexity and diversity, grammaticality, sentence complexity, lexical diversity, lexical errors, some

measures of productivity (MLU). Note that some measures straddle the micro- and macrolinguistic levels, such as cohesion (reference and conjunction use).

2. Macrolinguistic (or macrostructural): beyond sentence-level processes that relate to the overall content of the discourse; central theme, "gist" (e.g., global coherence), informativeness, completeness.

3. Superstructure: the overall organization of the discourse: story grammar, organization, structured event complex.

Transcription-based analysis

Some measures combine information from more than one level, for example, efficiency, which can be measured as correct information units per minute (CIU/min): whether the information is "correct" or not is a macrolinguistic decision, whereas the speed component (number of units per minute) is a microlinguistic measure. Differences in the discourse of non-brain-injured adults compared to adults with TBI have been found in all three levels, but in general the "macro"-level measures are more salient for identification and characterization of non-aphasic disruptions in discourse (Coelho, 2002). Microlinguistic levels of analysis are more common and perhaps more useful in aphasia, and as Steel and Togher (2018) noted that they "may be less relevant for other assessment purposes after TBI . . . and may not be a priority for use in intervention" (Steel & Togher, 2018, p. 51). Table 9.1 contains the most common microlinguistic and macrolinguistic discourse analysis methods, most of which require orthographic transcription. Non-transcription-based and holistic measures are described afterward. On a practical note, transcription will be quicker and less effortful when the clinician is clear on the methodology for segmenting language samples (using T-units or C-units). A T-unit ("minimal terminable unit") is defined as one main clause plus any subordinate clause or non-clausal structure that is attached to or embedded in the sentence (Hunt, 1965); a T-unit is similar to a sentence but prevents the problem of continuous joining of clauses. A C-unit (communication unit) is an independent clause with its subordinate clauses and modifiers (Loban, 1976). C-units are different from "utterances" because they provide more information for syntactic analysis, and unlike T-units, C-units can include partial sentences or single-word responses (e.g., "yes," "ok," "tired."). So the purpose of the analysis may drive the analysis type.

There are several other transcription-based analysis methods that do not fit under the discourse characteristics listed in Table 9.1, many of which are specific to the discourse genre being studied, for example:

- Topic management (avoiding repetitions, disruptive topic shifts, diversions) for conversation and personal narratives (Dijkstra et al., 2004)
- Quality or "Story Goodness Index" for narratives (Coelho et al., 2012; Lê et al., 2011; Lindsey et al., 2019)

- Monitoring Indicators of Scholarly Language (MISL) for written expository discourse (Gillam et al., 2017)
- Index of Narrative Microstructure (INMIS) for personal or fictional narratives (Justice et al., 2006).
- Curtin University Discourse Protocol (CUDP; Whitworth et al., 2015); and Curtin University Discourse Protocol-Adolescent (CUDP-A; Hill et al., 2020) assess discourse across genres, focusing on analysis of cohesion and coherence.

Non-transcription-based analysis

Despite the advantages of transcription-based measures, there are many non-transcription-based methods of analysis that provide additional important or unique information. Non-transcription-based methods can also allow incorporating the individual's own perception of their discourse, and such self-reporting of deficits and outcomes are central to person- or family-centered care (Boyle, 2020). The World Health Organization (WHO) uses a model of health and functioning that integrates those two domains in the International Classification of Functioning, Disability and Health (ICF; World Health Organization, 2001), and WHODAS 2.0 (World Health Organization, 2010), and recommends centering the patient perspective. This is best accomplished with patient questionnaires and family-centered input, such as the *La Trobe Communication Questionnaire* (LCQ; Douglas et al., 2000, 2007b).

Iwashita and Sohlberg (2019) compared two clinical rating scales of "dyadic interaction"; the *Pragmatics Rating Scale (PRS)* and the *Profile of Pragmatic Impairment in Communication (PPIC),* and found comparable clinical results but higher "clinical feasibility" in the PRS, as measured by mean completion time per sample and ratings on a clinical feasibility survey. Kim et al. (2020) devised a method of assessing discourse in people with aphasia that does not require transcription and coding. The authors measured function word use (e.g., pronouns, determiners, prepositions, conjunctions, adverbs, verb inflections, and auxiliary verbs) and created a "core function word" list by the ranking top 25 most frequent function words used by typical controls used while describing two wordless picture books (Kim et al., 2020). By comparing core function word use between controls and PWA, they found that the age- and education-matched healthy controls performed significantly better on core function word production than PWA. This type of analysis tool may have applicability for measuring function word use in discourse use in general, beyond those aphasic impairments. Another type of transcription-free discourse analysis can be conducted using modification of the *Montréal Protocol for the Evaluation of Communication (MEC;* Kim, J. et al., 2019). This is a self-reported subjective rating of discourse (SR-D) developed for adults with amnestic mild cognitive impairment (aMCI) that has been compared to objective discourse measures in the genres of picture description, dialogue, and procedural discourse. Using just ten items from this scale related to cognitive dysfunction and language processing

Table 9.1 Selective list of discourse characteristics and analysis methods.

Discourse characteristic	Description	Units of analysis
Microlinguistic Fluency	Speed, presence of pauses or mazes	Total time (Matsuoka et al., 2012) T-units per minute (Scott & Windsor, 2000) Words/minute (speech rate) Percent T-units with mazes (Galetto et al., 2013) Pause time (Peach, 2013)
Lexical diversity (also referred to as semantic complexity)	The diversity of words and vocabulary	Number of different words (NDW) per 100 words (Scott & Windsor, 2000) Number of different word roots (NDW) in the first 50 words (Koutsoftas & Gray, 2012) Type-token ratio (TTR) Propositional density (Stark, 2019)
Productivity (also "amount of talk," AOT)	The overall amount of discourse	C-units per narrative (Ghayoumi Anaraki et al., 2014) Total number of words (TNW) or total number of T-units (Justice et al., 2006; Scott & Windsor, 2000)
Cohesion (also referred to as local coherence)	Use of lexical or grammatical ties to connect sentences with each other in a passage	Cohesive ties per C-unit = Cohesive adequacy (Peach & Coelho, 2016) % cohesion errors (Galetto et al., 2013)
Efficiency	The combination of speed and content accuracy	correct information units (CIUs) per minute (Matsuoka et al., 2012; Milman et al., 2020; Nicholas & Brookshire, 1993) T-units with core or supplemental elements/total T-units (Cannizzaro et al., 2016)

Macrolinguistic

Term	Definition	Measure
Coherence (also called global coherence)	The relation of sentences to the overall theme (i.e., not tangential, incongruent, repetitive)	4-point global coherence rating scale (*Wright et al., 2014; see Table 9.2 of that article*)
Informativeness (also called completeness, content accuracy)	The number or percent of words that convey accurate/relevant lexical information	% lexical information units (Galetto et al., 2013; Marini et al., 2017) % thematic units produced (Kintz et al., 2018)
Completeness	Presence of essential elements in the discourse	# essential plot elements (Canfield et al., 2016) number of essential steps (in procedural discourse; Snow et al., 1997). Main event analysis, or main concept analysis (Capilouto et al., 2005; Dalton et al., 2020; Nicholas & Brookshire, 1995)

Superstructure

Term	Definition	Measure
Organization (story grammar)	The organization and logical relationships between characters and events	Story grammar: number of complete episodes (Cannizzaro & Coelho, 2002; Roth & Spekman, 1986) Proportion of T-units within episode structure (TUP): number of T-units that convey an essential episode component, divided by total number of T-units (Cannizzaro et al., 2016; Cannizzaro & Coelho, 2013; Galetto et al., 2013) Six-traits writing rubric (Koutsoftas & Gray, 2012) T-units within episode (Coelho, 2002)

Note: Mazes are speech disruptions such as filled pauses, partial or whole-word repetitions, and revisions (Loban, 1976).

(i.e., word-finding problems/incorrect choice of words, no self-correction of word errors, imprecise expression of ideas, inappropriate topic switches, lack of verbal initiative, excessive talking, repetitiveness, interruptions, loses track of conversation, speech rate too slow), this scale significantly differentiates the discourse of persons with and without mild cognitive impairment (Kim, J. et al., 2019). As memory impairment is a chief complaint and prevalent neuropsychological feature post TBI, and often implicated in disrupted discourse, this abbreviated tool holds promise for transcription free discourse assessment post-TBI.

Holistic analysis

In addition to the non-transcription-based and the transcription-based linguistic measures described earlier, there are holistic measures of discourse analysis. *Clinical Discourse Analysis* (CDA; Damico, 1991) is a conversational sampling procedure that can help analyze social communication, specifically conversation, at the descriptive level. It requires detailed interpretation, and the author is careful to point out that CDA

> is not a tool that can be employed solely to obtain quantitative data . . . interpretation requires a knowledge and analysis of complex conversational strategies and variables. . . . Data interpretation should be based on patterns not numbers.
>
> (Damico, 1997)

The Six Traits Writing Rubric (STWR; Koutsoftas & Gray, 2012) is another holistic measure that assesses written discourse in six traits: (1) Ideas and content, (2) Organization, (3) Voice, (4) Word choice, (5) Sentence fluency, (6) Conventions, and may be useful in assessing individuals who regularly use writing in their work or personal life. This is another excellent choice for discourse analysis when conversational abilities are prominently impaired.

Formulated discourse is highly responsive to the elicitation method

Confusion regarding discourse analysis may arise due to the variety of elicitation methods used, as well as the overly simplistic nature of some of the stimulus methods. For example, different elicitation methods usually elicit different genres of discourse, which in turn elicit different linguistic characteristics (e.g., story grammar, length, complexity, gist). Even within a single genre (such as "narrative"), there may be large differences between a personal narrative, a fictional narrative, and a "culturally entrenched" narrative such as retelling the *Cinderella* story (Armstrong, 2000, p. 885). Commonly used elicitation methods include picture and picture sequence descriptions (Capilouto et al., 2005; Coelho et al., 1994; Coelho, 1995; Nicholas & Brookshire, 1993), story generation based on a single picture, story retelling (Ulatowska et al., 1981; Williams et al., 1994), relating a well-known fictional narrative (commonly the *Cinderella* story; Byng et al., 1994), spontaneous prompts for personal narratives, "tell me about a memorable experience" (Ulatowska et al., 1981), or simple procedural tasks such as describing how to make a peanut butter sandwich, brush your teeth, or withdraw money from an ATM machine (Williams et al., 1994). Further, many elicitation methods are overly short and simple, meaning that all but the most severely impaired will experience a "ceiling" effect (Body & Perkins, 2004). When individuals perform above the ceiling level, the measures of discourse performance can have inadequate sensitivity and run the risk of type II errors. Simple tasks will elicit simple discourse, among all adults, with or without brain injury. Compare for example the procedural prompt, "explain how to make a peanut butter and jelly sandwich" versus common tenth-grade writing prompts: "Explain why some teens commit suicide; Explain how music affects your life; Explain why dealing with their parents' divorce can be difficult for many teens." Scott and Windsor (2000) noted that in school-aged children, expository discourse was shorter, less fluent (e.g., percent of T-units with mazes), more complex (e.g., words per T-unit), and more error prone than narrative discourse. Clinicians will want to use stimulus materials that elicit the problem being investigated and with prompts that have the complexity to reveal discourse impairments in the genres and levels that are appropriate for the client.

Regarding discourse measures, it has been reported that measures from both conversation (e.g., comments, and adequate-plus responses) and narration (e.g., T-units within episode structure) were able to discriminate between adults with brain injury and non-brain injured controls (Coelho et al., 2003). Several researchers have recommended that discourse not be measured using solely fictional narration or conversation genres (Malone et al., 2008; Nippold et al., 2008). Similarly, differences have been reported in the informativeness of discourse across multiple genres, which also argues in favor of multi-genre assessment (Cannizzaro & Stephens, 2019). These investigators also found a negative relationship between discourse efficiency and neurovascular activation, suggesting that discourse formulation, like certain motor movements, becomes less "effortful" as efficiency increases (Cannizzaro & Stephens, 2019). Therefore, discourse efficiency may be a particularly useful measure in adults with TBI, and is measurable across genres.

To address the importance of recognizing the diversity of discourse forms produced by adolescents, Hill et al. (2020) developed the *Curtin University Discourse Protocol-Adolescent* (CUDP-A). This tool examines discourse in four genres (i.e., recount, expository, persuasive, and narrative) and this format facilitates differentiation of typical spoken discourse skills from those of clinical populations, including those with acquired brain injury or developmental disorders (Hill et al., 2020). Wallis and colleagues used a moral dilemma task in which participants responded to short stories (a single paragraph of about 8–10 sentences) that contained a moral dilemma for one of the characters (Wallis et al., 2021); these discourse samples were analyzed for form (verbal productivity and syntactic complexity), content (semantic diversity and word percentages in three semantic domains: affective, social, and cognitive), and language use based on Bloom's revised taxonomy of thinking (Level 1: remembering/understanding; level 2: Applying/analyzing; level 3: Evaluating/creating). Although there were no differences between younger and older adolescents in the language form or content, there was a difference in language use; younger adolescents demonstrated a significantly higher proportion of utterances at Level 1 (remembering and understanding), while the older age group produced a higher proportion at Level 3 (evaluating and creating). These findings all support the contention that discourse performance is influenced by elicitation task and analysis measures selected. These factors need consideration when interpreting findings of analyses.

Recommendations for practicing clinicians: options for efficient assessment and effective treatment

The assessment of discourse following TBI should examine discourse across genres, primarily oral discourse production but also extending to written discourse and comprehension, if appropriate and relevant for the client. In addition, information should be gathered from patient self-report, close other report, and clinically measured tools. There are valid and reliable options that do not rely on orthographic transcription, but clinicians should not shy away from transcription-based measures. Such measures, with minor modifications, are clinically feasible and do not take more time to transcribe, analyze, and interpret than other standardized language tests. An international group of researchers and clinicians (i.e., INCOG) convened to develop clinical practice guidelines for cognitive rehabilitation post-traumatic brain injury (Togher, Wiseman-Hakes et al., 2014). The INCOG expert panel provided guidelines for treatment of discourse after brain injury. This group consensus suggests that intervention should consider premorbid communication status, be individualized to the person's needs, goals, and skills, provide training in use of assistive technology where appropriate; include training of communication partners, and occur in context to minimize the need for generalization, that is, be contextualized and involve personally relevant materials (Steel et al., 2021). Note that although there are no omnibus norm-referenced tests of discourse-level communication after TBI, empirically derived combinations of tools can provide time-effective assessment and treatment monitoring in adults and adolescents. As is often the case in the field of communication sciences and disorders, much of the research on discourse impairment has been focused on assessment rather than intervention. Table 9.2 contains a suggested checklist for a sequence of actions and tools for assessment and treatment.

Regarding discourse treatment, there are several published approaches that target communication beyond the word and sentence level. These procedures include an integrated treatment of fluency and word retrieval of target words in the context of sentences (Milman et al., 2020), an intervention addressing

Table 9.2 Selected discourse assessment and treatment approaches.

Assessment and treatment approaches	References
1. Use the Cognitive Communication Checklist for Acquired Brain Injury (CCCABI) screening, identification, and referral tool.	(MacDonald, 2021)
2. Use a self-report and other-report measure (e.g., La Trobe Communication Questionnaire).	(Douglas et al., 2007a)
3. Assess at least three genres of discourse (conversation, expository, procedural, persuasive, personal narrative, fictional narrative).	(Hill et al., 2020; Pritchard et al., 2018)
4. Use transcription-based measures see transcription and analysis checklists in appendices of Whitworth et al., 2015.	(Heilmann et al., 2010; Miller & Iglesias, 2020)
5. Use TBI Bank (https://tbi.talkbank. org/) from within TalkBank (https:// talkbank.org/). Clinicians can use it to transcribe faster and more accurately, and run multiple analyses with a click.	(MacWhinney, 2019; Togher, Elbourne et al., 2014)
6. Analyze the selected genres for relevant communication characteristics: fluency, lexical diversity, cohesion, coherence, productivity, informativeness, efficiency, organization, completeness, or other (see Table 9.1).	(Bryant et al., 2016, 2017) for overview.
7. For patients who are greater than 3 months post-injury, assess health-related quality of life, using for example the QOLIBRI.	(von Steinbüchel et al., 2010)
8. In planning treatment, use the cognitive-communication competence model that summarizes the complex array of influences on communication to provide a holistic view of communication competence after ABI.	(MacDonald, 2017)
9. Determine the communication characteristic(s) needing treatment, and choose a treatment that addresses that characteristic. For example, Cannizzaro and Coelho described a treatment of organization (story grammar).	(Cannizzaro & Coelho, 2002)
10. Refer to the two excellent reviews of interventions using impairment-specific and context-sensitive approaches.	(Finch et al., 2016; Steel et al., 2021)

emotion processing (Radice-Neumann et al., 2009), a project-based treatment of communication after ABI (Behn et al., 2019), Group Interactive Structured Treatment (GIST): an intervention targeting social competence after brain injury (Hawley & Newman, 2010), Metacognitive Strategy Instruction

(MSI; Copley et al., 2015), a Communication-specific Coping Intervention (CommCope-I) targeting coping in the context of communication breakdown (Douglas et al., 2019), Communication partner training, which was shown to improve communication interactions in two randomized controlled trials (Behn et al., 2012; Togher et al., 2013), and Cognitive Pragmatic Treatment (Bosco et al., 2018; Parola et al., 2019), a social communication program with components that target discourse. It is important to emphasize that there is no one treatment that is appropriate for all individuals with discourse deficits. Intervention decisions should be based on careful and thorough assessments, the individual's communicative strengths and weaknesses, their personal history, and everyday communicative needs.

Conclusion

The practicing clinician has long faced a cloud of uncertainty when attempting to assess and treat discourse-level communication impairments. Discourse is wide-ranging, context-specific, heterogeneous, and currently there is no single omnibus assessment that could purport to be representative of complex interactive communication in real-world pragmatic contexts. It is likely that discourse is best assessed and treated using empirically derived combinations of tools including the insight of the patient and others in their close circle. This will allow areas of impairment that have previously been endured in isolation to be recognized, assessed, and appropriately treated.

References

Aboud, K. S., Bailey, S. K., Del Tufo, S. N., Barquero, L. A., & Cutting, L. E. (2019). Fairy tales versus facts: Genre matters to the developing brain. *Cerebral Cortex (New York, NY: 1991)*, *29*(11), 4877–4888. https://doi.org/10.1093/cercor/bhz025

Al-Hassani, A., Strandvik, G. F., El-Menyar, A., Dhumale, A. R., Asim, M., Ajaj, A., Al-Yazeedi, W., & Al-Thani, H. (2018). Functional outcomes in moderate-to-severe traumatic brain injury survivors. *Journal of Emergencies, Trauma, and Shock*, *11*(3), 197–204. https://doi.org/10.4103/JETS.JETS_6_18

American Speech-Language Hearing Association (ASHA). (2003). *Technical report: Evaluating and treating communication and cognitive disorders*. American Speech-Language-Hearing Association. www./policy/tr2003-00137/

Anderson, S. A. S., Hawes, D. J., & Snow, P. C. (2016). Language impairments among youth offenders: A systematic review. *Children and Youth Services Review*, *65*, 195–203. https://doi.org/10.1016/j.childyouth.2016.04.004

Armstrong, E. (2000). Aphasic discourse analysis: The story so far. *Aphasiology*, *14*(9), 875–892. https://doi.org/10.1080/02687030050127685

Behn, N., Marshall, J., Togher, L., & Cruice, M. (2019). Feasibility and initial efficacy of project-based treatment for people with ABI. *International Journal of Language & Communication Disorders*, *54*(3), 465–478. https://doi.org/10.1111/1460-6984.12452

Behn, N., Togher, L., Power, E., & Heard, R. (2012). Evaluating communication training for paid carers of people with traumatic brain injury. *Brain Injury*, *26*(13–14), 1702–1715. https://doi.org/10.3109/02699052.2012.722258

Bloom, L., & Lahey, M. (1978). *Language development and language disorders*. Wiley.

Body, R., & Perkins, M. R. (2004). Validation of linguistic analyses in narrative discourse after traumatic brain injury. *Brain Injury*, *18*(7), 707–724. https://doi.org/10.1080/0269 9050310001596914

Bosco, F. M., Parola, A., Angeleri, R., Galetto, V., Zettin, M., & Gabbatore, I. (2018). Improvement of communication skills after traumatic brain injury: The efficacy of the cognitive pragmatic treatment program using the communicative activities of daily living. *Archives of Clinical Neuropsychology*, *33*(7), 875–888. https://doi.org/10.1093/arclin/acy041

Boyle, M. (2020). Choosing discourse outcome measures to assess clinical change. *Seminars in Speech and Language*, *41*(1), 1–9. https://doi.org/10.1055/s-0039-3401029

Brown, J., & Knollman-Porter, K. (2019). Evaluating cognitive-linguistic postconcussion in adults: Contributions of self-report and standardized measures. *Topics in Language Disorders*, *39*(3), 239–256. https://doi.org/10.1097/TLD.0000000000000186

Brown, R. (1973). *A first language: The early stages*. Harvard University Press.

Bryant, L., Ferguson, A., & Spencer, E. (2016). Linguistic analysis of discourse in aphasia: A review of the literature. *Clinical Linguistics & Phonetics*, *30*(7), 489–518. https://doi.org /10.3109/02699206.2016.1145740

Bryant, L., Spencer, E., & Ferguson, A. (2017). Clinical use of linguistic discourse analysis for the assessment of language in aphasia. *Aphasiology*, *31*(10), 1105–1126. https://doi.org /10.1080/02687038.2016.1239013

Byng, S., Nickels, L., & Black, M. (1994). Replicating therapy for mapping deficits in agrammatism: Remapping the deficit? *Aphasiology*, *8*, 315–341. https://doi.org/10.1080/ 02687039408248663

Canfield, A. R., Eigsti, I.-M., de Marchena, A., & Fein, D. (2016). Story goodness in adolescents with autism spectrum disorder (ASD) and in optimal outcomes from ASD. *Journal of Speech, Language, and Hearing Research: JSLHR*, *59*(3), 533–545. https://doi. org/10.1044/2015_JSLHR-L-15-0022

Cannizzaro, M. S., & Coelho, C. A. (2002). Treatment of story grammar following traumatic brain injury: A pilot study. *Brain Injury*, *16*(12), 1065–1073. https://doi. org/10.1080/02699050210155230

Cannizzaro, M. S., & Coelho, C. A. (2013). Analysis of narrative discourse structure as an ecologically relevant measure of executive function in adults. *Journal of Psycholinguistic Research*, *42*(6), 527–549. https://doi.org/10.1007/s10936-012-9231-5

Cannizzaro, M. S., Dumas, J., Prelock, P., & Newhouse, P. (2012). Organizational structure reduces processing load in the prefrontal cortex during discourse processing of written text: Implications for high-level reading issues after TBI. *Perspectives on Neurophysiology and Neurogenic Speech and Language Disorders*, *22*(2), 67–78. https://doi.org/10.1044/nnsld22.2.67

Cannizzaro, M. S., & Stephens, S. R. (2019). Discourse formulation and neurovascular activation across four genres. *Clinical Archives of Communication Disorders*, *4*(1), 10–20. https:// doi.org/10.21849/cacd.2019.00017

Cannizzaro, M. S., Stephens, S. R., Breidenstein, M., & Crovo, C. (2016). Prefrontal cortical activity during discourse processing: An observational fNIRS study. *Topics in Language Disorders*, *36*(1), 65–79. https://doi.org/10.1097/TLD.0000000000000082

Capilouto, G., Wright, H. H., & Wagovich, S. A. (2005). CIU and main event analyses of the structured discourse of older and younger adults. *Journal of Communication Disorders*, *38*(6), 431–444. https://doi.org/10.1016/j.jcomdis.2005.03.005

Centers for Disease Control and Prevention. (2015). *Report to congress on traumatic brain injury in the United States: Epidemiology and rehabilitation* (pp. 1–72). CDC. www.cdc.gov/trau maticbraininjury/pdf/tbi_report_to_congress_epi_and_rehab-a.pdf

Coelho, C. A. (1995). Discourse production deficits following traumatic brain injury: A critical review of the recent literature. *Aphasiology, 9*(5), 409–429. https://doi.org/10.1080/02687039508248707

Coelho, C. A. (2002). Story narratives of adults with closed head injury and non-brain-injured adults. *Journal of Speech, Language, and Hearing Research, 45*(6), 1232–1248. https://doi.org/10.1044/1092-4388(2002/099)

Coelho, C. A. (2007). Management of discourse deficits following traumatic brain injury: Progress, caveats, and needs. *Seminars in Speech and Language, 28*(2), 122–135. https://doi.org/10.1055/s-2007-970570

Coelho, C. A., Grela, B., Corso, M., Gamble, A., & Feinn, R. (2005). Microlinguistic deficits in the narrative discourse of adults with traumatic brain injury. *Brain Injury, 19*(13), 1139–1145. https://doi.org/10.1080/02699050500110678

Coelho, C. A., Lê, K., Mozeiko, J., Krueger, F., & Grafman, J. (2012). Discourse production following injury to the dorsolateral prefrontal cortex. *Neuropsychologia, 50*(14), 3564–3572. https://doi.org/10.1016/j.neuropsychologia.2012.09.005

Coelho, C. A., Liles, B. Z., Duffy, R. J., Clarkson, J. V., & Elia, D. (1994). Longitudinal assessment of narrative discourse in a mildly aphasic adult. *Clinical Aphasiology, 22*, 145–155.

Coelho, C. A., Youse, K., Le, K., & Feinn, R. (2003). Narrative and conversational discourse of adults with closed head injuries and non-brain-injured adults: A discriminant analysis. *Aphasiology, 17*(5), 499–510. https://doi.org/10.1080/02687030344000111

Copley, A., Smith, K., Savill, K., & Finch, E. (2015). Does metacognitive strategy instruction improve impaired receptive cognitive-communication skills following acquired brain injury? *Brain Injury, 29*(11), 1309–1316. https://doi.org/10.3109/02699052.2015.1043343

Crewe-Brown, S. J., Stipinovich, A. M., & Zsilavecz, U. (2011). Communication after mild traumatic brain injury—a spouse's perspective. *Journal of Communication Disorders—Die Suid-Afrikaanse Tydskrif Vir Kommunikasieafwykings, 1*, 48–55.

Crozier, S., Sirigu, A., Lehéricy, S., van de Moortele, P. F., Pillon, B., Grafman, J., Agid, Y., Dubois, B., & LeBihan, D. (1999). Distinct prefrontal activations in processing sequence at the sentence and script level: An fMRI study. *Neuropsychologia, 37*(13), 1469–1476. https://doi.org/10.1016/s0028-3932(99)00054-8

Dalton, S. G. H., Hubbard, H. I., & Richardson, J. D. (2020). Moving toward non-transcription based discourse analysis in stable and progressive aphasia. *Seminars in Speech and Language, 41*(1), 32–44. https://doi.org/10.1055/s-0039-3400990

Damico, J. S. (1991). Clinical discourse analysis: A functional approach to language assessment. In C. S. Simon (Ed.), *Communication skills and classroom success: Assessment and therapy methodologies for language and learning disabled students*. Thinking Publications.

Damico, J. S. (1997). *Clinical discourse analysis.* https://userweb.ucs.louisiana.edu/~jsd6498/damico/damico-cda.html

Dijkstra, K., Bourgeois, M. S., Allen, R. S., & Burgio, L. D. (2004). Conversational coherence discourse analysis of older adults with and without dementia. *Journal of Neurolinguistics, 17*(4), 263–283. https://doi.org/10.1016/S0911-6044(03)00048-4

Dikmen, S., Machamer, J., & Temkin, N. (2017). Mild traumatic brain injury: Longitudinal study of cognition, functional status, and post-traumatic symptoms. *Journal of Neurotrauma, 34*(8), 1524–1530. https://doi.org/10.1089/neu.2016.4618

Dipper, L., Marshall, J., Boyle, M., Hersh, D., Botting, N., & Cruice, M. (2021). Creating a theoretical framework to underpin discourse assessment and intervention in aphasia. *Brain Sciences, 11*(2). https://doi.org/10.3390/brainsci11020183

Douglas, J. M., Bracy, C. A., & Snow, P. C. (2007a). Measuring perceived communicative ability after traumatic brain injury: Reliability and validity of the La Trobe communication questionnaire. *The Journal of Head Trauma Rehabilitation, 22*(1), 31–38. https://doi.org/10.1097/00001199-200701000-00004

Douglas, J. M., Bracy, C. A., & Snow, P. C. (2007b). Exploring the factor structure of the La Trobe communication questionnaire: Insights into the nature of communication deficits following traumatic brain injury. *Aphasiology, 21*(12), 1181–1194. https://doi.org/10.1080/02687030600980950

Douglas, J. M., Bracy, C. A., & Snow, P. C. (2016). Return to work and social communication ability following severe traumatic brain injury. *Journal of Speech, Language, and Hearing Research: JSLHR, 59*(3), 511–520. https://doi.org/10.1044/2015_JSLHR-L-15-0025

Douglas, J. M., Knox, L., De Maio, C., Bridge, H., Drummond, M., & Whiteoak, J. (2019). Effectiveness of communication-specific coping intervention for adults with traumatic brain injury: Preliminary results. *Neuropsychological Rehabilitation, 29*(1), 73–91. https://doi.org/10.1080/09602011.2016.1259114

Douglas, J. M., O'Flaherty, C. A., & Snow, P. C. (2000). Measuring perception of communicative ability: The development and evaluation of the La Trobe communication questionnaire. *Aphasiology, 14*(3), 251–268. https://doi.org/10.1080/026870300401469

Doyle, P. J., McNeil, M. R., Park, G., Goda, A., Rubenstein, E., Spencer, K., Carroll, B., Lustig, A., & Szwarc, L. (2000). Linguistic validation of four parallel forms of a story retelling procedure. *Aphasiology, 14*(5–6), 537–549. https://doi.org/10.1080/026870300401306

Eggins, S., & Martin, J. R. (1997). Genres and registers of discourse. In T. van Dijk (Ed.), *Discourse as structure and process: Discourse studies: A multidisciplinary introduction* (Vol. 1, pp. 230–256). Sage. https://doi.org/10.4135/9781446221884

Elbourn, E., Kenny, B., Power, E., & Togher, L. (2019). Psychosocial outcomes of severe traumatic brain injury in relation to discourse recovery: A longitudinal study up to 1 year post-injury. *American Journal of Speech-Language Pathology, 28*(4), 1463–1478. https://doi.org/10.1044/2019_AJSLP-18-0204

Ferstl, E. C., Neumann, J., Bogler, C., & von Cramon, D. Y. (2008). The extended language network: A meta-analysis of neuroimaging studies on text comprehension. *Human Brain Mapping, 29*(5), 581–593. https://doi.org/10.1002/hbm.20422

Ferstl, E. C., & von Cramon, D. Y. (2001). The role of coherence and cohesion in text comprehension: An event-related fMRI study. Brain Research. *Cognitive Brain Research, 11*(3), 325–340.

Finch, E., Copley, A., Cornwell, P., & Kelly, C. (2016). Systematic review of behavioral interventions targeting social communication difficulties after traumatic brain injury. *Archives of Physical Medicine and Rehabilitation, 97*(8), 1352–1365. https://doi.org/10.1016/j.apmr.2015.11.005

Frith, M., Togher, L., Ferguson, A., Levick, W., & Docking, K. (2014). Assessment practices of speech-language pathologists for cognitive communication disorders following traumatic brain injury in adults: An international survey. *Brain Injury, 28*(13–14), 1657–1666. https://doi.org/10.3109/02699052.2014.947619

Fromm, D., Forbes, M., Holland, A., & MacWhinney, B. (2020). Using AphasiaBank for discourse assessment. *Seminars in Speech and Language, 41*(1), 10–19. https://doi.org/10.1055/s-0039-3399499

Galetto, V., Andreetta, S., Zettin, M., & Marini, A. (2013). Patterns of impairment of narrative language in mild traumatic brain injury. *Journal of Neurolinguistics, 26*(6), 649–661. https://doi.org/10.1016/j.jneuroling.2013.05.004

Galski, T., Tompkins, C., & Johnston, M. V. (1998). Competence in discourse as a measure of social integration and quality of life in persons with traumatic brain injury. *Brain Injury*, *12*(9), 769–782.

Ghayoumi Anaraki, Z., Marini, A., Yadegari, F., Mahmoodi Bakhtiari, B., Fakharian, E., Rahgozar, M., & Rassouli, M. (2014). Narrative discourse impairments in Persian-speaking persons with traumatic brain injury: A pilot study. *Folia Phoniatrica et Logopaedica: Official Organ of the International Association of Logopedics and Phoniatrics (IALP)*, *66*(6), 273–279. https://doi.org/10.1159/000371443

Gillam, R. B., & Pearson, N. A. (2017). *Test of narrative language* (2nd ed.). Pro-Ed. www.proedinc.com/Products/14560/tnl2-test-of-narrative-languagesecond-edition.aspx

Gillam, S. L., Gillam, R. B., Fargo, J. D., Olszewski, A., & Segura, H. (2017). Monitoring indicators of scholarly language: A progress-monitoring instrument for measuring narrative discourse skills. *Communication Disorders Quarterly*, *38*(2), 96–106. https://doi.org/10.1177/1525740116651442

Hawley, L. A., & Newman, J. K. (2010). Group interactive structured treatment (GIST): A social competence intervention for individuals with brain injury. *Brain Injury*, *24*(11), 1292–1297. https://doi.org/10.3109/02699052.2010.506866

Heilmann, J., Miller, J. F., Nockerts, A., & Dunaway, C. (2010). Properties of the narrative scoring scheme using narrative retells in young school-age children. *American Journal of Speech-Language Pathology*, *19*(2), 154–166. https://doi.org/10.1044/1058-0360(2009/08-0024)

Hill, E., Claessen, M., Whitworth, A., & Boyes, M. (2020). Profiling variability and development of spoken discourse in mainstream adolescents. *Clinical Linguistics & Phonetics*, 1–21. https://doi.org/10.1080/02699206.2020.1731607

Hill, E., Whitworth, A., Boyes, M., Ziegelaar, M., & Claessen, M. (2021). The influence of genre on adolescent discourse skills: Do narratives tell the whole story? *International Journal of Speech-Language Pathology*, 1–11. https://doi.org/10.1080/17549507.2020.1864016

Holland, A. L. (1982). When is aphasia aphasia? The problem of closed head injury. *Clinical Aphasiology: Proceedings of the Conference 1982*, 345–349. http://aphasiology.pitt.edu/746/

Hunt, K. W. (1965). *Grammatical structures written at three grade levels*. NCTE Research Report No. 3. National Council of Teachers of English.

Iwashita, H., & Sohlberg, M. M. (2019). Measuring conversations after acquired brain injury in 30 minutes or less: A comparison of two pragmatic rating scales. *Brain Injury*, *33*(9), 1219–1233. https://doi.org/10.1080/02699052.2019.1631487

Jacoby, N., & Fedorenko, E. (2020). Discourse-level comprehension engages medial frontal Theory of Mind brain regions even for expository texts. *Language, Cognition and Neuroscience*, *35*(6), 780–796. https://doi.org/10.1080/23273798.2018.1525494

Justice, L. M., Bowles, R. P., Kaderavek, J. N., Ukrainetz, T. A., Eisenberg, S. L., & Gillam, R. B. (2006). The index of narrative microstructure: A clinical tool for analyzing school-age children's narrative performances. *American Journal of Speech-Language Pathology*, *15*(2), 177–191. https://doi.org/10.1044/1058-0360(2006/017)

Kim, B. S., Kim, Y. B., & Kim, H. (2019). Discourse measures to differentiate between mild cognitive impairment and healthy aging. *Frontiers in Aging Neuroscience*, *11*, 221. https://doi.org/10.3389/fnagi.2019.00221

Kim, H., Kintz, S., & Wright, H. H. (2020). Development of a measure of function word use in narrative discourse: Core lexicon analysis in aphasia. *International Journal of Language & Communication Disorders*. https://doi.org/10.1111/1460-6984.12567

Kim, J., Shim, J., & Yoon, J. H. (2019). Subjective rating scale for discourse: Evidence from the efficacy of subjective rating scale in amnestic mild cognitive impairments. *Medicine*, *98*(2), e14041. https://doi.org/10.1097/MD.0000000000014041

Kintz, S., Hibbs, V., Henderson, A., Andrews, M., & Wright, H. H. (2018). Discourse-based treatment in mild traumatic brain injury. *Journal of Communication Disorders, 76,* 47–59. https://doi.org/10.1016/j.jcomdis.2018.08.001

Kopelman, M., Wilson, B. A., & Baddeley, A. (1990). *Autobiographical memory interview (AMI).* Pearson. www.pearsonclinical.co.uk/Psychology/AdultCognitionNeuropsychol ogyandLanguage/AdultMemory/AutobiographicalMemoryInterview(AMI)/Autobiogra phicalMemoryInterview(AMI).aspx

Koutsoftas, A. D., & Gray, S. (2012). Comparison of narrative and expository writing in students with and without language-learning disabilities. *Language, Speech, and Hearing Services in Schools, 43*(4), 395–409. https://doi.org/10.1044/0161-1461(2012/11-0018)

Lê, K., Coelho, C., Mozeiko, J., & Grafman, J. (2011). Measuring goodness of story narratives. *Journal of Speech, Language, and Hearing Research: JSLHR, 54*(1), 118–126. https://doi.org/10.1044/1092-4388(2010/09-0022)

Liles, B. Z. (1985). Cohesion in the narratives of normal and language-disordered children. *Journal of Speech and Hearing Research, 28*(1), 123–133. https://doi.org/10.1044/jshr.2801.123

Lindsey, A., Hurley, E., Mozeiko, J., & Coelho, C. (2019). Follow-up on the story goodness index for characterizing discourse deficits following traumatic brain injury. *American Journal of Speech-Language Pathology, 28*(1S), 330–340. https://doi.org/10.1044/2018_AJSLP-17-0151

Loban, W. (1976). *Language development: Kindergarten through grade twelve.* NCTE Committee on Research Report No. 18. National Council of Teachers of English. https://eric.ed.gov/?id=ED128818

Lundine, J. P., & Barron, H. D. (2019). Microstructural and fluency characteristics of narrative and expository discourse in adolescents with traumatic brain injury. *American Journal of Speech-Language Pathology, 28*(4), 1638–1648. https://doi.org/10.1044/2019_AJSLP-19-0012

Lundine, J. P., & Hall, A. (2020). Using nonstandardized assessments to evaluate cognitive-communication abilities following pediatric traumatic brain injury. *Seminars in Speech & Language, 41*(2), 170–182. https://doi.org/10.1055/s-0040-1701685

MacDonald, S. (2017). Introducing the model of cognitive-communication competence: A model to guide evidence-based communication interventions after brain injury. *Brain Injury, 31*(13–14), 1760–1780. https://doi.org/10.1080/02699052.2017.1379613

MacDonald, S. (2021). The cognitive-communication checklist for acquired brain injury: A means of identifying, recording, and tracking communication impairments. *American Journal of Speech-Language Pathology, 30*(3), 1074–1089. https://doi.org/10.1044/2021_AJSLP-20-00155

MacWhinney, B. (2019). Understanding spoken language through talkbank. *Behavior Research Methods, 51*(4), 1919–1927. https://doi.org/10.3758/s13428-018-1174-9

Malone, T., Miller, J., Andriacchi, K., Heilmann, J., Nockerts, A., & Schoonveld, L. (2008). *Let me explain: Teenage expository language samples.* ASHA Convention. www.asha.org/Events/convention/handouts/2008/1614_Nockerts_Ann/

Mar, R. A. (2011). The neural bases of social cognition and story comprehension. *Annual Review of Psychology, 62,* 103–134. https://doi.org/10.1146/annurev-psych-120709-145406

Marcotte, K., Sanchez, E., Arbour, C., Brambati, S. M., Bedetti, C., Martineau, S., Descoteaux, M., & Gosselin, N. (2020). Long-term discourse outcomes and their relationship to white matter damage in moderate to severe adulthood traumatic brain injury. *Brain and Language, 204,* 104769. https://doi.org/10.1016/j.bandl.2020.104769

Marini, A., Zettin, M., Bencich, E., Bosco, F. M., & Galetto, V. (2017). Severity effects on discourse production after TBI. *Journal of Neurolinguistics, 44*, 91–106. https://doi.org/10.1016/j.jneuroling.2017.03.005

Matsuoka, K., Kotani, I., & Yamasato, M. (2012). Correct information unit analysis for determining the characteristics of narrative discourse in individuals with chronic traumatic brain injury. *Brain Injury, 26*(13–14), 1723–1730. https://doi.org/10.3109/02699 052.2012.698789

McCabe, A., Bliss, L., Barra, G., & Bennett, M. (2008). Comparison of personal versus fictional narratives of children with language impairment. *American Journal of Speech-Language Pathology, 17*(2), 194–206. https://doi.org/10.1044/1058-0360(2008/019)

McNeil, M. R., Doyle, P. J., Fossett, T. R. D., Park, G. H., & Goda, A. J. (2001). Reliability and concurrent validity of the information unit scoring metric for the story retelling procedure. *Aphasiology, 15*(10–11), 991–1006. https://doi.org/10.1080/02687040143 000348

Merritt, D. D., & Liles, B. Z. (1987). Story grammar ability in children with and without language disorder: Story generation, story retelling, and story comprehension. *Journal of Speech and Hearing Research, 30*(4), 539–552. https://doi.org/10.1044/jshr.3004.539

Meulenbroek, P., & Turkstra, L. S. (2016). Job stability in skilled work and communication ability after moderate-severe traumatic brain injury. *Disability and Rehabilitation, 38*(5), 452–461. https://doi.org/10.3109/09638288.2015.1044621

Miller, J., Andriacchi, K., & Nockerts, A. (2016). Using language sample analysis to assess spoken language production in adolescents. *Language, Speech, and Hearing Services in Schools, 47*(2), 99–112. https://doi.org/10.1044/2015_LSHSS-15-0051

Miller, J., & Iglesias, A. (2020). *Systematic analysis of language transcripts (SALT)* (Version 20) [Computer software]. SALT Software, LLC. https://saltsoftware.com/

Milman, L., Anderson, E., Thatcher, K., Amundson, D., Johnson, C., Jones, M., Valles, L., & Willis, D. (2020). Integrated discourse therapy after glioblastoma: A case report of face-to-face and tele-neurorehabilitation treatment delivery. *Frontiers in Neurology, 11*, 583452. https://doi.org/10.3389/fneur.2020.583452

Müller, N., Guendouzi, J. A., & Wilson, B. (2009). Discourse analysis and communication impairment. In *The handbook of clinical linguistics* (pp. 1–31). John Wiley & Sons, Ltd. https://doi.org/10.1002/9781444301007.ch1

Nicholas, L. E., & Brookshire, R. H. (1993). A system for quantifying the informativeness and efficiency of the connected speech of adults with aphasia. *Journal of Speech and Hearing Research, 36*(2), 338–350.

Nicholas, L. E., & Brookshire, R. H. (1995). Presence, completeness, and accuracy of main concepts in the connected speech of non-brain-damaged adults and adults with aphasia. *Journal of Speech and Hearing Research, 38*(1), 145–156. https://doi.org/10.1044/jshr.3801.145

Nippold, M. A., Frantz-Kaspar, M. W., Cramond, P. M., Kirk, C., Hayward-Mayhew, C., & MacKinnon, M. (2014). Conversational and narrative speaking in adolescents: Examining the use of complex syntax. *Journal of Speech, Language, and Hearing Research, 57*(3), 876–886. https://doi.org.ezproxy.uvm.edu/10.1044/1092-4388(2013/13-0097)

Nippold, M., Mansfield, T., Billow, J., & Tomblin, B. (2008). Expository discourse in adolescents with language impairments: Examining syntactic development. *American Journal of Speech-Language Pathology, 17*(4), 356–366. https://doi.org/10.1044/1058-0360(2008/07-0049)

Oetting, J. B., Cleveland, L. H., & Cope, R. F. (2008). Empirically derived combinations of tools and clinical cutoffs: An illustrative case with a sample of culturally/linguistically diverse children. *Language, Speech, and Hearing Services in Schools, 39*(1), 44–53. https://doi.org/10.1044/0161-1461(2008/005)

Parola, A., Bosco, F. M., Gabbatore, I., Galetto, V., Zettin, M., & Marini, A. (2019). The impact of the cognitive pragmatic treatment on the pragmatic and informative skills of individuals with traumatic brain injury (TBI). *Journal of Neurolinguistics, 51*, 53–62. https://doi.org/10.1016/j.jneuroling.2018.12.003

Peach, R. K. (2013). The cognitive basis for sentence planning difficulties in discourse after traumatic brain injury. *American Journal of Speech-Language Pathology, 22*(2), S285–S297. https://doi.org/10.1044/1058-0360(2013/12-0081)

Peach, R. K., & Coelho, C. A. (2016). Linking inter- and intra-sentential processes for narrative production following traumatic brain injury: Implications for a model of discourse processing. *Neuropsychologia, 80*, 157–164. https://doi.org/10.1016/j.neuropsychologia.2015.11.015

Peach, R. K., & Hanna, L. E. (2021). Sentence-level processing predicts narrative coherence following traumatic brain injury: Evidence in support of a resource model of discourse processing. *Language, Cognition and Neuroscience*, 1–17. https://doi.org/10.1080/23273798.2021.1894346

Piaget, J. (1926). *The language and thought of the child*. Harcourt, Brace, & Company.

Ponsford, J. L., Downing, M. G., Olver, J., Ponsford, M., Acher, R., Carty, M., & Spitz, G. (2014). Longitudinal follow-up of patients with traumatic brain injury: Outcome at two, five, and ten years post-injury. *Journal of Neurotrauma, 31*(1), 64–77. https://doi.org/10.1089/neu.2013.2997

Pritchard, M., Hilari, K., Cocks, N., & Dipper, L. (2017). Reviewing the quality of discourse information measures in aphasia. *International Journal of Language & Communication Disorders, 52*(6), 689–732. https://doi.org/10.1111/1460-6984.12318

Pritchard, M., Hilari, K., Cocks, N., & Dipper, L. (2018). Psychometric properties of discourse measures in aphasia: Acceptability, reliability, and validity. *International Journal of Language & Communication Disorders, 53*(6), 1078–1093. https://doi.org/10.1111/1460-6984.12420

Radice-Neumann, D., Zupan, B., Tomita, M., & Willer, B. (2009). Training emotional processing in persons with brain injury. *The Journal of Head Trauma Rehabilitation, 24*(5), 313–323. https://doi.org/10.1097/HTR.0b013e3181b09160

Roth, F. P., & Spekman, N. J. (1986). Narrative discourse: Spontaneously generated stories of learning-disabled and normally achieving students. *Journal of Speech and Hearing Disorders, 51*, 8–23.

Scott, C. M., & Windsor, J. (2000). General language performance measures in spoken and written narrative and expository discourse of school-age children with language learning disabilities. *Journal of Speech, Language, and Hearing Research: JSLHR, 43*(2), 324–339. https://doi.org/10.1044/jslhr.4302.324

Sherratt, S. (2007). Multi-level discourse analysis: A feasible approach. *Aphasiology, 21*(3–4), 375–393. https://doi.org/10.1080/02687030600911435

Snow, P. (2019). Speech-language pathology and the youth offender: Epidemiological overview and roadmap for future speech-language pathology research and scope of practice. *Language, Speech, and Hearing Services in Schools, 50*(2), 324–339. https://doi.org/10.1044/2018_LSHSS-CCJS-18-0027

Snow, P., Douglas, J., & Ponsford, J. (1997). Procedural discourse following traumatic brain injury. *Aphasiology, 11*(10), 947–967. https://doi.org/10.1080/02687039708249421

Spaulding, T. J., Plante, E., & Farinella, K. A. (2006). Eligibility criteria for language impairment: Is the low end of normal always appropriate? *Language, Speech, and Hearing Services in Schools, 37*(1), 61–72. https://doi.org/10.1044/0161-1461(2006/007)

Stark, B. C. (2019). A comparison of three discourse elicitation methods in aphasia and age-matched adults: Implications for language assessment and outcome. *American Journal of Speech-Language Pathology, 28*(3), 1067–1083. https://doi.org/10.1044/2019_AJSLP-18-0265

Steel, J., Elbourn, E., & Togher, L. (2021). Narrative discourse intervention after traumatic brain injury: A systematic review of the literature. *Topics in Language Disorders*, *41*(1), 47–72. https://doi.org/10.1097/TLD.0000000000000241

Steel, J., & Togher, L. (2018). Social communication assessment after TBI: A narrative review of innovations in pragmatic and discourse assessment methods. *Brain Injury*, 1–14. https://doi.org/10.1080/02699052.2018.1531304

Stout, C. E., Yorkston, K. M., & Pimentel, J. I. (2000). Discourse production following mild, moderate, and severe traumatic brain injury. *Journal of Medical Speech-Language Pathology*, *8*(1), 15–25.

Thordardottir, E. (2015). *French language samples: Does length matter?* Symposium on Research in Child Language Disorders. www.srcld.org/Archive/PresentationDetail. aspx?SUBID=3136

Togher, L., Elbourne, E., Power, E., Kenny, B., McDonald, S., Tate, R., Turkstra, L., Holland, A., Fromm, D., Forbes, M., & MacWhinney, B. (2014). *TBI bank is a feasible assessment protocol to evaluate the cognitive communication skills of people with severe TBI during the subacute stage of recovery.* https://tbi.talkbank.org/posters/14Presentation-Togher.pdf

Togher, L., McDonald, S., Tate, R., Power, E., & Rietdijk, R. (2013). Training communication partners of people with severe traumatic brain injury improves everyday conversations: A multicenter single blind clinical trial. *Journal of Rehabilitation Medicine*, *45*(7), 637–645. https://doi.org/10.2340/16501977-1173

Togher, L., Wiseman-Hakes, C., Douglas, J., Stergiou-Kita, M., Ponsford, J., Teasell, R., Bayley, M., Turkstra, L. S., & INCOG Expert Panel. (2014). INCOG recommendations for management of cognition following traumatic brain injury, part IV: Cognitive communication. *The Journal of Head Trauma Rehabilitation*, *29*(4), 353–368. https://doi. org/10.1097/HTR.0000000000000071

Tremblay, P., & Dick, A. S. (2016). Broca and Wernicke are dead, or moving past the classic model of language neurobiology. *Brain and Language*, *162*, 60–71. https://doi. org/10.1016/j.bandl.2016.08.004

Ulatowska, H. K., North, A. J., & Macaluso-Haynes, S. (1981). Production of narrative and procedural discourse in aphasia. *Brain and Language*, *13*(2), 345–371. https://doi. org/10.1016/0093-934x(81)90100-0

von Steinbüchel, N., Wilson, L., Gibbons, H., Hawthorne, G., Höfer, S., Schmidt, S., Bullinger, M., Maas, A., Neugebauer, E., Powell, J., von Wild, K., Zitnay, G., Bakx, W., Christensen, A. L., Koskinen, S., Formisano, R., Saarajuri, J., Sasse, N., Truelle, J. L., & QOLIBRI Task Force. (2010). Quality of life after brain injury (QOLIBRI): Scale validity and correlates of quality of life. *Journal of Neurotrauma*, *27*(7), 1157–1165. https://doi. org/10.1089/neu.2009.1077

Wallis, A. K., Westerveld, M. F., Waters, A. M., & Snow, P. C. (2021). Investigating adolescent discourse in critical thinking: Monologic responses to stories containing a moral dilemma. *Language, Speech, and Hearing Services in Schools*, 1–14. https://doi. org/10.1044/2020_LSHSS-20-00134

Whitworth, A., Claessen, M., Leitão, S., & Webster, J. (2015). Beyond narrative: Is there an implicit structure to the way in which adults organise their discourse? *Clinical Linguistics & Phonetics*, *29*(6), 455–481. https://doi.org/10.3109/02699206.2015.1020450

Williams, S. E., Li, E. C., Della Volpe, A., & Ritterman, S. I. (1994). The influence of topic and listener familiarity on aphasic discourse. *Journal of Communication Disorders*, *27*(3), 207–222.

Wood, J. N., & Grafman, J. (2003). Human prefrontal cortex: Processing and representational perspectives. *Nature Reviews: Neuroscience*, *4*(2), 139–147. https://doi.org/10.1038/ nrn1033

World Health Organization (WHO). (2001). *International classification of functioning, disability and health (ICF)*. www.who.int/standards/classifications/international-classification-of-functioning-disability-and-health

World Health Organization (WHO). (2010). *Measuring health and disability: Manual for WHO disability assessment schedule WHODAS 2.0* (T. B. Üstün, Ed.). World Health Organization.

Worrall, L., Sherratt, S., Rogers, P., Howe, T., Hersh, D., Ferguson, A., & Davidson, B. (2011). What people with aphasia want: Their goals according to the ICF. *Aphasiology, 25*(3), 309–322. https://doi.org/10.1080/02687038.2010.508530

Wright, H. H., Koutsoftas, A. D., Capilouto, G. J., & Fergadiotis, G. (2014). Global coherence in younger and older adults: Influence of cognitive processes and discourse type. *Aging, Neuropsychology, and Cognition, 21*(2), 174–196. https://doi.org/10.1080/13825585.2013.794894

Ylvisaker, M., Szekeres, S., & Feeney, T. (2008). Communication disorders associated with traumatic brain injury. In R. Chapey (Ed.), *Language intervention strategies in aphasia and related neurogenic communication disorders* (5th ed., pp. 879–962). Lippincott, Williams & Wilkins.

10 Prosody: Linguistic and clinical perspectives

Jennifer Cole, Allison Hilger, and Shivani Patel

Abstract

Prosody is sometimes described as the musical quality of speech, and though it involves melodic and rhythmic dimensions of sound that are also primary characteristics of music, it is far from ornamental and has critical roles signaling linguistic structure in continuous speech, and conveying meaning related to a speaker's communicative intentions. This chapter reviews the phonological and phonetic characteristics of prosody in relation to their linguistic function, with reference to English, and the physiological requirements for the expression of prosody in speech, and then reviews some of the more common patterns of atypical prosody associated with structural and/or neurological impairment in adult special populations. The chapter highlights methods for assessing prosody and current approaches to treatment, and discusses some of the consequences of atypical prosody for social interaction.

Statement to the reader

As a clinician, you may often note disrupted or atypical prosody in the presence of structural or neurological impairment in adults, impacting linguistic communication and social interaction. But *what exactly are the acoustic and articulatory characteristics of prosody, and why is it that prosodic impairments can disrupt communication?* This chapter addresses these questions from the perspective of current linguistic theory and introduces current approaches to the assessment and treatment of deficits in the production of prosody. A discussion of the key role of prosody in successful communication and social interaction highlight the importance of addressing prosody in the clinical domain.

Introduction

Prosody refers to the patterning of pitch, timing, loudness, voice quality, and timbre across the syllables of a spoken word, phrase, sentence, or larger discourse

DOI: 10.4324/9781003045519-12

unit. Prosodic patterning is rich in its potential to convey *linguistic* meaning related to the interpretation of words, sentences and discourse, and *paralinguistic* meaning related to the speaker's psychological state, social identity, and the communicative setting. Prosody is inherent to speech and a property of every spoken language. At the same time, languages differ from one another in their prosodic systems, with perceptually salient differences in the melodic and rhythmic aspects of speech, and in the mapping from prosodic expressions to linguistic meaning. The distinct prosodic patterns used in a given language, and even in a particular dialect, are part of what a child learns in the normal course of development. Deviations from community norms in the production of prosodic patterns, or in the perception and interpretation of those patterns, can impact communication outcomes.

This chapter presents an overview of prosody as expressed in typical speaker–hearer populations, considering the kinds of linguistic and paralinguistic information that prosody conveys, the phonological and phonetic encoding of prosody, and the physiological mechanisms involved in the production of prosody. These topics provide the foundation for the analysis of atypical prosody and prosodic adaptation in special adult populations, and for the development of approaches to prosodic assessment and interventions. We conclude with a discussion of prosody as it relates more broadly to interactive social behavior. Throughout the chapter, reference is made to the prosodic patterns of American English, some of which generalize to other dialects of English. But it is important to bear in mind that prosodic patterns and their function in conveying linguistic meaning are known to differ across languages, and therefore identifying typical or atypical prosody must be done with reference to the norms of a specific speech community.

The functions of prosody in conveying linguistic and non-linguistic information

Prosodic encoding of structure in word, sentence, and discourse-level juncture

A core function of prosody is the encoding of linguistic structure, on analogy with the function of punctuation, font emphasis (italic, bold), space between words, and paragraph indentation in written language. In some languages, prosodic patterns operating at the word-level function to mark word boundaries, for example, through stress assigned to the syllable that sits at or near the initial or final word boundary. English has an especially complex system of word stress, with stress placed at or near the right edge of a word, but subject to numerous constraints on syllable and morphological structure (Fudge, 2015). It's important to note that not all languages distinguish stressed and unstressed syllables within words, and among those that do not are many of the so-called tone or pitch-accent languages, in which tone features are part of a phonological make-up of the word (i.e., along with its consonants and vowels, as part of its dictionary specification), for example, Mandarin, Thai, and Vietnamese

(Gussenhoven, 2004). Yet other languages appear not to have any system of prosodic marking at the word level, for example, Indonesian (Gordon, 2014).

While word-level prosody is not universal among languages, to the best of our knowledge, all languages use prosody to mark structure at the phrase level (1), and to identify structural relations among successive phrases in complex sentences (2, from Ladd, 2008).

(1) [*When Lily awakened*] [*the baby was crying*]
(2) i. [[A and B] but C]] *"Warren is a stronger campaigner, and Ryan has more popular policies, but Allen has a lot more money."*
     ii. [A [but B and C]] *"Warren is a stronger campaigner, but Ryan has more popular policies, and Allen has a lot more money."*

Prosodic phrases are composed in relation to syntactic structure, though they are not necessarily direct extensions of syntactic phrases (Shattuck-Hufnagel & Turk, 1996). Typically, a prosodic juncture (the boundary between successive prosodic phrases) must be located at a syntactic boundary (e.g., a noun phrase, verb phrase, prepositional phrase, or clause), but a single prosodic phrase may span two or more syntactic phrases, for example, including the subject noun phrase and the verb phrase in (3). It is also possible for a single syntactic phrase to be split into two or more prosodic phrases, as with the more complex verb phrase in (4). Prosodic phrasing reflects speech production planning (Krivokapić, 2014) such that the location of a prosodic phrase boundary between two words depends on the presence of a syntactic phrase boundary at that location, and on the length and complexity of the syntactic constituents preceding and following the syntactic juncture (Watson & Gibson, 2004). Moreover, although syntax constrains prosodic phrasing, speakers have substantial flexibility in the prosodic phrasing of a sentence, in both the number and extent of prosodic phrases, especially for complex or long sentences; non-grammatical factors such as speech rate and style also play a role (Gee & Grosjean, 1983).

(3) [Sam gave the man a ticket]
(4) [Sam gave a certificate of achievement] [to each child who completed the course]

Generally speaking, the presence of a prosodic phrase boundary is a fairly reliable cue for the presence of a syntactic constituent boundary at the same location. Indeed, a prosodic boundary located in a position that is not also a major syntactic boundary, as in (5ii), disrupts sentence processing, and in some instances, may result in faulty sentence interpretation, for example, (6ii) (Speer et al., 1996).

(5) i.   [George and Mary] [gave blood]
     ii. ?? [George] [and Mary gave blood]
(6) i.   [Whenever the guard checks] [the door is locked]
     ii. ?? [Whenever the guard checks the door] [is locked]

Looking above the level of the sentence, prosody further serves to convey dialogue structure in interactive speech. For instance, prosody functions as a resource for managing turn-taking in a conversation, and there are also distinct prosodic patterns used to signal the initiation, end, or continuation of topics (Ward, 2019). When the prosodic marking of the end of a conversational turn is not present, or if it occurs in other locations, it disrupts conversational flow. Such disruptions often result in increased talker overlap, or awkwardly long pauses before a change of talker turn.

Prosodic prominence

In addition to their grouping function, prosodic phrases also define a domain for prominence, a feature that identifies one or more elements within a prosodic domain as standing out relative to other elements. What it means to "stand out" depends on the level of prosodic structure under consideration. For languages with word-level prosody, word-level prominence corresponds to primary word-level stress, which is located relative to the left or right edge of the word according to language-specific constraints. In some languages, including English, additional syllables in a longer polysyllabic word may be designated as having a lower degree of prominence, realized as secondary stress. The location of primary word-level stress in English is important for accurate word recognition for native (English-speaking) listeners (Cutler & Clifton, 1984).

Prominence is also a feature of prosodic phrases, wherein one word in the phrase is assigned the primary phrasal stress, also termed *nuclear stress* or *nuclear prominence*. In languages with word-level stress, including English, phrasal prominence must be realized on a word that has word-level stress, which excludes stressless monosyllable "function" words (determiners, pronouns, prepositions, conjunctions). In these languages, a syllable that is marked for both word-level and phrasal stress has greater prominence than a syllable that has only word-level stress. In a parallel manner with word-level stress, phrasal stress is located relative to the edge of the prosodic phrase. In English, the rightmost stressable word is assigned phrasal prominence, as illustrated in (7) (the syllable with phrasal and word-level stress is marked by CAPS). In addition to the primary phrasal stress, English also allows for optional secondary prominences on stressable words in *prenuclear* position (preceding the nuclear stress), which are particularly common in phrase-initial position, as illustrated in (8), with optional prenuclear prominences on *Sam* and *usually*, and nuclear phrasal prominence on *tickets*.

(7) i.   [Sam gave the man the TICKet]
     ii. [Sam gave the TICKet to him]
(8) [SAM/Sam was USually/usually the one to buy the **TICK**ets]

Because every stressable word in a sentence is eligible to realize phrasal prominence, the occurrence of a stressable word with phrasal stress, by itself, does not provide information about sentence structure. All possible assignments of phrasal prominence to stressable words are prosodically well-formed. But as we will see next, in English the location of the primary phrasal stress encodes *information structure* distinctions related to focus and the status of a word as introducing "new" or "given" information relative to the discourse context, and a mismatch between phrasal prominence and the information structure context can impair sentence comprehension.

Pragmatic meaning

Beyond its structure-marking function, in English, prosody also conveys pragmatic meaning (i.e., meaning related to the context of an utterance) through intonation, which is the specification of tone features associated with prominent words and the edges of prosodic phrases. English is not alone in conveying pragmatic meaning through intonation, but the richness of the system is a hallmark of English and other West Germanic languages. Two distinct pragmatic functions are encoded through intonation in English: information structure and speech act meaning. Information structure relates to *reference*—the entity (physical or abstract) in the world that a linguistic expression refers to—and covers notions like corrective or contrastive focus (9) and the status of a referent as discourse-new or discourse-given (10) (Brazil, 1980; Hirschberg, 2015; Westera et al., 2020). English marks information structure distinctions through the phonetic implementation of phrasal stress and in the choice of tone features (as described earlier) associated with words that have corrective focus (the bolded word in 9i) or contrastive focus (9ii), words that convey the answer to a question (i.e., narrow focus, 9iii), and for words that introduce new information to the discourse (10i). If a discourse-given word occurs in the default (phrase-final) position for nuclear stress (the underlined *bears* in 10ii), it will typically not be assigned nuclear stress, which instead shifts leftward to the nearest stressable word (*see*).

(9)   i.   Speaker A: I think Sam is going to the meeting tomorrow.
            Speaker B: No, **Sue** was asked to go instead of Sam.
      ii. Speaker A: Sue hates to travel so I was surprised she volunteered when Sam was unable to go to the meeting.
            Speaker B: Well, Sue was **asked** to go in his place.
      iii. Speaker A: Sam had to cancel, so who will go to the meeting tomorrow?
            Speaker B: **Sue** was asked to go in his place.
(10) i.   (The guidebook says wildlife is abundant in this park . . .) I don't see any **bears**.
      ii. (The guidebook says bears live around here . . ..) I don't **see** any <u>bears</u>.

As with prosodic boundaries, listeners also pay attention to phrasal stress in sentence comprehension. In particular, the absence of phrasal stress on the rightmost stressable word in the prosodic phrase is a strong cue that that word is discourse-given. Likewise, the location of primary phrasal stress on a word in non-final position, especially when the final word is discourse-new, leads listeners to interpret the non-final word as focused, as in (9ii, iii). As illustrated earlier, under typical conditions, the prominence status of a word is congruent with the prior discourse context that establishes focus and givenness. But in the event of a mismatch, e.g., where phrasal stress is realized on a phrase-final word that is discourse-given (e.g., if phrasal stress is on "bears" in 10ii), listeners can be confused about the intended referent of the expression. Faced with a speaker who is unreliable in producing prominence patterns that are congruent with the discourse context, listeners rapidly adapt by disregarding phrasal stress as an interpretive cue to focus or givenness (Roettger & Franke, 2019).

Speech act meaning (also called *illocutionary force*) concerns the speaker's communicative goal (e.g., to assert, inquire, request, contradict). English conveys speech act meaning through the choice of sentence type (e.g., declarative, wh-question, imperative) paired with *nuclear tune*, which is the pitch melody spanning the nuclear stress to the end of the intonational phrase. For example, a declarative sentence with a falling tune is the typical way to express an assertion, but the same sentence paired with a rising tune can be used to seek confirmation or to inquire. Contemporary linguistic accounts of English intonation derive these tunes from a sequence of tone features marking the nuclear stress and prosodic phrase boundary (Gussenhoven, 2004; Ladd, 2008).

Paralinguistic meaning related to social factors and speaker affect

Evaluating prosody for its function in marking linguistic structure and conveying pragmatic meaning is complicated by the fact that the speech channel simultaneously conveys information about the speaker's affect, in terms of emotion, attitude, and mood. There is an expansive literature on affective prosody (also known as *emotional* prosody) showing that variation in pitch, tempo, and other acoustic-prosodic parameters correlates with enacted or perceived distinctions in speaker affect along dimensions such as arousal/potency and valence (Bänziger & Scherer, 2005). To date there is little research examining linguistic and emotional prosody together to understand how they contribute to convey meaning, independently or jointly, in any given utterance. Yet, since similar acoustic patterns are seen in linguistic and emotional prosodic expression, this is a question that is important for anyone evaluating prosody in a research or clinical setting, and an area in need of further research.

The social context in which an utterance occurs also influences a speaker's choice of prosodic expression. In contexts of interactive communication, social factors may play a role in listeners' interpretation of pragmatic meaning conveyed through prosody. Prosody can index a speaker's social affiliation, illustrated for example in the distinct prosodic patterns associated with ethnic or regional dialects, gender, or sexual orientation (Holliday, 2021). Another dimension of social meaning tied to prosody is politeness, where higher pitch, slower speech rate, and increased vowel (or syllable) duration are associated with perceived politeness (Navarro & Nebot, 2014).

Prosody in phonological representations and its phonetic expression

Prosodic structure is part of the phonological representation of words and phrases. At the word level, prosodic structure consists of "metrical feet" that bundle successive syllables together and which determine the placement of stress. In English, the metrical foot may include two syllables, with stress on the leftmost of the pair; primary stress goes on the rightmost foot in the word, and in longer words a secondary stress is possible on other feet, subject to constraints on rhythmic stress alternation. At the phrase level, there is a hierarchy of prosodic phrases, with smaller *intermediate* phrases (ip) that are combined into larger *intonational* phrases (IP), as illustrated in Fig. 10.1.[1] At each level of prosodic structure, one element is designated as prominent. In the intermediate phrase, prominence is on the rightmost stressable word, which marks the location of the nuclear (phrasal) stress (*students* and *daily* in Fig. 10.1). The perceptually strongest prominence in the intonational phrase is the nuclear stressed word of the rightmost intermediate phrase, *daily* in Fig. 10.1 (Cole et al., 2010, 2019). The nuclear prominence in the intermediate phrase is marked with an obligatory pitch accent—a low or high tone feature associated with the stressed syllable (annotated L* or H*).[2] There are also optional prenuclear pitch accents on earlier stressed words. The right edge of the intermediate and intonational phrases is marked with tone features (annotated H- or L-, for intermediate phrases, and H% or L% for intonational phrases). These edge-marking tones combined with the preceding nuclear pitch accent together derive the typical intonation pattern of English: a perceptually salient, dynamic pitch movement at the end of a phrase. Since the end of a sentence tends also to be the end of an intermediate phrase and intonational phrase, the nuclear "tune" in English tends to occur at the end of a sentence. This pattern is overridden in sentences that mark narrow, corrective or contrastive focus on a word located earlier in the sentence (as in 9, above), in which case the nuclear pitch accent is located on the focused word, with loss of prominence ("deaccenting") on any following word.

Prosodic structure and associated intonational features (pitch accents, boundary tones) are phonetically expressed through variation in articulation and corresponding variation in acoustic parameters. The details of this phonetic spell-out vary across languages, but generally speaking, prominence is associated with phonetic enhancement, and boundaries are associated with lengthening and pauses. These phonetic effects of prosody come about due to changes in laryngeal settings, oral aperture, the volume of airflow across the glottis, and in the timing of speech gestures (e.g., tongue body raising, lip closure). Articulatory studies of English show that phonetic enhancement associated

---

1. This model is based on the work of Pierrehumbert (1980), and is couched within Autosegmental-Metrical theory, a phonological theory of prosody, tone and intonation. See Ladd (2008).
2. The inventory of pitch accents in English also includes a downstepped high (!H*), and several accents composed of a two-tone sequence, such as L+H* (Ladd, 2008).

| H* | !H* | | H* | Pitch accent |
| | | L- | | L- H% | Boundary tone |

IP[ip[The music students]ip ip[practiced daily]ip]IP.

Figure 10.1 Prosodic structure and intonational features for a spoken production of the sentence *The music students practiced daily.*

with prominence is implemented with hyper-articulation (Byrd & Krivokapić, 2021; de Jong, 1995), increased airflow, and regular (modal) as opposed to irregular (non-modal) phonation, and laryngeal adjustments involved in the realization of high- or low-pitch targets in the spell-out of the pitch accents. Different articulatory adjustments are involved in the production of prosodic boundaries. A gradual slowing down of articulatory gestures occurs immediately preceding a prosodic phrase boundary, with maximal effects of lengthening on the final syllable. This is accompanied by hypoarticulation—a reduction in the magnitude of articulatory gestures, especially those in non-prominent syllables. Younger American English speakers increasingly also deploy irregular (creaky) phonation at the end of an intonational phrase, in the presence of low boundary tones.

The articulatory effects just described give rise to corresponding acoustic effects of prosody, with prominence manifest in increased intensity and duration, spectral measures (e.g., formants) reflecting gestures at more peripheral locations in the oral cavity (Cho, 2005), and spectral envelope measures of increased vocal effort (Sluijter & van Heuven, 1996). Accompanying these are dynamic patterns of fundamental frequency (f_0) change, producing pitch contours that implement the high and low tones of pitch accents when present. Each of these acoustic effects contributes to making the prominent element stand out perceptually (Cole et al., 2010, 2019). Acoustic correlates of prosodic phrase boundaries are lengthened duration and reduced intensity of the phrase-final syllable (or longer pre-boundary interval), and irregular pitch periods perceived as creaky voice. F_0 correlates of boundaries depend on the tone features associated with the boundary, resulting in a pitch rise, fall, or sustained pitch level from the preceding (nuclear) pitch accent.

Physiological requirements for prosody

The control of pitch, loudness, and timing for prosody in speech requires highly precise coordination among the speech subsystems: respiration, phonation, resonance, and articulation (Kent et al., 1989). While accurate prosodic production mainly relies on the subsystems of respiration and phonation, resonance and articulation also play important roles. In this section, we briefly summarize the anatomy and physiology of each subsystem and their roles in the production of prosody.

Respiration is the driving force of speech production (Bunn & Mead, 1971). Intensity and fundamental frequency (f_0) are directly influenced by air pressure from exhalation (Huber, 2008; Titze, 1989). Speech timing is influenced by the location of pauses and breath during speech (Wang et al., 2010). In resting breathing, there is a relatively regular pattern of inspiration and expiration; the diaphragm is the primary muscle involved with little need for accessory muscle involvement. This breathing pattern is vastly modified when speaking (Hixon et al., 1973; Hoit et al., 1989). Speech production requires a long exhale and a short inhale. The exhale must be controlled so that alveolar air pressure can be modified for phonation.

For prosody, speakers make subtle changes in alveolar air pressure to alter vocal intensity (Huber, 2008), for example in a loud restaurant, or to increase intensity at a more local scale for phrasal stress and boundary. Neurological impairment can disrupt respiratory coordination and result in poor loudness control. For example, ataxic dysarthria due to cerebellar damage is characterized by explosive loudness bursts, which result from the lack of control over alveolar air pressure during exhalation (Kent et al., 2000). Hypokinetic dysarthria due to Parkinson's disease is also associated with poor loudness control, character-ized by reduced loudness with little variation in intensity during speech due to multiple factors including air leakage through bowed vocal folds, lack of control over exhalation, speaking into the expiratory reserve volume, and inhaling to an inadequate inspiratory volume (Huber & Darling-White, 2017).

Respiratory control is required for appropriate phrasing and timing in speech. The length of a prosodic phrase is dependent on the degree of respira-tory support (Russell & Stathopoulos, 1988). Being able to produce a longer and slower exhale, for example, allows a speaker to produce more words per phrase before needing to pause to take a breath. When respiratory support is reduced due to physiological or neurological injury, speakers often need to take a breath at every pause and to pause more frequently (Huber, 2008). Accord-ingly, pauses frequently occur at unusual locations in speech. These atypical pauses can be perceived as unintended phrasal boundaries, leading to shorter prosodic phrases and misinterpretations of prosodic meaning.

Although f_0, the acoustic correlate of pitch, is mainly controlled at the laryngeal level, respiration also plays an important role. Indeed, control of f_0 exemplifies the precise coordination between the phonatory and respiratory systems (Titze, 1989). F_0 is influenced by the degree of subglottal pressure. When respiratory–phonatory coordination is disrupted, there may be inade-quate subglottal pressure to effectively set the vocal folds into vibration, leading to reduced vocal quality and poor control of f_0. Greater detail of pitch control will be provided in the next subsection on phonation.

Phonatory control is needed for prosodic aspects of f_0, intensity, and vocal quality. Disruption to laryngeal coordination and respiratory–phonatory coor-dination is common in neurological injury, resulting in variable pitch and loud-ness production and poor vocal quality. Changes in vocal fold movement alter the degree of glottal closure and frequency of vibration, leading to perceptual changes in vocal quality, pitch, and, to a lesser extent, intensity.

Although the respiratory and phonatory subsystems are the primary sys-tems of prosodic control, resonance and articulation also play notable roles.

Physiological and neurological impairments can impact the control and coordination of the velum, resulting in hypo- or hyper-nasal sounding speech. While nasality in speech does not directly influence the production of vocal intensity and fundamental frequency, it can influence the perception of loudness and pitch. For example, hyper-nasal speech is often perceived as monotone and flat intonation (Tardif et al., 2018).

Similar to resonance, articulation has little direct impact on the control of intensity and fundamental frequency when compared with respiration and phonation, but it does play an important role in timing in speech. The timing of articulatory movements is modified to lengthen or shorten syllable and word duration in speech, which influences the perception of word-level and phrasal stress (de Jong et al., 1993). Stressed syllables are produced with lengthened vowel duration and hyperarticulation. Imprecise articulation, one of the most common characteristics in motor speech disorders, impacts the perception of timing, word-level stress, and phrasal stress.

Characteristics of atypical prosody in adult special populations

The production of prosody in speech is accomplished through precise coordination both within and across speech subsystems, which can be disrupted when there is structural and/or neurological impairment. In this section, we describe the characteristics of atypical prosody in dysarthria, apraxia of speech, right hemisphere disorder, and autism spectrum disorder in adults.

Dysarthria

Dysarthria is defined as an impairment in the execution of speech (Yorkston et al., 1999). It is differentiated from other motor speech impairments involved in the planning and programming of speech (i.e., apraxia of speech). Six subtypes of dysarthria were delineated in the classic 1969 study by Darley, Aronson, and Brown based on collections of perceived articulatory, phonatory, and prosodic errors (Darley et al., 1969). While there is variability within each dysarthria subtype, all subtypes have the potential for prosodic impairment, some more directly, such as ataxic dysarthria, and some more indirectly, such as spastic dysarthria.

Ataxic dysarthria is associated with ataxia, or damage to the cerebellum or cerebellar pathways (Kent et al., 2000) and is characterized by both articulatory and prosodic errors. Articulatory errors include irregular consonant production and vowel distortions, and prosodic errors include explosive loudness, variable pitch, a word-by-word cadence, and equal and excess stress patterns. These speech errors result from disruption to the timing, scaling, and coordination of speech movements in the cerebellum (Ackermann, 2008). For example, explosive loudness results from poor control over alveolar air pressure in conjunction with the onset of phonation. The resulting lack of loudness and pitch control create perceptual confusion in identification of pitch accents and phrasal boundaries.

Both hyperkinetic and hypokinetic dysarthrias are associated with basal ganglia impairment (Spencer & Rogers, 2005; Zyski & Weisiger, 1987). The basal ganglia are important neural structures for the control and inhibition of movement, reflected in the differential impairment in hyperkinetic and hypokinetic dysarthria. Hyperkinetic dysarthria is characterized by a disinhibition of movement, resulting in involuntary movement in the body. In speech production, both articulation and prosody are interrupted by abnormal, involuntary movement. Speakers with hyperkinetic dysarthria often speak in short phrases as a compensatory technique to attempt to produce a complete message prior to an involuntary movement. The shorter phrasing results in variable rate of speech, strained voice, and reduced phrasal stress. When an involuntary movement occurs during speech, it can cause articulatory breakdown, variations in pitch and loudness, and hypernasality.

Hypokinetic dysarthria, associated with Parkinson's Disease, is characterized by inhibition of movement, resulting in difficulty in preparing, maintaining, and switching motor programs. In speech, inhibition of movement is reflected in a flat intonation, reduced emotional prosody, and lack of range of motion for articulation. Counterintuitively, the reduction in range of motion results in a rapidly increased rate of speech. Therefore, prosody in hypokinetic dysarthria is exhibited by rapid speech and flat intonation. Because of the lack of variation in pitch, loudness, and syllable duration, perceptual identification of stress and prosodic boundaries is difficult. Speakers with hypokinetic dysarthria are often misperceived as being bored, angry, or disinterested when the speaker may actually feel much differently (Pell et al., 2006).

Both spastic and unilateral upper motor neuron (UUMN) dysarthrias are associated with damage to the upper motor neuron pathways in the cortex usually due to stroke, tumor, or degenerative disease such as primary lateral sclerosis (Duffy, 2013). Spastic dysarthria is associated with bilateral upper motor neuron damage, whereas UUMN dysarthria is associated with unilateral damage. The bilateral damage in spastic dysarthria typically results in a more severe speech impairment, characterized by slow rate of speech, imprecise consonants, strained vocal quality, spasticity, monopitch, and monoloudness. Prosody in spastic dysarthria will be influenced mostly by the slow rate of speech and lack of control over pitch and loudness. The impairments in pitch, loudness, and vocal quality in spastic dysarthria arise from spasticity in the vocal folds. During phonation, the vocal folds are hyper-adducted, leading to the strained vocal quality and difficulty in modulating pitch and loudness. Prosody is sometimes affected in UUMN dysarthria but usually at a mild severity level, with articulatory breakdown, slow rate of speech, mild hypernasality, and mildly strained phonation. Each of these characteristics can affect the perception of phrasal stress and boundaries in speech. UUMN dysarthria is commonly co-occurring with aphasia and apraxia of speech due to the locus of impairment.

Flaccid dysarthria is the final dysarthria subtype, associated with damage to the lower motor neuron pathways (Duffy, 2013). The site of lesion can occur at four levels within these pathways: the brainstem, cranial or spinal nerves, neuromuscular junction, or muscle. The presentation of flaccid dysarthria has considerable variability depending on the site of lesion. For example, if cranial nerve seven (CN VII) is damaged, the resulting facial paralysis will cause considerable articulatory error. However, if cranial nerve ten (CN X) is damaged, the resulting vocal fold weakness or paralysis will affect vocal quality. Prosody may be impaired in flaccid dysarthria depending on the site of lesion and the severity of damage. If articulation is considerably disrupted, then phrasal stress will be impacted by variable syllable lengthening. If phonation is impaired, then voice quality, pitch, and loudness may become more variable in speech.

Apraxia of speech (AOS)

Apraxia of speech (AOS) is a disorder affecting the ability to plan and program motor plans for speech (Yorkston et al., 1999). Unlike dysarthria, which can occur from damage to multiple parts of the brain, AOS always results from pathology to the left cerebral hemisphere typically from stroke or tumor. The specific neural areas usually affected in AOS are Broca's Area (i.e., the inferior frontal gyrus) and the Supplemental Motor Area. AOS commonly co-occurs with aphasia (usually Broca's Aphasia) and UUMN dysarthria.

The planning and programming impairments in AOS cause both articulatory and prosodic disruption. For articulation, consonant and vowel distortions and substitutions are common. These articulatory errors can impact the perception of word-level and phrasal stress because of disruption in syllable lengthening for stress. Prosodic disruption in AOS includes slow rate, syllable segregation, and error in stress assignment. Pitch and loudness control are only affected in AOS in the context of speech production. Individuals with AOS are able to sing with appropriate pitch and loudness control. Because AOS is a disorder of planning and programming speech, and not a disorder of the execution of speech, the impairments are isolated to the context of speech. Therefore, pitch, loudness, and timing are only affected when speaking and not during other tasks involving vocalization.

Right hemisphere disorder (Aprosodia)

Aprosodia, the lack of prosody (rather than disrupted prosody described in dysarthria and AOS), can result from damage to the right hemisphere (Duffy, 2013). In aprosodia, prosody is flat and robotic-like, with significant monotony in pitch, loudness, and duration. Damage to the right hemisphere can cause aprosodia because of the role of the right hemisphere in emotional and affective components of behavior. Therefore, right hemisphere disorder results in a lack of expressive or affective prosody in speech. Their lack of affective prosody is generally not reflective of their true emotional state.

Autism spectrum disorder (ASD) in adults

While ASD is primarily characterized by deficits in social communication and restricted/repetitive behaviors (American Psychiatric Association, 2013), deficits in prosody are among the first detectable characteristics to create an impression of "oddness" among typically developing individuals (Mesibov, 1992; Van Bourgondien & Woods, 1992). Prosodic differences observed in autistic adults generally impact a range of characteristics, including intonation, stress patterns, speech rate, affective quality, and loudness (Baltaxe et al., 1984; Baltaxe & Simmons, 1985; Baron-Cohen & Staunton, 1994; Fay, 1969; Patel et al., 2020; Pronovost et al., 1966; Shriberg et al., 2001). Notably, there is substantial variation in the prosodic patterns of individuals with ASD such that differences in any of the observed characteristics (e.g., intonation) may be described as being too flat/monotone for a subset of individuals yet too variable/sing-songy for yet another subset. Autistic adults show reduced affective prosody recognition (Globerson et al., 2015). An important point is that while commonly noted among autistic individuals, prosodic differences are not a defining characteristic of the disorder, meaning that a subset of individuals with ASD may present with fairly typical receptive and expressive prosody. Preliminary research suggests that atypical sensory-motor integration, particularly between the auditory (sensory) and vocal (motor) systems contributes to atypical expressive prosody among individuals with ASD (Patel et al., 2019).

Linguistically informed approaches to assessment and treatment

Assessment and treatment of prosody in adults is a difficult task (Peppé, 2009). Prosody is highly variable among individual speakers and norms for typical prosody have not yet been objectively delineated. In this section, we propose strategies for assessment and treatment of prosody based on linguistic theory and physiological knowledge of the speech impairments.

Assessment

Assessment of prosodic impairment in adults should include estimates of the severity of the impairment, the subsystems that could be contributing to the impairment, and the accuracy and appropriateness of various aspects of prosody. While there are some formal assessments of prosody, issues with validity and efficiency limit the use of these assessments (Peppé, 2009). Current standardized assessments that include prosody are often used mainly with Right Hemisphere Disorder. Some of these assessments include the Burns Brief Inventory of Communication and Cognition: Right Hemisphere Inventory (BBI-RHI; Burns, 1997), Mini Inventory of Right Brain Injury (MIRBI-2, Pimental & Knight, 2000), Montreal Protocol for the Evaluation of Communication (Protocol MEC; Australasian Society for the Study of Brain Impairment & Joanette, 2015), and the RIC Evaluation of Communication Problems in Right Hemisphere Dysfunction (RICE-2; Halper et al., 1991). However, the norms for typical prosody have not yet been objectively established. Therefore, we propose the use of a combination of perceptual and acoustic measures to determine the severity and features of the prosodic impairment. Detailing these characteristics will allow clinicians to set up goals for treatment.

The first goal in assessment will be to collect observations of which prosodic features are disrupted. Prosodic features to observe include the following:

- Rate of speech
- Length of phrasing
- Location of pauses
- Breathing patterns during speech
- Overall loudness
- **Perceptual salience of word-level and phrasal stress**
- **Perceptual salience of prosodic phrase boundary**
- **Expression of emotion during speech**

We focus on the bolded items in the above list of features and how to use linguistically informed assessment to examine prosodic impairment.

Phrasal stress is perceptually salient when there is a change in pitch, increased loudness, lengthened word duration, and hyperarticulation. The clinician should listen to the client's speech in sentence production, passage reading, and spontaneous speech to identify stressed words. When prosody is highly variable, such as in ataxic or hyperkinetic dysarthria, it can be difficult to identify the stressed word when pitch, loudness, and timing vary during the production of each word. Likewise, when prosody has too little variation, such as in hypokinetic dysarthria or right hemisphere disorder, there is little information in pitch, loudness, and timing to identify which word is stressed. In addition to perceptual evaluation, visual inspection of spectrograms and pitch contours in the acoustic speech signals are used to examine patterns of pitch and loudness variation. Visual inspection can be carried out using software such as Praat (Boersma & Weenink, 2016) and Audacity (Audacity, 2014).

Word-level stress is assessed in a similar manner. A common characteristic of dysarthria and AOS is stress on the wrong syllable in a multisyllabic word. To assess word-level stress, the client should produce multisyllabic words in isolation, sentences, and paragraphs to determine whether breakdown occurs at different levels of task complexity.

Prosodic phrase boundaries are perceptually salient when there is a decrease in loudness, lengthening of the final word, a reset in pitch, and/or a pause. The clinician should listen to the client speaking and reading to perceptually identify phrasal boundaries, followed by visual inspection of the acoustic signal to locate and measure the duration of breaks in speech that mark pauses. Breathing patterns should also be noted to assess if the client takes a breath at every break or pauses in the middle of a word or phrase to breathe.

If it is not easy to identify where stress and prosodic boundaries are occurring in speech, then it is likely that the client is not effectively controlling pitch, loudness, and timing for prosodic expression. The next step is to identify which speech subsystems are contributing to the lack of prosodic control. Lack of control in coordination of the respiratory and phonatory subsystems is the most likely cause of prosodic impairment in adults; however, nasality and articulatory errors can also be contributing factors. Understanding the contribution of these speech subsystems to prosodic control will be important for guiding treatment goals.

Severity of prosodic impairment can be assessed by determining the number of prosodic features that are disrupted and how much they impede the perceptual salience of phrasal stress and prosodic boundaries. For example, a person with ataxic dysarthria will have a severe prosodic impairment if they are speaking in two-word phrases where each word is lengthened with a large change in pitch and loudness. For this client, it will be very difficult to identify stress and boundaries and to make accurate interpretations of prosodic meaning. Alternatively, a person with flaccid dysarthria will have a mild prosodic impairment if articulatory errors from muscle weakness disrupt the timing of multisyllabic words but phrasing, pitch, and loudness are all perceived as normal.

Expression of emotion during speech should also be included as part of an assessment of prosody. Despite the lack of standardized protocols for assessment of emotional prosody, clinicians may conduct an informal assessment of emotional expression by instructing clients to produce target phrases, sentences, and/or passages while conveying a particular emotion. It is often beneficial to have caregivers or family/friends of the patient provide input on the patient's expression of emotion in the case of acquired disorders as they may be able to provide important information about the patient's baseline expression of emotion during speech.

Generally, tools for the assessment of prosody are far more limited than tools to assess other aspects of speech and language (e.g., vocabulary, syntax). As such, assessment of prosody often relies on clinician ratings and judgment. The Prosody Voice Screening Profile (PVSP; Shriberg et al., 1990) may be used to guide assessment of a speaker's phrasing, rate, stress, loudness, pitch, and voice quality. It uses cut-off scores to rate a speaker's prosody as typical across these areas and provides over 200 samples of speech to compare speaker vocalizations against. While adult samples are included, the majority of the samples are produced by children. There is a clear need for additional assessment tools focused on prosody in adults to promote standardization within the field.

Treatment

There are few evidence-based interventions for prosodic impairment, and most of these interventions treat prosody indirectly. For example, Lee Silverman Voice Treatment (LSVT) focuses on increasing vocal loudness in dysarthria (Sapir et al., 2006). Many studies have measured improvements in pitch and timing in speech as well (Levy et al., 2020). Given the limited number of treatment studies on prosodic impairment, linguistically informed observations of the perceptual salience of stress and boundaries are useful to guide treatment.

A scaffolding approach for education and treatment of prosodic control is one recommended approach. The clinician should describe how pitch, loudness, and timing are used in speech to emphasize the stressed word relative to surrounding words. Then, the clinician may demonstrate exaggerated phrasal stress and ask the client to identify the stressed word, with attention to changes in pitch, loudness, and timing to build perceptual skills. The same approach can be used for prosodic phrase boundaries. At the end of this stage, the client should be able to consistently identify phrasal stress and prosodic boundaries in the clinician's speech and describe how pitch, loudness, and timing are being used.

The next step is to use short, simple, structured sentences for the client to practice emphasizing the stressed word and pausing appropriately for prosodic boundaries. Information from the speech evaluation should be applied at this level to determine which speech subsystems are contributing to the prosodic impairment. If poor respiratory control is contributing to bursts in loudness, then the client can practice control of expiration during short sentences to modulate loudness for the stressed word. Additionally, planning out the locations of pauses and breaths during this structured task will assist with producing phrasal boundaries. If hypernasality is resulting in poor expiratory control, then options such as a palatal lift should be investigated. Common subsystem impairments contributing to prosodic deficit include weakness and/or incoordination in the respiratory, phonatory, or resonatory systems. Acoustic biofeedback may be beneficial for allowing the client to visualize changes in pitch and loudness for the stressed word. Principles of motor learning for increased volume of practice trials and variable feedback should be applied to improve generalizability and learning. At the end of this level, the client should be able to consistently produce salient phrasal stress and boundaries in short, simple sentences.

The scaffolding approach proceeds by increasing the complexity of the speech stimuli until the client is able to start implementing the strategies in spontaneous speech. At each level, the clinician must provide verbal comments and biofeedback. For this approach to succeed, the client must have the cognitive ability to consciously change their speech patterns, which requires significant cognitive load. If cognition is impaired, then it is possible that other programs like LSVT may be more beneficial. Another potential approach would be to use minimal pairs for intonation to treat distinctions between statements versus questions in English, for example.

Intervention for autistic adults may also draw upon the techniques described earlier. While a given client's focus (e.g., intonation pattern, stress, rate, loudness) in therapy may vary, intervention focused on prosodic production typically includes an emphasis on expression as well as self-monitoring to promote generalization of skills. Several studies, both within and outside the area of speech and language, support the use of visual aids to promote communication skills in individuals with ASD (Elwell, 2019; Kidder & McDonnell, 2017). In line with this research, visual aids representing a particular prosodic characteristic may be used during intervention. For example, a clinician may underline or ask the patient to underline the stressed portion of a word when targeting word-level stress. Additionally, audio recording the client's production of targets, listening together, and discussing the sample together may provide more concrete feedback than verbal feedback alone. Devoting time to develop a client's awareness of their own prosodic differences and the ability to rate changes in their productions within sessions may be particularly important in supporting generalization of skills.

Social factors: association between prosody and interactional dynamics

Prosody plays an important role in interactive speech, through its dual functions of signaling linguistic structure and pragmatic meaning. To put it simply, *how* something is said impacts the interpretation of the *what* was said (Couper-Kuhlen & Selting, 1996). As such, prosodic deficits have the potential to significantly disrupt overall social interactions and thereby warrant assessment and intervention. Prosody is especially important in conversation for turn management (Levinson, 2016; Ward, 2019). Within an utterance, a speaker may mark the location of a potential turn transition by slower tempo, rising or falling pitch movements, lower intensity, hypoarticulation, creaky voice, and silent pause or audible exhalation at the end of an utterance. A different set of prosodic patterns, for example, sustained mid-level pitch, are used to signal that a speaker intends to hold the floor beyond the current utterance. A speaker who flouts these prosodic conventions to signal turn-taking may be seen by their interlocutor as uncooperative, or attempting to dominate the conversation.

Considering the important role of prosody in social interactions, there is a burgeoning interest in prosodic entrainment, a phenomenon by which a speaker converges to the prosodic patterns of their conversation partner. Prosodic entrainment can be seen in converging speech rate, voice quality, pause behavior, and pitch patterns and other features over the course of an interaction. Stronger entrainment reflects mutual positive attitudes of the interlocutors and is positively correlated with perceived social attractiveness, mutual likability, competence, and supportiveness (Beňuš, 2014). Entrainment between conversation partners is associated with smoother and more successful interactions, with shorter gaps between turns, fewer interruptions and less overlap, and increased objective ratings of success (Levitan et al., 2012).

Atypical prosody arising from prosodic deficits associated with neurological function may impair the speaker's ability to entrain. Likewise, a speaker whose conversation partner exhibits atypical prosody may have difficulty entraining to the novel or irregular prosodic patterns. Deficits in prosodic entrainment are observed in adolescents and young adults with autism (Patel et al., 2022), and in adults with dysarthria (Borrie et al., 2015). Difficulties in assessment have essentially ruled out a focus on prosodic entrainment in clinical practice, although recent developments in the acoustic measurement and modeling of prosody may stimulate new interest in clinical applications (Borrie et al., 2015; Patel et al., 2022).

Conclusion

It is fair to say that prosody is the interface that links linguistic structure, discourse meaning, speaker stance, and social dynamics through the modulation of the melodic, rhythmic, and energy elements in speech. This chapter has reviewed the function of prosody in marking juncture between words and phrases, and in conveying pragmatic meaning related to reference and speech acts. Prosody was characterized in phonological representation in terms of the prominences and boundaries of hierarchically organized prosodic structures (words and phrases), and phonetically described in speech articulation and acoustics. Physiological requirements for prosody were reviewed for an understanding of how and why prosody deficits may arise in populations with structural or neurological impairment affecting speech, as illustrated in brief for atypical prosody in dysarthria, apraxia of speech, right hemisphere disorder, and autism spectrum disorder in adults. Approaches to clinical assessment and intervention were reviewed, with an emphasis on approaches that are informed by linguistic research on prosody. Finally, a case was made for a focus on prosody in the clinical domain based on its importance for successful communication and social interaction, as seen in behaviors related to conversational turn management and entrainment.

References

Ackermann, H. (2008). Cerebellar contributions to speech production and speech perception: Psycholinguistic and neurobiological perspectives. *Trends in Neurosciences, 31*(6), 265–272. https://doi.org/10.1016/j.tins.2008.02.011

American Psychiatric Association. (2013). *Diagnostic and statistical manual of mental disorders* (5th ed.).

Audacity, T. (2014). *Audacity.* https://www.audacityteam.org/2014/?p=t

Australasian Society for the Study of Brain Impairment, & Joanette, Y. (2015). *Montreal protocol for the evaluation of communication (MEC): Manual; 1 stimulus book; 25 copies of the informant questionnaire; 25 copies of the interviewer questionnaire; 5 copies of the response booklet; 1 memory stick with 2 audio files, informant questionnaire, interviewer questionnaire, response booklet.* ASSBI Resources.

Baltaxe, C. A. M., & Simmons, J. Q. (1985). Prosodic development in normal and autistic children. In *Communication problems in autism* (pp. 95–125). Springer. https://doi.org/10.1007/978-1-4757-4806-2_7

Baltaxe, C. A. M., Simmons, J. Q., & Zee, E. (1984). Intonation patterns in normal, autistic and aphasic children. *Proceedings of the Tenth International Congress of Phonetic Sciences,* 713–718.

Bänziger, T., & Scherer, K. R. (2005). The role of intonation in emotional expressions. *Speech Communication, 46*(3–4), 252–267.

Baron-Cohen, S., & Staunton, R. (1994). Do children with autism acquire the phonology of their peers? An examination of group identification through the window of bilingualism. *First Language, 14*(42–43), 241–248. https://doi.org/10.1177/014272379401404216

Beňuš, Š. (2014). Social aspects of entrainment in spoken interaction. *Cognitive Computation, 6*(4), 802–813. https://doi.org/10.1007/s12559-014-9261-4

Boersma, P., & Weenink, D. (2016). *Praat software.* University of Amsterdam. www.fon.hum.uva.nl/praat

Borrie, S. A., Lubold, N., & Pon-Barry, H. (2015). Disordered speech disrupts conversational entrainment: A study of acoustic-prosodic entrainment and communicative success in populations with communication challenges. *Frontiers in Psychology.* https://doi.org/10.3389/FPSYG.2015.01187

Brazil, D. (1980). *Discourse intonation and language teaching.* ERIC.

Bunn, J. C., & Mead, D. (1971). Control of ventilation during speech. *Journal of Applied Physiology, 31*(6).

Burns, M. S. (1997). *Burns brief inventory of communication and cognition.* Psychological Corporation.

Byrd, D., & Krivokapić, J. (2021). Cracking prosody in articulatory phonology. *Annual Review of Linguistics, 7*(1), 31–53. https://doi.org/10.1146/annurev-linguistics-030920-050033

Cho, T. (2005). Prosodic strengthening and featural enhancement: Evidence from acoustic and articulatory realizations of /a,i/ in English. *The Journal of the Acoustical Society of America, 117*(6), 3867–3878. https://doi.org/10.1121/1.1861893

Cole, J., Hualde, J. I., Smith, C. L., Eager, C., Mahrt, T., & Napoleão de Souza, R. (2019). Sound, structure and meaning: The bases of prominence ratings in English, French and Spanish. *Journal of Phonetics, 75*, 113–147. https://doi.org/10.1016/j.wocn.2019.05.002

Cole, J., Mo, Y., Hasegawa-Johnson, M. 2010. Signal-based and expectation-based factors in the perception of prosodic prominence. *Laboratory Phonology.* 1: 425–452. https://doi.org/10.1515/labphon.2010.022

Couper-Kuhlen, E., & Selting, M. (1996). *Prosody in conversation: Interactional studies.* Cambridge University Press.

Cutler, A., & Clifton, C. (1984). The use of prosodic information in word recognition. In *Attention and performance X: Control of language processes* (pp. 183–196). http://pubman.mpdl.mpg.de/pubman/item/escidoc:69901:6/component/escidoc:69902/cc_chapErlbaum.pdf

Darley, F. L., Aronson, A. E., & Brown, J. R. (1969). Differential diagnostic patterns of dysarthria. *Journal of Speech and Hearing Research, 12*(2), 246–269.

de Jong, K. J. (1995). The supraglottal articulation of prominence in English: Linguistic stress as localized hyperarticulation. *The Journal of the Acoustical Society of America, 97*(1), 491–504. https://doi.org/10.1121/1.412275

de Jong, K. J., Beckman, M. E., & Edwards, J. (1993). The interplay between prosodic structure and coarticulation. *Language and Speech, 36*(2–3), 197–212. https://doi.org/10.1177/002383099303600305

Duffy, J. R. (2013). *Motor speech disorders-e-book: Substrates, differential diagnosis, and management.* Elsevier Health Sciences.

Elwell, E. (2019). *The impact of using visual supports to increase independence for students with autism that require very substantial support in a vocational classroom.* http://hdl.handle.net/11603/13868

Fay, W. H. (1969). On the basis of autistic echolalia. *Journal of Communication Disorders, 2*(1), 38–47. https://doi.org/10.1016/0021-9924(69)90053-7

Fudge, E. (2015). *English word-stress.* Routledge.

Gee, J. P., & Grosjean, F. (1983). Performance structures: A psycholinguistic and linguistic appraisal. *Cognitive Psychology*, *15*(4), 411–458. https://doi.org/10.1016/0010-0285(83)90014-2

Globerson, E., Amir, N., Kishon-Rabin, L., & Golan, O. (2015). Prosody recognition in adults with high-functioning autism spectrum disorders: From psychoacoustics to cognition. *Autism Research*, *8*(2), 153–163. https://doi.org/10.1002/aur.1432

Gordon, M. (2014). Disentangling stress and pitch-accent: A typology of prominence at different prosodic levels. *Word Stress: Theoretical and Typological Issues*, 83–118.

Gussenhoven, C. (2004). *The phonology of tone and intonation*. Cambridge University Press.

Halper, A. S., Bums, M. S., Chemey, L. R., & Mogil, S. I. (1991). *RIC evaluation of communication problems in right hemisphere dysfunction-revised (RICE-2)*. Aspen Publishers.

Hirschberg, J. (2015). *Pragmatics and prosody* (Y. Huang, Ed., Vol. 1). Oxford University Press. https://doi.org/10.1093/oxfordhb/9780199697960.013.28

Hixon, T. J., Goldman, M. D., & Mead, J. (1973). Kinematics of the chest wall during speech production: Volume displacements of the rib cage, abdomen, and lung. *Journal of Speech and Hearing Research*, *16*(1), 78–115. https://doi.org/10.1044/jshr.1601.78

Hoit, J. D., Hixon, T. J., Altman, M. E., & Morgan, W. J. (1989). Speech breathing in women. *Journal of Speech and Hearing Research*, *32*(2), 353–365. https://doi.org/10.1044/jshr.3202.353

Holliday, N. (2021). Prosody and sociolinguistic variation in American Englishes. In *Annual review of linguistics* (Vol. 7, pp. 55–68). Annual Reviews Inc. https://doi.org/10.1146/annurev-linguistics-031220-093728

Huber, J. E. (2008). Effects of utterance length and vocal loudness on speech breathing in older adults. *Respiratory Physiology and Neurobiology*, *164*(3), 323–330. https://doi.org/10.1016/j.resp.2008.08.007

Huber, J. E., & Darling-White, M. (2017). Longitudinal changes in speech breathing in older adults with and without Parkinson's disease. *Seminars in Speech and Language*, *38*(3), 200–209. https://doi.org/10.1055/s-0037-1602839

Kent, R. D., Kent, J. F., Duffy, J. R., Thomas, J. E., Weismer, G., & Stuntebeck, S. (2000). Ataxic dysarthria. *Journal of Speech, Language, and Hearing Research*, *43*(1–5), 1275–1289. https://doi.org/10.1044/jslhr.4305.1275

Kent, R. D., Weismer, G., Kent, J. F., & Rosenbek, J. C. (1989). Toward phonetic intelligibility testing in dysarthria. *Journal of Speech and Hearing Disorders*, *54*(4), 482–499. https://doi.org/10.1044/jshd.5404.482

Kidder, J. E., & McDonnell, A. P. (2017). Visual aids for positive behavior support of young children with autism spectrum disorders. *Young Exceptional Children*, *20*(3), 103–116. https://doi.org/10.1177/1096250615586029

Krivokapić, J. (2014). Gestural coordination at prosodic boundaries and its role for prosodic structure and speech planning processes. In *Philosophical transactions of the royal society B: Biological sciences* (Vol. 369, Issue 1658). Royal Society of London. https://doi.org/10.1098/rstb.2013.0397

Ladd, D. R. (2008). *Intonational phonology*. Cambridge University Press.

Levinson, S. C. (2016). Turn-taking in human communication–origins and implications for language processing. *Trends in Cognitive Sciences*, *20*(1), 6–14.

Levitan, R., Gravano, A., Willson, L., Beňuš, Š., Hirschberg, J., & Nenkova, A. (2012). *Acoustic-prosodic entrainment and social behavior* (pp. 11–19). NAACL HLT 2012–2012 Conference of the North American Chapter of the Association for Computational Linguistics: Human Language Technologies, Proceedings of the Conference. www.mturk.com

Levy, E. S., Moya-Galé, G., Chang, Y. H. M., Freeman, K., Forrest, K., Brin, M. F., & Ramig, L. A. (2020). The effects of intensive speech treatment on intelligibility in Parkinson's disease: A randomised controlled trial. *eClinicalMedicine, 24*, 100429. https://doi.org/10.1016/j.eclinm.2020.100429

Mesibov, G. B. (1992). Treatment issues with high-functioning adolescents and adults with autism. In *High-functioning individuals with autism* (pp. 143–155). Springer. https://doi.org/10.1007/978-1-4899-2456-8_8

Navarro, A. H., & Nebot, A. C. (2014). On the importance of the prosodic component in the expression of linguistic im/politeness. *Journal of Politeness Research, 10*(1), 5–27. https://doi.org/10.1515/pr-2014-0002

Patel, S. P., Cole, J., Lau, J. C., Fragnito, G., & Losh, M. (2022). Verbal entrainment in autism spectrum disorder and first-degree relatives. *Scientific Reports, 12*(1), 1–14.

Patel, S. P., Kim, J. H., Larson, C. R., & Losh, M. (2019). Mechanisms of voice control related to prosody in autism spectrum disorder and first-degree relatives. *Autism Research, 12*(8), 1192–1210. https://doi.org/10.1002/aur.2156

Patel, S. P., Nayar, K., Martin, G. E., Franich, K., Crawford, S., Diehl, J. J., & Losh, M. (2020). An acoustic characterization of prosodic differences in autism spectrum disorder and first-degree relatives. *Journal of Autism and Developmental Disorders, 50*, 3032–3045. https://doi.org/10.1007/s10803-020-04392-9

Pell, M. D., Cheang, H. S., & Leonard, C. L. (2006). The impact of Parkinson's disease on vocal-prosodic communication from the perspective of listeners. *Brain and Language, 97*(2), 123–134. https://doi.org/10.1016/j.bandl.2005.08.010

Peppé, S. J. E. (2009). Why is prosody in speech-language pathology so difficult? *International Journal of Speech-Language Pathology, 11*(4), 258–271. https://doi.org/10.1080/17549500902906339

Pimental, P., & Knight, J. (2000). *MIRBI-2: The mini inventory of right brain injury*. Pro-Ed.

Pronovost, W., Wakstein, M. P., & Wakstein, D. J. (1966). A longitudinal study of the speech behavior and language comprehension of fourteen children diagnosed atypical or autistic. *Exceptional Children, 33*(1), 19–26. https://doi.org/10.1177/001440296603300104

Roettger, T. B., & Franke, M. (2019). Evidential strength of intonational cues and rational adaptation to (un-)reliable intonation. *Cognitive Science, 43*(7), e12745. https://doi.org/10.1111/COGS.12745

Russell, N. K., & Stathopoulos, E. (1988). Lung volume changes in children and adults during speech production. *Journal of Speech and Hearing Research, 31*(2), 146–155. https://doi.org/10.1044/jshr.3102.146

Sapir, S., Olson Ramig, L., & Fox, C. (2006). The Lee Silverman voice treatment ® for voice, speech and other orofacial disorders in patients with Parkinson's disease. *Future Neurology, 5*, 563–570. https://doi.org/10.2217/14796708.1.5.563

Shattuck-Hufnagel, S., & Turk, A. E. (1996). A prosody tutorial for investigators of auditory sentence processing. *Journal of Psycholinguistic Research, 25*(2), 193–247. https://doi.org/10.1007/BF01708572

Shriberg, L. D., Paul, R., McSweeny, J. L., Klin, A., Cohen, D. J., & Volkmar, F. R. (2001). Speech and prosody characteristics of adolescents and adults with high-functioning autism and Asperger syndrome. *Journal of Speech, Language, and Hearing Research, 44*(5), 1097–1115. https://doi.org/10.1044/1092-4388(2001/087)

Shriberg, L. D., Kwiatkowski, J., & Rasmussen, C. (1990). *Prosody-voice screening profile (PVSP): Scoring forms and training materials*. Communication Skill Builders.

Sluijter, A. M., & van Heuven, V. J. (1996). Spectral balance as an acoustic correlate of linguistic stress. *Journal of the Acoustical Society of America, 100*(4(1)), 2471–2485. https://doi.org/10.1121/1.417955

Speer, S. R., Kjelgaard, M. M., & Dobroth, K. M. (1996). The influence of prosodic structure on the resolution of temporary syntactic closure ambiguities. *Journal of Psycholinguistic Research*, *25*(2).

Spencer, K. A., & Rogers, M. A. (2005). Speech motor programming in hypokinetic and ataxic dysarthria. *Brain and Language*, *94*(3), 347–366. https://doi.org/10.1016/j.bandl.2005.01.008

Tardif, M., Berti, L. C., Marino, V. C. D. C., Pardo, J., & Bressmann, T. (2018). Hypernasal speech is perceived as more monotonous than typical speech. *Folia Phoniatrica et Logopaedica*, *70*(3–4), 183–190. https://doi.org/10.1159/000492385

Titze, I. R. (1989). On the relation between subglottal pressure and fundamental frequency in phonation. *Citation: The Journal of the Acoustical Society of America*, *85*, 901. https://doi.org/10.1121/1.397562

Van Bourgondien, M. E., & Woods, A. V. (1992). Vocational possibilities for high-functioning adults with autism. In *High-functioning individuals with autism* (pp. 227–239). Springer. https://doi.org/10.1007/978-1-4899-2456-8_12

Wang, Y. T., Green, J. R., Nip, I. S. B., Kent, R. D., & Kent, J. F. (2010). Breath group analysis for reading and spontaneous speech in healthy adults. *Folia Phoniatrica et Logopaedica*, *62*(6), 297–302. https://doi.org/10.1159/000316976

Ward, N. G. (2019). *Prosodic patterns in English conversation*. Cambridge University Press.

Watson, D., & Gibson, E. (2004). The relationship between intonational phrasing and syntactic structure in language production. *Language and Cognitive Processes*, *19*(6), 713–755. https://doi.org/10.1080/01690960444000070

Westera, M., Goodhue, D., & Gussenhoven, C. (2020). Meanings of tones and tunes. In *The Oxford handbook of language prosody* (pp. 443–453). Oxford University Press.

Yorkston, K., Beukelman, D., Strand, E., & Bell, K. (1999). *Management of motor speech disorders in children and adults*. Pro-ed. Inc.

Zyski, B. J., & Weisiger, B. E. (1987). Identification of dysarthria types based on perceptual analysis. *Journal of Communication Disorders*, *20*(5), 367–378. https://doi.org/10.1016/0021-9924(87)90025-6

11 Sociolinguistics

The linguistics of accentedness: How phonetics, phonology, and sociolinguistic considerations impact clinical intervention of accent modification

Naomi Gurevich and Talia Bugel

Abstract

Speaking with a foreign accent is not an impairment and cannot be reduced to articulation errors. Accents are often critical to the cultural and linguistic identity of the speakers. Native sound inventories and rules, group identity, and language attitudes can all influence the perception of accentedness by a listener. These considerations also affect listeners' perception of the accented speaker's intelligibility. Although clinicians are regularly taught to distinguish between language learning and disorders in children, the considerations of fully developed phonologies and cultural identifications of adults are rarely addressed in communication disorders curricula. Clinicians are therefore often not adequately prepared to work with accent modifications clients. In this chapter, we outline the phonetic and phonological bases of accentedness, as well as the sociolinguistic factors that contribute to a complex phenomenon that doesn't fit the typical diagnose-then-treat paradigm. Clinical implications for accent modification practice are addressed, and suggestions for a culturally-aware paradigm for the assessment and treatment of such clients are presented.

Statement to the reader

As a clinician, it is likely clear to you that speaking with a foreign accent is a communication *difference*, not a *disorder*. However, when it comes to working with accent modification clients, you may have little training on how to assess and treat without relying on a disorder-driven model that requires determining the severity of the difficulty so that it can be reduced through intervention. In this chapter we explain why the disorder-driven model is not suited for accent modification and provide you with the basic knowledge about what foreign

DOI: 10.4324/9781003045519-13

accents are using simple and well-defined terminology. We also provide the clinician with two tools: One to help collect accent-related data in order to initiate intervention, and the other to help baseline and track progress of a condition whose severity is not always proportional to the impact it may have on a speaker.

Introduction

A trained speech-language pathologist (SLP) might approach an accent-modification client using a diagnose-then-treat paradigm, drawing on the clinical skillset related to filling in missing phonemes for school-age populations, or related to supporting intelligibility, for example, when treating dysarthria. The clinician might assess a client's speech and generate an inventory of mispronunciations, then target these for articulation intervention. In doing so, this clinician would be treating accented speech as a disorder of misarticulation, which by extension implies the thicker the current accent, the greater the impact on a client's life. Further, the clinician may assume a client's motivation to modify their accent demonstrates negative feelings about their current one. In this chapter, we dispel these assumptions and offer a multilinguistically aware paradigm for assessment and treatment of accent modification that combines the SLP's skillset with phonetic, phonological, and sociolinguistic considerations. We offer two tools to help clinicians plan and carry out intervention: An intake form to help identify a pattern of misarticulations, and an accent impact index to support collecting client-reported outcomes. These tools are language-neutral, which means they can be used with clients regardless of their native or target languages.

What is accented speech?

Technically, all speech is accented. All languages, and language varieties, are accented: Given the internal changes in languages due to both linguistic and sociohistorical conditions that include among them influences from language contact (Wolfram, 1991), each group has a different way of speaking. Some differences are more noticeable (e.g., across linguistically distant languages, such as English and Korean) while others are barely perceptible to listeners who are not fluent in the language being spoken (e.g., across regional varieties of one language). "Accent is the map which listeners perceive through their ears" (Esling, 1999, p. 169). To wit, accents may tell listeners where speakers were born, where they have lived, what social groups they belong to, even how old they are. However, speakers of a specific language variety do not generally consider their own speech accented (Esling, 1999). As such when we think of accents we really think of "foreign" accents. The question then is, what is a "foreign" accent?

Interference from a speaker's native or previously learned languages (hereafter referred to as *influencing* languages, or ILs) may present as a foreign accent in a target language (TL). The foreign accent may make it difficult for others to understand the speaker, and may affect the speaker's communication in vocational and social activities (American Speech-Language-Hearing Association (ASHA), 2010). A foreign accent, or accentedness, is related to intelligibility and comprehensibility, but several studies have shown that the interaction among these three measures is not always direct (Franklin et al., 2016). *Accentedness* is a measure of the extent of the foreign accent in one's speech, or how much listeners perceive one's speech to be different from their own variety (Derwing & Munro, 2005). *Intelligibility* is a measure of how much of a person's speech, often interpreted as the acoustic signal, can be understood by a listener (Franklin et al., 2016; Yorkston et al., 1996). And *comprehensibility* is a measure of how easy accented speech is to understand (Hansen Edwards et al., 2018; Isaacs & Trofimovich, 2012; Munro & Derwing, 1999), which is a slightly different definition than used in Communication Sciences and Disorders (CSD) literature where *comprehensibility* is defined as a holistic measure of overall communicative effectiveness (Gurevich & Scamihorn, 2017; Yorkston et al., 1996).

All three of these interrelated measures are also subjective. Although the physical properties of sound, the acoustics, can be analyzed using objective tools, listener interpretation of acoustic signals (intelligibility) is sensitive to context, situation, topic, and familiarity with the speaker (D'Innocenzo et al., 2006; Hustad & Cahill, 2003; Liss et al., 2002; Utianski et al., 2011; Ziegler & Zierdt, 2008). Similarly, the measure of accentedness is subjective and complex, and can be affected by factors ranging from linguistic considerations, to language attitudes and shared experiences, and it is not always predictable from the speakers' intelligibility (Hansen Edwards et al., 2018) or comprehensibility (Isaacs & Trofimovich, 2012). Speech-based biases can have significant consequences for individuals (Lindberg & Trofimovich, 2020). For example, studies show that accented instructors are regularly evaluated more negatively, including in terms of intelligibility and comprehensibility (Hendriks et al., 2021). Multiple studies show there is a clear bias against certain accents, for example, seeing an Asian face can make listeners perceive speech as more accented and less intelligible (Rubin, 1992; Rubin et al., 1999; Rubin & Smith, 1990; Yi et al., 2014, 2013; Zheng & Samuel, 2017). Another example of linguistic prejudice is faced by Spanish-influenced English speaking students in the United States, whose work (including writing exhibiting no Spanish influence) was rated lower than that of native English speakers (Ford, 1984). Even the attitudes of speakers, for example, toward their listeners, toward the non-native language they are using, or toward a situation, can affect how accented, intelligible, or proficient the speakers are perceived to be (Hutchinson et al., 2019).

Writing a goal to reduce accentedness in order to increase intelligibility and comprehensibility may seem clinically sound based on experience with disordered speech such as dysarthria. However, not only is the relationship among these measures indirect, but there is also another caveat. Accentedness is essentially a measure of the listener's perspective: their perception of how different a speaker's accent is from their own. Moreover, the speaker's view of how much their own accent impacts their life may not be proportional to the degree of their accentedness. In our own research, we found that while one accented speaker may have little trouble with intelligibility or comprehensibility yet desire more native-like proficiency, another speaker may have difficulty being understood by unfamiliar listeners and yet have no desire to change their own pronunciation. An SLP experienced with acquired cognitive-communication disorders often targets awareness of impairments in their plan of care as part of the diagnose-then-treat paradigm. A well-meaning clinician might consider increasing a client's awareness of the impact of their accent on a listener's ability to understand them. In doing so, again, the accent is treated as a disorder, and the treatment target favors the listeners (their ability to understand the speech) rather than the speaker. The speaker is the client, and a client-focused approach must primarily consider the impact their accent has on their life. In taking on accent modification clients, we must stop thinking in terms of "severity of accentedness" (a disorder-focused approach) and start thinking in terms of "experience of the speaker," which necessarily involves not only the phonetic and phonological bases of accents, but also sociolinguistic factors such as language and group identities and attitudes.

The linguistics of a "foreign" accent: phonetics and phonology

As we are discussing the SLP's role in accent modification, not a language teacher's role in improving overall proficiency with a new language, we will focus on how languages sound. In other words, in addressing the sounds of "foreign" accents we will consider phonetics and phonology.

Phonetics involves articulation of sounds and the acoustic properties of sounds (phones) of all human languages. These are universal properties, related to the shared anatomy of speakers and to physical properties of sounds. Whether /t/ is produced in English, Russian, or Bengali, it is an oral (velum closed) voiceless (abducted vocal folds) plosive (produced by blocking the airflow, then releasing it) produced at the alveolar place of articulation (with the tongue blade at the alveolar ridge), and subject to coarticulation. Likewise, the vocal tract is in similar positions when producing a high front vowel /i/, resulting in a low first formant and a high second formant, regardless of the language. *Phonology* is language-specific, and it includes the organization and the rules of sounds in a given language. Not all phones of all human languages play a role in individual languages. A subset of these phones hold meaning in a given language (are phonemic) and the inventory of phonemes in a language make up its sound system. Additionally, there are rules that govern the use of sounds in each language. The sound systems of languages and phonological rules are two primary sources of speech that sounds accented.[1]

---

1. Interestingly, while several studies have shown that consonants are particularly critical to word-level intelligibility in speech perception and in language acquisition (e.g., Fogerty et al., 2012; Hochmann et al., 2011; Toro et al., 2008), when it comes to accentedness, vowels contribute to measures of both accentedness and intelligibility (e.g., Alexander et al., 2008).

Sound systems

Although in theory all speakers are able to produce all phones in human languages, very early in our development (as early as 6 months old) we stop attending to differences between sounds that are not phonemic in our language (Kuhl, 2004; Kuhl et al., 1992). By age five most children acquire 93% of the phonemes of their language (McLeod & Crowe, 2018), and once their native sound system is mastered, it becomes difficult for speakers to acquire new non-native patterns (Dobel et al., 2009; Kuhl, 2004). In simple terms we can think of speakers transitioning from having access to all phones to getting accustomed to using and attending only to their own language's phonemes and the rules that govern the use of these phonemes.

How does this result in accented speech? Languages differ in their phonemic inventories. A sound that is used in one language (e.g., /ɣ/ in Greek and Navajo, or /ɦ/ in Hebrew and Nepali) is not used in others (e.g., neither of these phones are phonemic in English). The mismatch of phonemes across languages means that a native speaker of one language may have little experience with producing non-native sounds that are phonemic in another language. For example, an American English speaker learning Greek or Hebrew may have a difficult time producing /ɣ/ or /ɦ/. This new language learner might make a distorted attempt to produce the voiced velar or glottal voiced fricative or might substitute familiar phonemes from American English that seem closest to the target ones in place and manner of articulation. For example, the closest voiced velar in the inventory of English phonemes is /g/, so the Greek "I love you" (σ'αγαπώ) /saɣa'po/ might be produced as [saga'po] (or more likely [sa'gapo] because English speakers are not used to stressing the final syllable). The closest glottal fricative among English phonemes is the voiceless counterpart /h/ which is not a Hebrew phoneme, and accordingly, "love" (אוהב) /ʔo'ɦev/ might be produced as /ʔo'hev/ (or more likely [o'hev] because English speakers are more used to word-initial vowels).

The choice of native phoneme to fill in for a non-native one depends on the phonology of one's native language, which includes not just the organization and phonotactic rules of the language, but also phoneme frequency and functional load (these concepts are discussed in the Gurevich and Kim chapter in this book). For example, neither Russian nor Hebrew phonemes include /θ/, and both include /s/ and /t/. A Russian speaker is more likely to substitute the sibilant for the dental voiceless fricative, and the open back vowel for the /æ/ ("bathroom"/'bæθrum/['bɑsrum]) while a Hebrew speaker is more likely to select the alveolar stop ("bathroom"/'bæθrum/['bɑtrum]).

Comparing the TL phonemic inventory with the IL inventory allows the identification of TL phonemes missing from the IL and has a strong potential for predicting how some of the missing phonemes will be handled (then easily confirmed by listening to the accented speech). Moreover, this strategy can support initial goals that address filling in missing TL phonemes and can help bring up awareness for the client of the cause of some of their mispronunciations (filling in IL phonemes for missing TL ones). Filling in missing phonemes is within the SLP's skillset, but clinicians should not assume all inventory mismatches will lead to misarticulations and remember that comparing inventories is suggested only as a starting point to help identify potential problems that can be easily confirmed or ruled out by listening to the client.

To summarize, one primary source of accented speech is that the phonemic mismatch between the TL and the IL results in inventory gaps which are replaced either by IL sounds not in the TL (like /ɦ/>[h] in Hebrew in the example above) or by other TL sounds (like /θ/>[s/t] in English in the example above).

Phonological rules

Whether speakers are aware of these or not (usually not), all languages have phonological rules. An example from English is the aspiration of stressed-syllable-initial voiceless plosives (e.g., "cat" /kæt/ [kʰæt]) or voicing of the plural/3rd person singular/possessive suffix "s" when it follows a voiced sound (e.g., "cats" [kʰæts] versus "bees" [biz]). Proficient (or native) speakers of English apply these rules automatically, but a non-native speaker must learn these rules and the contexts where they apply, and subsequently learn to apply them regularly. When a rule is not applied, the listeners notice: Imagine someone saying [dɑgs] instead of [dɑgz] for "dogs" in American English; despite sounding a bit strange the meaning might be clear to some, while others might perceive the word as [dɑks] "docs." A non-native speaker must also inhibit the rules of their native language (their IL), something that is difficult to do considering most speakers are not aware that they are applying these rules. English speakers have a difficult time inhibiting the aspiration of stressed-syllable-initial voiceless plosives, and for example, Talia /talʲja/ (the first name of one of the authors in Spanish) is often produced as [tʰalʲja] by U.S. speakers or interpreted as [dalʲja] when the author's native pronunciation is heard. Another example of misapplication of IL rules in the TL comes from Greek speakers of English. In Modern Greek the /s/ is voiced to [z] before most voiced consonants, for example /svino/ > [zvino] "extinguish," and /kosmos/ > [kozmos] "world" and /kosmos mu/ > [kozmozmu][2] "my world." Greek speakers often apply this rule when speaking English, for example pronouncing "smile" as [zmaɪl].

The second main source of accented speech is the misapplication of phonological rules by either underapplying TL rules or overapplying IL rules. Prosodic elements of speech such as stress and intonation are also language-specific and rule-governed, and as such play an important role in accentedness (e.g., the preference for avoiding word-final stress in English illustrated in the Greek "I love you" /saɣaˈpo/ to [saˈgapo] example from the Sound Systems section). Clinicians that have had sufficient linguistic training to distinguish cross-linguistic prosodic features and misapplication of native prosodies should certainly approach this component of speech to guide initial accent modification

---

2. This example shows that this is a *synchronic* rule in Greek. Speakers don't simply learn the word /kozmoz/; the word-final /s/ is voiceless except when followed by the voiced /m/.

goals if indicated for the individual speaker. This, however, may not be in every clinician's skillset given that our attention to prosody within graduate SLP curricula (in the United States) is limited to impairments related to motor-speech disorders such as speech rate, ability to indicate stress, and ability to vary pitch. Clinicians can make use of free software that can help them and their clients analyze intonation patterns and other acoustic components of speech (e.g., PRAAT (Boersma & Weenink, 2020) or WASP (Huckvale, 2020)). It is also worth mentioning that when it comes to reducing accentedness, prosodic training was found to be effective, but did not appear to be more effective than phoneme-focused training (Behrman, 2014). For additional reading on prosody refer to two chapters devoted to this topic in this volume: Thorson's chapter with application to pediatric populations (Chapter 3), and Cole et al.'s chapter with applications to adult populations (Chapter 10).

The linguistics of a "foreign" accent: sociolinguistics

Sociolinguistics is the study of how social factors impact the use of language and influence language change and language shift. These factors include all the information that can be learned from one's speech independently from the content of what is said. This may include the accent, the choice of words, the sentence organization, and whether the speaker switches from one language to another or not. Language attitudes are among the dominant extralinguistic factors that may reflect, among other things, the values that groups of people assign to a language, a language variety, or to a group that speaks it.

In the introduction we noted that the measure of accentedness is subjective and complex. The relevant phonological factors were discussed in the previous section, and now we turn our attention to the sociolinguistic information that contributes to this subjectivity and bias. In a landmark study in the field of social psychology, Lambert and colleagues (1960) developed the matched-guise technique that brought attention to the effect of social stereotypes on how spoken language is perceived. The experiment involved English and French students in Quebec who were asked to listen to recordings of French and English speakers and rate them on scales of positive-to-negative traits such as likeability, reliability, education, and intelligence. The English speakers were consistently rated higher on positive adjectives by both English- and French-speaking students. However, the English and French speakers in the recordings were always the same bilingual individuals, speaking under two guises, so every student heard the exact same speaker in both languages, delivering the same message. This showed that the students' reactions to the recordings were influenced solely by the language spoken and revealed how the (social, cultural, educational, political, economic) status of a language in a specific community impacts how its speakers are perceived (in this case in 1960s Quebec, reflecting the lower status of French in Canada vis-à-vis English at the time).

In the face of bias, we would expect speakers of a lower status or stigmatized group to want to move out of it and into the prestigious group, by learning the language or affecting the accent of the more prestigious variety. This does happen. For example, Labov (1966) described sales attendants in three department stores in New York modifying their production of /r/ to match their clients' pronunciation. However, research shows that in fact large scale movement of speakers across groups of differing levels of prestige are often countered by the forces of group identity, representing the speakers' sense of belonging and their need for acceptance. Conversely, group identity tied to a particular language variety may also involve shunning new members, closing rank against speakers from other groups (e.g., Labov, 1963). French may have been stigmatized in Canada in the 1960s, but its historical prestige in Europe may have contributed to the group identity of its speakers in Quebec at the time, reducing their desire to cross group boundaries. A more recent example of this was presented by MacGregor-Mendoza (2015), who found that Spanish-speaking immigrants from the Latin American educated elites chose to maintain Spanish, despite the stigmatized status of the language in the United States. And just as the status of a language can affect perception of its speakers, the status of the speakers can influence the relative status of a language or language variety (Giles & Niedzielski, 1999; Lodge, 1999). For example, vis-à-vis Indigenous languages of Latin America, Spanish is prestigious, given the higher socio-economic status of its speakers. Meanwhile, the lower socio-economic status of Spanish-speakers in the United States makes Spanish a stigmatized language. As such, in the United States, speakers of English with Spanish accents are regularly subjected to biases (e.g., Brennan & Brennan, 1981; Ford, 1984; Galindo, 1995; Hosoda et al., 2012).

In a seminal study at Martha's Vineyard, Labov (1963) examined the possibility and social motivation of adopting accents of language varieties different than one's own. Men from the island who worked on the mainland would use the mainland's accent on their return home. This was seen as a way of achieving higher status by showing worldliness. However, when tourists arrived at Martha's Vineyard for summer vacations, the island men would revert to their distinctive island accents to show they are local. This influential work showed how speakers who can manipulate their accents can use this skill to their advantage to communicate selective information about themselves.

With all this in mind, when working with accent modification clients, it is important to take into account a native speaker's attachment to their language or language variety and the role their language plays in terms of their own identity. The fact a speaker wants to improve their accent in their TL does not necessarily mean the speaker wants to move out of their old group and into a new one. A speaker may wish to feel accepted by a new group (e.g., a job where they have to speak the TL) while simultaneously wishing to avoid, even fearing, rejection by their existing group (i.e., the community of speakers of their IL). A client's own goals for working on their accent may be affected by multiple considerations related to their own individual, familial, and community experiences that they may not be able to articulate (and in some cases may not even be fully aware of). A prepared clinician will realize that their own experience with language varieties may bear no resemblance to the client's and be prepared to allow the client to educate them rather than them educating the client.

SLPs are used to teaching communication strategies, and to helping clients generalize these beyond the treatment sessions. From this perspective, the diagnose-then-treat paradigm suggests that wider implementation of a strategy, in more situations, more often, and with less cuing, is optimal. For accent modification clients, generalization must take a different meaning. The situational contexts in which speakers may wish to use modified accents may not be predictable by a bystander (or by a clinician). Accent modification intervention involves helping speakers control the influence that the sound system of their IL exerts over their TL, so they can switch among sound systems as needed (whether in isolated situations, for specific purposes, or in general). In helping speakers gain control of accents, clinicians should always remember that spoken language is part of one's identity, and it communicates to the world who the speaker is. Modifying how one sounds can affect this identity, and how a person presents themselves to the world, and it is up to that person to judge which situations they want to "generalize" the results of accent modification intervention to.

Application: Two tools

Given that the clinician is not expected to have experience with the TL/IL of each client, some tools may be needed to help organize data collection, what to pay attention to, and what to ask. The resources in this chapter help the clinician identify intervention targets but do not provide intervention strategies (such as discrimination followed by practice with minimal pairs) as these are well within a clinician's training (e.g., Schmidt, 1997). We offer two tools, both provided in the Appendix: (1) A client intake form that helps to focus on sound patterns, not "disorders," that can be used to prioritize and motivate initial intervention goals, and (2) an accent-impact index that we are developing to help support the need for client-reported outcomes.

Accent modification intake form

In this section, we outline an approach that explicitly targets comparing and contrasting the TL and IL sound systems to help clients recognize the pattern of sound-use that shapes their "foreign" accent. As previously noted, speakers are not typically aware of the phonological sound and rule systems in their own languages, much less how these differ between their TL and ILs. Increasing familiarity with the linguistic components of one's native and new languages has been shown to assist in language learning. This is supported by Contrastive Analysis theory, applied to language learning as far back as the 1940s (Khansir & Pakdel, 2019; Wardhaugh, 1970). It was also applied in educational settings to help children transition to a standard dialect for use in the schools (e.g., Taylor, 1989). This method was found to be more effective than traditional approaches that did not involve contrastive analysis (Rickford, 2005).

The purpose of this form is to help the clinician and client compare the inventories of the TL and the ILs to identify *potential* sources of mismatches. The client's production can then confirm or rule out these areas as sources of accentedness. The form also helps guide the clinician and client in identifying potential mismatches of phonological rules between the TL and IL. This is a more complex endeavor given that (1) there are no known lists of all phonological rules for every language; and (2) speakers are not typically aware of knowing or implementing these rules (e.g., English speakers are not typically aware they aspirate the stressed-syllable initial voiceless plosives). Given this lack of explicit awareness of automatically applying the phonological rules of our native language, it is difficult for speakers to inhibit use of these rules even when speaking a different language. A Greek speaker can easily produce the voiceless /s/ in many contexts and is unlikely to notice regularly voicing it before nasals (pronouncing "smile" as [zmaɪl]). Drawing attention to this systematic voicing of /s/ when speaking English can facilitate a conscious inhibition of this synchronic sound change. Similarly, if English speakers are made aware of the systemic aspiration of /p, t, k/ in stressed syllable-initial positions, they can focus on inhibiting this rule when speaking a different language.

Example of Use. As instructed in the form, highlight the cells of all TL phonemes, cross-out the ones that aren't used in the ILs, and circle IL sounds not in the TL. See Figure 11.1 example for English as the TL and Hebrew as the IL. In this figure the English phonemes are in the highlighted (gray) cells. The five English consonants that are not used in Hebrew (w, θ, ð, ɹ, ŋ), and eight vowels (ɪ, e, æ, ə, ɜ, ʊ, ʌ, ɔ) are crossed out. The four Hebrew phonemes (all consonants: ɾ, x, ʁ, ɦ) that are not used in English are all circled. Sounds in white cells are irrelevant (they are not used in either language).

A Hebrew speaker who finds the alveolar approximant /ɹ/ difficult (that is not to say all Hebrew speakers will have this issue) may replace it with a retroflex flap /ɽ/. Likewise, the English glottal voiceless fricative /h/ is likely to be replaced by the Hebrew voiced counterpart /ɦ/. Experience with Hebrew speakers of English leads us to assume /θ, ð/ will be replaced with /t, d/ until the dental fricatives are mastered, and the approximant /w/ is often replaced by /v/ (and sometimes vocalized to /u/). American vowels are reduced to their closest corner vowels /i, ɛ, u, o, ɑ/. Some examples of how this will affect words are "hard" (/hɑɹd/) may be produced as [ɦɑɽd], and "heard" (/hɜrd/) may be produced as [ɦɛɽd]. The word "cat," which native speakers produce as [kʰæt], may be pronounced as [kɛt], which to an American ear without the aspiration may sound more like [gɛt]. Again, these are hypothetical examples assuming a speaker who has yet to master any of the new TL phonemes, when in fact many speakers will have quickly mastered the new consonants. Listening to the client's speech and asking them their concerns would easily help establish which of these hypothetical issues, if any, exists for a given client.

To summarize, the filled-out inventory provides a roadmap for starting to collect data: The TL phonemes that are crossed out have the greatest potential for production problems. Listen to the client's speech and determine which of these, if any, may pose difficulty. The circled IL phonemes *may* help predict which sounds

Consonants

	Bilabial	Labiodental	Dental	Alveolar	Postalveolar	Retroflex	Palatal	Velar	Uvular	Pharyngeal	glottal
Plosive	p b			t d		ʈ ɖ	c ɟ	k g	q ɢ		ʔ
Nasal	m	ɱ		n		ɳ	ɲ	ŋ	ɴ		
Trill	ʙ			r					ʀ		
Tap/flap				ɾ		ɽ					
Fricative	ɸ β	f v	θ ð	s z	ʃ ʒ	ʂ ʐ	ç ʝ	x ɣ	χ ʁ	ħ ʕ	h ɦ
Lateral fricative				ɬ ɮ							
Approximant	ʋ	ʋ				ɻ	j	ɰ			
Lateral approximant				l		ɭ	ʎ	ʟ			

Vowels

	Front		Central		Back	
Close	i	y	ɨ	ʉ	ɯ	u
Close-mid	e	ø	ɘ	ɵ	ɤ	o
Open-mid	ɛ	œ	ɜ	ɞ	ʌ	ɔ
Open	a	ɶ	a		ɑ	ɒ

Figure 11.1 Example of Hebrew-to-English Inventory

will be selected by the speaker to replace any missing TL phonemes (or help explain why those are the sounds being used). Also, look for patterns: are certain phonemes only problematic in specific words or locations, or across the board?

Accent Impact Index

We are in the process of developing a resource to support collecting client-reported outcomes, which are a crucial component of client-centered approaches to intervention (Yorkston & Baylor, 2019).[3] The version of our index included in this chapter is from the qualitative assessment stage (the review of items).[4] As discussed in this chapter, each speaker's experience is different, and the "thickness" or salience of one's accent is not necessarily proportional to the impact the accent has on one's life. Moreover, it is difficult to predict what situations or contexts a speaker may have difficulty with. In contrast to disorders, a speaker may also have experience with benefitting from their accent and may only seek to control it better rather than eliminate it. The questionnaire we developed encourages clients to reflect on their needs for accent modification, helps develop appropriate, informed goals for this intervention, and provides a tool for measuring baseline and tracking progress.

In "scoring" the responses, it is important to remember that there is no "within normal limits (WNL)" analog in the accent impact index, and there is no basis for comparing the scores across speakers/clients. The client responses only relate to their individual experiences and are not externally measurable. That is, there are no associations between score ranges and any measure of severity (because accentedness is not a disorder). Each client's score can only function as a baseline for that individual. And with this in mind, the more items included in the index, the more personalized the picture that emerges for each individual. For this reason, clients should be encouraged to add their own items to the index that can, in turn, be included in baselining and measuring progress of the intervention. There is, however, one measure addressed in our index that lends itself to the traditional clinical evaluate-and-treat paradigm: being understood by digital assistants such as Siri or Alexa. This measure relies exclusively on the processing of acoustic signals and as such is technically purely a matter of intelligibility and can have a severity rating as well as an objective way to assess it (how much of the person's speech can be understood by the program). Our ongoing research suggests this is a commonly selected target for accent intervention by speakers. The chapter on the Phonetics and Phonology of Intelligibility (Chapter 6 by Gurevich and Kim) has resources that may be of use for targeting this specific goal.

3. Note that typically clinical tools for collecting client-reported outcomes are based on the World Health Organization's International Classification of Functioning, Disability, and Health (e.g., the Overall Assessment of the Speaker's Experience of Stuttering (OASES) (Yaruss & Quesal, 2006) or the Voice Handicap Index (VHI) (Jacobson et al., 1997)). However, given that accentedness is not a disorder, definitions of disability have no relevance to the client's perspective or expected outcomes.
4. You are welcome to use the resource in its current form; feel free to contact the authors for updated versions.

Example of Use. With respect to interpretation of scores, not count-ing custom client items, the highest score possible is 136,[5] and the lowest is 0. Given that scores are determined by each client's experience, there is no basis for comparison across clients: a client with a score of 97 may not have a higher impact on their life than a client with a score of 35, and the client with the score of 35 may in fact have a higher motivation for accent modification (our experience shows that speakers with minimal accent are often the most motivated to remove it; to control it better). With this in mind, each indi-vidual's total is their baseline before intervention that can be compared to post-intervention totals to measure progress. Such progress would be reflected in a lower overall score on the index.

We end with an example of the optional "Custom Client Ratings" section of the Accent Impact Index. These customized items were written by a university professor who speaks with an accent:

My accent . . .	never	rarely	sometimes	often	always
Interferes with my comfort level when lecturing	0	1	2	3	4
Interferes with my ability to explain difficult concepts to class	0	1	2	3	4
Is blamed by students when they don't understand a concept	0	1	2	3	4
Is responsible for lower ratings on my teaching evaluations	0	1	2	3	4
Makes students feel I am less approachable	0	1	2	3	4
Makes colleagues feel I am less approachable	0	1	2	3	4
Subtotal 5: Add up each column, then provide sum: [____]					

Summary

Although most clinicians possess the skills needed to work with accent modifi-cation clients, they may not be accustomed to working with clients whose needs do not fit the typical disorder diagnose-then-treat model. To be both client-centered and effective, clinicians need to understand the unique complexity of the phonetic and phonological bases of accentedness as well as the sociolinguis-tic factors that contribute to its impact on speakers, resulting in an impact that is unique to each individual and is not always proportional to the "thickness" of one's accent. In this chapter we addressed these considerations and offer novel tools to help the clinician initiate accent modification intervention and track its progress by way of an index focused on client-reported outcomes.

5. There are a total of 33 items, 32 of them have a maximum score of 4, and one of them has a maxi-mum score of 8. As such, the highest possible score is 136.

Appendix 11.1

Accent modification intake form

This form can be used to identify potential sources of accentedness to guide targets for intervention involving most languages (and can be adapted to include all).

Target language (TL): _____

Influencing languages (ILs): _____

Step 1: Sound systems

Use the Consonant and Vowel charts to compare the phonemic inventories of the TL and ILs.

Instructions[6]: (1) Highlight the cells of all phonemes in the client's TL. (2) Cross-out highlighted phonemes missing from the client's ILs. (3) Circle phonemes in the ILs that are not highlighted (see example in chapter).

Resulting charts: The resulting charts help identify mismatches between the TL and ILs:

(1) Crossed-out highlighted sounds are new to the speaker; potential articulation targets
(2) If any circled sounds are used to replace crossed-out sounds, focus on those new TL sounds first
(3) Sounds that are neither highlighted nor circled can be ignored (they are neither targets nor potential errors)

Collect additional information:

(1) Ask the client which sounds seem to them most problematic or difficult.
(2) Ask the client if there are specific words or phrases that are difficult.

---

6. Sources for phonemic inventories of multiple languages: (1) The speech accent archive at George Mason University: accent.gmu.edu (2) American Speech-Language-Hearing Association (ASHA) Multicultural tools: www.asha.org/practice/multicultural/phono

Appendix Table 11.1

Consonants

	Bilabial	Labiodental	Dental	Alveolar	Postalveolar	Retroflex	Palatal	Velar	Uvular	Pharyngeal	glottal
Plosive	p b			t d		ʈ ɖ	c ɟ	k ɡ	q ɢ		ʔ
Nasal	m	ɱ		n		ɳ	ɲ	ŋ	ɴ		
Trill	ʙ			r					ʀ		
Tap/flap				ɾ		ɽ					
Fricative	ɸ β	f v	θ ð	s z	ʃ ʒ	ʂ ʐ	ç ʝ	x ɣ	χ ʁ	ħ ʕ	h ɦ
Lateral fricative				ɬ ɮ							
Approximant	w	ʋ		ɹ		ɻ	j	ɰ			
Lateral approximant				l		ɭ	ʎ	ʟ			

Appendix Table 11.2

Vowels

	Front		Central		Back	
Close	i	y	ɨ	ʉ	ɯ	u
	ɪ	ʏ				ʊ
Close-mid	e	ø	ɘ	ɵ	ɤ	o
				ə		
Open-mid	ɛ	œ	ɜ	ɞ	ʌ	ɔ
		æ		a		
Open	a	ɶ		ɐ	ɑ	ɒ

Step 2: Phonological rules[7]

Attend to patterns of usage to determine which TL rules are not being followed or IL rules that are not being inhibited. Are there sound substitutions or distortions at systematic locations? For example, is the speaker able to produce a voiceless /s/ but is voicing it to /z/ some of the time? If so, it is likely to be context-specific (due to misapplication of an IL rule).

Instructions: (1) Use the chart from step 1 to mark TL phonemes that are inconsistent. (2) Make two lists: one of words where these phonemes are produced accurately, and one of the words where there is distortion or substitution. (3) Look for generalizations (e.g., is distortion limited to certain word positions or proximity to other phonemes?). (4) Once the cause of the problem is identified (the triggering environment) it can be targeted for focused intervention. Alternatively, a client can be asked to develop these lists outside of treatment sessions to initiate this step.

Collect additional information:

(1) Stress pattern—attend to misapplication of lexical stress (putting stress on the wrong syllable in a word)
(2) Intonation pattern—attend to non-TL patterns (consider using acoustic analysis software to provide visual feedback)

---

7. This step is significantly more difficult for clinicians without formal training in Phonology and is complicated by the fact that there are no easily accessible references for cross-linguistic phonological rules. However, clinicians are trained to attend to patterns of speech and to recognize phonetic categories of sounds. As such, with practice and by working collaboratively with the client, this step is doable.

Appendix 11.2
Accent Impact Index

Background information

This section is not scored

What languages do you speak and how often?

Appendix Table 11.3

Language	Daily	Occasionally	Rarely	Never

Indicate which is/are responsible for your accent and which is/are impacted by it.

Appendix Table 11.4

Influencing Language (IL)—the accent source	Target Language (TL)—the one impacted

Language/accent attitudes

This section is not scored, and is not the target of accent modification intervention

☐ My accent makes me unique
☐ My accent is part of who I am
☐ My accent makes me interesting
☐ My accent helps start conversations, socialize
☐ My community of speakers with a similar accent to mine is (e.g., just me, my family, my neighborhood, etc.): _____
_____

☐ In the community where I live/work/socialize my accent is generally viewed (positively, negatively, neutral): _____
_____

☐ My accent may communicate something about me that I want to reveal. Please provide details: _____
_____

☐ My accent may communicate something about me that I do not want to reveal. Please provide details: _____
_____

Speaker's awareness of accent impact

Appendix Table 11.5

My accent . . .	never	rarely	some-times	often	always
Is noticeable to me	0	1	2	3	4
Is distracting to me	0	1	2	3	4
Is more noticeable to me when I hear a recording of my speech (e.g., voicemail greeting)	0	1	2	3	4
Is under my control as needed for specific situations/purposes	4	3	2	1	0
Is more noticeable when I'm rushed or stressed	0	1	2	3	4
My accent . . .	agree		undecided		disagree
Is the final aspect of the target language I'm learning and the only clue that I'm not a native speaker	4	3	2	1	0
Negatively impacts my self-image	4	3	2	1	0
Reduces my self-confidence	4	3	2	1	0
Is something I want to be better able to control	4	3	2	1	0
Subtotal 1: Add up each column, then provide sum: [____]					

Speaker's judgment of listeners' impression

Appendix Table 11.6

My accent . . .	never	rarely	sometimes	often	always
Is noticeable to others (e.g., gets comments)	0	1	2	3	4
Makes me seem less proficient in the target language	0	1	2	3	4
Makes people treat me differently than they treat others	0	1	2	3	4
My accent . . .	agree		undecided		disagree
Is distracting to *familiar* people I interact with	4	3	2	1	0
Is distracting to *unfamiliar* people I interact with	4	3	2	1	0
Makes me sound *more* knowledgeable	0	1	2	3	4
Makes me sound *less* knowledgeable	4	3	2	1	0
My accent . . .	more negatively		same		more positively
Leads people to perceive me differently than how I perceive myself [if no, mark 2=same]	4	3	2	1	0
Subtotal 2: Add up each column, then provide sum: [____]					

Communicative effectiveness & intelligibility

Appendix Table 11.7

My accent . . .	never	rarely	sometimes	often	always
Makes it difficult for *familiar* people to understand me	0	1	2	3	4
Makes it difficult for *unfamiliar* people to understand me	0	1	2	3	4
Leads to miscommunications/ misunderstandings	0	1	2	3	4
Is blamed for miscommunications/ misunderstandings	0	1	2	3	4
Leads to having to repeat myself	0	1	2	3	4
Gets in the way of using digital assistants (e.g., Siri or Alexa) or speech-to-text applications	0	2	4	6	8
Subtotal 3: Add up each column, then provide sum: [____]					

Activity and participation

Appendix Table 11.8

My accent . . .	never	rarely	sometimes	often	always
Disrupts my professional life (e.g., school, work)	0	1	2	3	4
Disrupts my social life (with friends, acquaintances)	0	1	2	3	4
Disrupts my personal life (with family, partner)	0	1	2	3	4
Disrupts my daily life (e.g., shopping, hobbies)	0	1	2	3	4
Leads to me avoiding specific situations	0	1	2	3	4
Affects my job performance	0	1	2	3	4
Is blamed when someone doesn't understand what I said even when fully intelligible (i.e., they can repeat verbatim what I said)	0	1	2	3	4
Gets in the way of me fitting in	0	1	2	3	4
Helps me fit into various groups/ communities	4	3	2	1	0
My accent . . .	more negatively		unchanged		more positively
Is responsible for the way my ability to do my job is evaluated: Because of my accent this ability is perceived	4	3	2	1	0
Subtotal 4: Add up each column, then provide sum: [____]					

Scoring

Add the four subtotals from the tables above: [____] + [____] + [____] + [____] = **Total** _____

Custom client ratings (optional)

Given the breadth of differing experiences in accented speakers, custom client-developed concerns (e.g., for specific situations) can make the index more meaningful. These client-developed ratings should be added to the total above for baseline pre/post intervention.

Appendix Table 11.9

My accent . . .	never	rarely	sometimes	often	always
	0	1	2	3	4
	0	1	2	3	4
	0	1	2	3	4
	0	1	2	3	4
	0	1	2	3	4
Subtotal 5: Add up each column, then provide sum: [_____]					

Interpretation

There is no direct association between score ranges and client needs. Each individual's total is their baseline before intervention that can be compared to post-intervention totals to measure progress.

References

Alexander, J., Sidaras, S., & Nygaard, L. (2008). The contribution of vowel production to the intelligibility and accentedness of nonnative speech. *The Journal of the Acoustical Society of America, 123*, 3078. https://doi.org/10.1121/1.2932878

American Speech-Language-Hearing Association (ASHA). (2010). *Let's talk: Accent modification: Changing the way you speak*. ASHA.

Behrman, A. (2014). Segmental and prosodic approaches to accent management. *American Journal of Speech-Language Pathology, 23*(4), 546–561. https://doi.org/10.1044/2014_AJSLP-13-0074

Boersma, P., & Weenink, D. (2020). *PRAAT* (Version 6.1.40). University of Amsterdam. www.praat.org

Brennan, E. M., & Brennan, J. S. (1981). Accent scaling and language attitudes: Reactions to Mexican American English speech. *Language and Speech, 24*(3), 207–221. https://doi.org/10.1177/002383098102400301

Derwing, T. M., & Munro, M. J. (2005). Second language accent and pronunciation teaching: A research-based approach. *TESOL Quarterly, 39*(3), 379–397. https://doi.org/10.2307/3588486

D'Innocenzo, J., Tjaden, K., & Greenman, G. (2006). Intelligibility in dysarthria: Effects of listener familiarity and speaking condition. *Clinical Linguistics & Phonetics, 20*(9), 659–675. https://doi.org/10.1080/02699200500224272

Dobel, C., Lagemann, L., & Zwitserlood, P. (2009). Non-native phonemes in adult word learning: Evidence from the N400m. *Philosophical transactions of the Royal Society of London. Series B, Biological Sciences, 364*(1536), 3697–3709. https://doi.org/10.1098/rstb.2009.0158

Esling, J. H. (1999). Myth 20: Everyone has an accent except me. In L. Bauer & P. Trudgill (Eds.), *Language myths* (pp. 169–175). Penguin.

Fogerty, D., Kewley-Port, D., & Humes, L. E. (2012). The relative importance of consonant and vowel segments to the recognition of words and sentences: Effects of age and hearing loss. *The Journal of the Acoustical Society of America, 132*(3), 1667–1678. https://doi.org/10.1121/1.4739463

Ford, C. E. (1984). The influence of speech variety on teachers' evaluation of students with comparable academic ability. *TESOL Quarterly*, *18*(1), 25–40. https://doi.org/10.2307/3586333

Franklin, A. D., Oksanen, K. A., & Gilfert, K. E. (2016). Goodness and accentedness ratings of /hVt/ tokens by aware and naive listeners. *American Journal of Speech-Language Pathology*, *25*(4), 620–633. https://doi.org/10.1044/2016_AJSLP-15-0106

Galindo, D. L. (1995). Language attitudes toward Spanish and English varieties: A Chicano perspective. *Hispanic Journal of Behavioral Sciences*, *17*(1), 77–99. https://doi.org/10.1177/07399863950171005

Giles, W. H., & Niedzielski, N. (1999). Myth 11: Italian is beautiful, German is Ugly. In L. Bauer & P. Trudgill (Eds.), *Language myths* (pp. 85–93). Penguin.

Gurevich, N., & Scamihorn, S. L. (2017). Speech-language pathologists' use of intelligibility measures in adults with dysarthria. *American Journal of Speech-Language Pathology*, *26*(3), 873–892. https://doi.org/10.1044/2017_AJSLP-16-0112

Hansen Edwards, J. G., Zampini, M. L., & Cunningham, C. (2018). The accentedness, comprehensibility, and intelligibility of Asian Englishes. *World Englishes*, *37*(4), 538–557. https://doi.org/10.1111/weng.12344

Hendriks, B., van Meurs, F., & Usmany, N. (2021). The effects of lecturers' non-native accent strength in English on intelligibility and attitudinal evaluations by native and non-native English students. *Language Teaching Research*. https://doi.org/10.1177/1362168820983145

Hochmann, J. R., Benavides-Varela, S., Nespor, M., & Mehler, J. (2011). Consonants and vowels: Different roles in early language acquisition. *Developmental Science*, *14*(6), 1445–1458. https://doi.org/10.1111/j.1467-7687.2011.01089.x

Hosoda, M., Nguyen, L. T., & Stone-Romero, E. F. (2012). The effect of Hispanic accents on employment decisions. *Journal of Managerial Psychology*, *27*(4), 347–364. https://doi.org/10.1108/02683941211220162

Huckvale, M. (2020). *SFS/WASP*. University College London. www.phon.ucl.ac.uk/resource/sfs/wasp/

Hustad, K. C., & Cahill, M. A. (2003). Effects of presentation mode and repeated familiarization on intelligibility of dysarthric speech. *American Journal of Speech-Language Pathology*, *12*(2), 198–208. https://doi.org/10.1044/1058-0360(2003/066)

Hutchinson, A., Weirick, J., Ahn, S., & Dmitrieva, O. (2019). *Language attitudes affect perceived intelligibility, proficiency, and accentedness of non-native speech*. Proceedings of the 19th International Congress of Phonetic Sciences. www.researchgate.net/publication/335704320

Isaacs, T., & Trofimovich, P. (2012). Deconstructing comprehensibility. *Studies in Second Language Acquisition*, *34*(3), 475–505. https://doi.org/10.1017/S0272263112000150

Jacobson, B. H., Johnson, A., Grywalski, C., Silbergleit, A., Jacobson, G., Benninger, M. S., & Newman, C. W. (1997). The voice handicap index (VHI). *American Journal of Speech-Language Pathology*, *6*(3), 66–70. https://doi.org/10.1044/1058-0360.0603.66

Khansir, A. A., & Pakdel, F. (2019). Contrastive analysis hypothesis and second language learning. *Journal of ELT Research: The Academic Journal of Studies in English Language Teaching and Learning*, *4*(1), 35–43. https://doi.org/10.22236/JER_Vol4Issue1pp35-43

Kuhl, P. K. (2004). Early language acquisition: Cracking the speech code. *Nature Reviews Neuroscience*, *5*(11), 831–843. https://doi.org/10.1038/nrn1533

Kuhl, P. K., Williams, K. A., Lacerda, F., Stevens, K. N., & Lindblom, B. (1992). Linguistic experience alters phonetic perception in infants by 6 months of age. *Science*, *255*(5044), 606–608. www.jstor.org/stable/2876832

Labov, W. (1963). The social motivation of a sound change. *Word*, *19*(3), 273–309. https://doi.org/10.1080/00437956.1963.11659799

Labov, W. (1966). *The social stratification of "r" in New York City department stores.* Center for Applied Linguistics.

Lambert, W. E., Hodgson, R. C., Gardner, R. C., & Fillenbaum, S. (1960). Evaluational reactions to spoken languages. *The Journal of Abnormal and Social Psychology, 60*(1), 44–51. https://doi.org/10.1037/h0044430

Lindberg, R., & Trofimovich, P. (2020). Second language learners' attitudes toward French varieties: The roles of learning experience and social networks. *The Modern Language Journal, 104*(4), 822–841. https://doi.org/10.1111/modl.12674

Liss, J. M., Spitzer, S. M., Caviness, J. N., & Adler, C. (2002). The effects of familiarization on intelligibility and lexical segmentation in hypokinetic and ataxic dysarthria. *Journal of the Acoustical Society of America, 112*(6), 3022–3030. https://doi.org/10.1121/1.1515793

Lodge, A. (1999). Myth 4: French is a logical language. In L. Bauer & P. Trudgill (Eds.), *Language myths* (pp. 23–31). Penguin.

MacGregor-Mendoza, P. (2015). Son importantes los dos: Language use and attitudes among wives of Mexican profesionistas on the U.S.-Mexico border. In K. Potowski & T. Bugel (Eds.), *Sociolinguistic change across the Spanish-speaking world* (pp. 147–186). Peter Lang. https://doi.org/10.3726/978-1-4539-1409-0

McLeod, S., & Crowe, K. (2018). Children's consonant acquisition in 27 languages: A cross-linguistic review. *American Journal of Speech-Language Pathology, 27*(4), 1546–1571. https://doi.org/10.1044/2018_AJSLP-17-0100

Munro, M. J., & Derwing, T. M. (1999). Foreign accent, comprehensibility, and intelligibility in the speech of second language learners. *Language Learning, 49*(Suppl 1), 285–310. https://doi.org/10.1111/0023-8333.49.s1.8

Rickford, J. R. (2005). Using the vernacular to teach the standard. In J. D. Ramirez, T. G. Wiley, G. D. Klerk, E. Lee, & W. E. Wright (Eds.), *Ebonics: The urban education debate* (2nd ed., pp. 18–40). Multilingual Matters Ltd. https://doi.org/10.21832/9781853597985

Rubin, D. L. (1992). Nonlanguage factors affecting undergraduates' judgments of nonnative English-speaking teaching assistants. *Research in Higher Education, 33*(4), 511–531. www.jstor.org/stable/40196047

Rubin, D. L., Ainsworth, S., Cho, E., Turk, D., & Winn, L. (1999). Are Greek letter social organizations a factor in undergraduates' perceptions of international instructors? *International Journal of Intercultural Relations, 23*(1), 1–12. https://doi.org/10.1016/S0147-1767(98)00023-6

Rubin, D. L., & Smith, K. A. (1990). Effects of accent, ethnicity, and lecture topic on undergraduates' perceptions of nonnative English-speaking teaching assistants. *International Journal of Intercultural Relations, 14*(3), 337–353. https://doi.org/10.1016/0147-1767(90)90019-S

Schmidt, A. M. (1997, Spring). Working with adult foreign accent: Strategies for intervention. *Contemporary Issues in Communication Science and Disorders, 24*, 47–56. https://doi.org/10.1044/cicsd_24_S_47

Taylor, H. U. (1989). *Standard English, Black English, and bidialectalism: A controversy.* Peter Lang.

Toro, J. M., Nespor, M., Mehler, J., & Bonatti, L. L. (2008). Finding words and rules in a speech stream: Functional differences between vowels and consonants. *Psychological Science, 19*(2), 137–144. https://doi.org/10.1111/j.1467-9280.2008.02059.x

Utianski, R. L., Lansford, K. L., Liss, J. M., & Azuma, T. (2011). The effects of topic knowledge on intelligibility and lexical segmentation in hypokinetic and ataxic dysarthria. *Journal of Medical Speech-Language Pathology, 19*(4), 25–36. https://pubmed.ncbi.nlm.nih.gov/24569812

Wardhaugh, R. (1970). The contrastive analysis hypothesis. *TESOL Quarterly, 4*(2), 123–130. https://doi.org/10.2307/3586182

Wolfram, W. (1991). *Dialects and American English*. Prentice Hall.

Yaruss, J. S., & Quesal, R. W. (2006). Overall assessment of the speaker's experience of stuttering (OASES): Documenting multiple outcomes in stuttering treatment. *Journal of Fluency Disorders, 31*(2), 90–115. https://doi.org/10.1016/j.jfludis.2006.02.002

Yi, H. G., Phelps, J. E., Smiljanic, R., & Chandrasekaran, B. (2013). Reduced efficiency of audiovisual integration for nonnative speech. *Journal of the Acoustical Society of America, 134*(5), El387–El393. https://doi.org/10.1121/1.4822320

Yi, H. G., Smiljanic, R., & Chandrasekaran, B. (2014). The neural processing of foreign-accented speech and its relationship to listener bias [Original Research]. *Frontiers in Human Neuroscience, 8*(768). https://doi.org/10.3389/fnhum.2014.00768

Yorkston, K. M., & Baylor, C. (2019). Patient-reported outcomes measures: An introduction for clinicians. *Perspectives of the ASHA Special Interest Groups, 4*(1), 8–15. https://doi.org/10.1044/2018_PERS-ST-2018-0001

Yorkston, K. M., Strand, E. A., & Kennedy, M. R. T. (1996). Comprehensibility of dysarthric speech. *American Journal of Speech-Language Pathology, 5*(1), 55–66. https://doi.org/10.1044/1058-0360.0501.55

Zheng, Y., & Samuel, A. G. (2017). Does seeing an Asian face make speech sound more accented? *Attention, Perception, & Psychophysics, 79*(6), 1841–1859. https://doi.org/10.3758/s13414-017-1329-2

Ziegler, W., & Zierdt, A. (2008). Telediagnostic assessment of intelligibility in dysarthria: A pilot investigation of MVP-online. *Journal of Communication Disorders, 41*(6), 553–577. https://doi.org/10.1016/j.jcomdis.2008.05.001

Index

Page numbers in *italics* refer to figures. Page numbers in **bold** refer to tables.

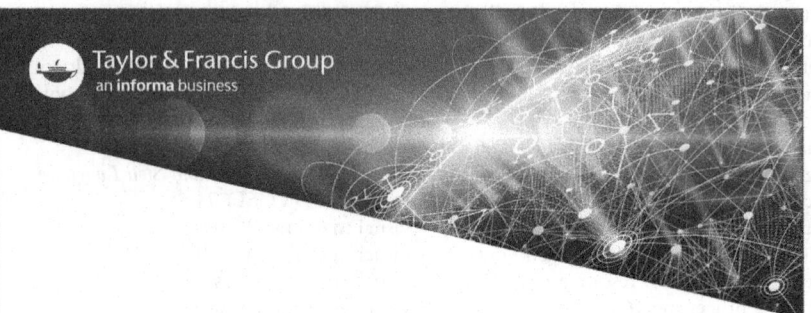
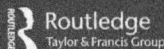
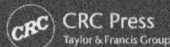